Case-based Reviews in
PEDIATRIC EMERGENCIES

Case-based Reviews in
PEDIATRIC EMERGENCIES

Academic Editor

Suraj Gupte MD FIAP FSAMS (Sweden) FRSTMH (London)
Professor and Head
Postgraduate Department of Pediatrics
Mamata Medical College and General and Super Specialty Hospitals
Khammam, Telangana, India
E-mail: drsurajgupte@gmail.com
Website: www.drsurajgupte.com

Editor: The Short Textbook of Pediatrics, Recent Advances in Pediatrics (Series), Textbook of Pediatric Emergencies, Neonatal Emergencies, Pediatric Nutrition, and Pediatric Gastroenterology, Hepatology and Nutrition, Pediatric Infectious Diseases, Influenza: Complete Spectrum, Clinical Problem Solving in Neonatal Emergences and Intensive Care, etc.

Author: Differential Diagnosis in Pediatrics, Instructive Case Studies in Pediatrics, Pediatric Drug Directory, Influenza, Perspectives in Influenza, Nutrition in Neonatal ICU, Speaking of Child Care, etc.

Chief Editor (Gastroenterology Section): International Journal of Gastroenterology, Hepatology, Transplant and Nutrition.

Co-editor: Asian Journal of Maternity and Child Health (Manila, Philippines).

Section and Guest Editor: Pediatric Today (New Delhi).

Editorial Advisor: Asian Journal of Pediatric Practice (New Delhi).

Editorial Advisory Board Member/Reviewer: Indian Journal of Pediatrics (New Delhi), Indian Pediatrics (New Delhi), Indian J Child Health (Gwalior), Synopsis (Detroit, USA), Maternal and Child Nutrition (Preston, UK), Journal of Infectious Diseases (Turkey), EC Pediatrics (London), Journal of Clinical Pediatrics, etc.

Examiner: Several Universities, including National Board of Examinations (NBE) for DNB, New Delhi; All India Institute of Medical Sciences (AIIMS), New Delhi; Postgraduate Institute of Medical Education and Research (PGIMER), Chandigarh; Sher-i-Kashmir Institute of Medical Sciences (SKIMS), Srinagar; Indira Gandhi Open University (IGNOU), New Delhi.

Pediatric Faculty Selection Expert: All India Institute of Medical Sciences (AIIMS), Punjab Public Service Commission, Jammu and Kashmir Public Service Commission, Union Public Service Commission.

Executive Editor
Novy Gupte MD

Foreword
Elizabeth Smith MRCP FRCP PhD

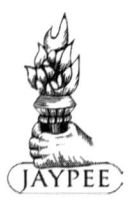

JAYPEE *The Health Sciences Publisher*
New Delhi | London | Panama

Jaypee Brothers Medical Publishers (P) Ltd

Headquarters
Jaypee Brothers Medical Publishers (P) Ltd
4838/24, Ansari Road, Daryaganj
New Delhi 110 002, India
Phone: +91-11-43574357
Fax: +91-11-43574314
Email: jaypee@jaypeebrothers.com

Overseas Offices

J.P. Medical Ltd
83 Victoria Street, London
SW1H 0HW (UK)
Phone: +44 20 3170 8910
Fax: +44 (0)20 3008 6180
Email: info@jpmedpub.com

Jaypee-Highlights Medical Publishers Inc
City of Knowledge, Bld. 237, Clayton
Panama City, Panama
Phone: +1 507-301-0496
Fax: +1 507-301-0499
Email: cservice@jphmedical.com

Jaypee Brothers Medical Publishers (P) Ltd
17/1-B Babar Road, Block-B, Shaymali
Mohammadpur, Dhaka-1207
Bangladesh
Mobile: +08801912003485
Email: jaypeedhaka@gmail.com

Jaypee Brothers Medical Publishers (P) Ltd
Bhotahity, Kathmandu, Nepal
Phone: +977-9741283608
Email: kathmandu@jaypeebrothers.com

Website: www.jaypeebrothers.com
Website: www.jaypeedigital.com

© 2018, Jaypee Brothers Medical Publishers

The views and opinions expressed in this book are solely those of the original contributor(s)/author(s) and do not necessarily represent those of editor(s) of the book.

All rights reserved. No part of this publication may be reproduced, stored or transmitted in any form or by any means, electronic, mechanical, photocopying, recording or otherwise, without the prior permission in writing of the publishers.

All brand names and product names used in this book are trade names, service marks, trademarks or registered trademarks of their respective owners. The publisher is not associated with any product or vendor mentioned in this book.

Medical knowledge and practice change constantly. This book is designed to provide accurate, authoritative information about the subject matter in question. However, readers are advised to check the most current information available on procedures included and check information from the manufacturer of each product to be administered, to verify the recommended dose, formula, method and duration of administration, adverse effects and contraindications. It is the responsibility of the practitioner to take all appropriate safety precautions. Neither the publisher nor the author(s)/editor(s) assume any liability for any injury and/or damage to persons or property arising from or related to use of material in this book.

This book is sold on the understanding that the publisher is not engaged in providing professional medical services. If such advice or services are required, the services of a competent medical professional should be sought.

Every effort has been made where necessary to contact holders of copyright to obtain permission to reproduce copyright material. If any have been inadvertently overlooked, the publisher will be pleased to make the necessary arrangements at the first opportunity.

Inquiries for bulk sales may be solicited at: jaypee@jaypeebrothers.com

Case-based Reviews in Pediatric Emergencies / Suraj Gupte

First Edition: **2018**

ISBN: 978-93-86322-50-0

Printed at Sanat Printers

Dedicated to

All those associated with achievement of excellence in management of pediatric emergencies

Contributors

Gautami Anand
Senior Fellow
Division of Pediatric Neurology
State University of New York
New York, New York, USA
Ch 21: Bacterial Meningitis

K Anitha
Assistant Professor (Ex)
Department of Pediatrics
MS Ramaiah Medical College and Teaching Hospital
Bangalore, Karnataka, India
Ch 40: Severe Acute Malnutrition

Anupam Bahe
Pediatric Intensivist
Continental Children's Center
Continental Hospitals
Hyderabad, Telangana, India
Ch 30: Severe Dengue

Harmesh S Bains
Professor and Head
Department of Pediatrics
Punjab Institute of Medical Sciences
Jalandhar, Punjab, India
Ch 12: Annular Pancreas

Anthony Block
Senior Consultant in Infectious Diseases
Advanced Medical Center
Liverpool, UK
Ch 32: Influenza

Meenakshi Bothra
Senior Resident, AIIMS
New Delhi, India
Ch 6: Diabetes Ketoacidosis

Robert Brakeman
Assistant Professor
Division of Pediatric Neurology
State University of New York
New York, New York, USA
Ch 21: Bacterial Meningitis

Rita Carswell
Senior Fellow in Pediatrics
Harvard Medical School
Boston, Massachusetts, USA
Ch 24: Acute Bronchiolitis

Biswaroop Chakrabarty
Assistant Professor
Child Neurology
Department of Pediatrics, AIIMS
New Delhi, India
Ch 19: Acute Flaccid Paralysis

Dinesh Chirla
Director
Intensive Care
Rainbow Children's Hospital
Hyderabad, Telangana, India
Ch 17: Raised Intracranial Pressure
Ch 27: Malignant Hypertension

Anjul Dayal
Pediatric Intensivist
Incharge, Continental Children's Center, Continental Hospitals
Hyderabad, Telangana, India
Ch 13: Traumatic Brain Injury
Ch 23: Acute Respiratory Distress Syndrome
Ch 26: Acute Severe Asthma
Ch 29: Congestive Heart Failure
Ch 30: Severe Dengue
Ch 31: Cerebral Malaria
Ch 44: Vasculitis Syndrome
Ch 45: Obstructive Sleep Apnea

Sheffali Gulati
Professor and Chief
Child Neurology
Department of Pediatrics, AIIMS
New Delhi, India
Ch 14: Acute Seizures
Ch 18: Acute Febrile Encephalopathy
Ch 19: Acute Flaccid Paralysis
Ch 20: Metabolic Crisis

Suraj Gupte
Professor and Head
Postgraduate Department of Pediatrics
Mamata Medical College and General and Super Specialty Hospitals
Khammam, Telangana, India
Ch 21: Bacterial Meningitis
Ch 24: Acute Bronchiolitis
Ch 25: Pneumonia
Ch 32: Influenza
Ch 39: Acute Pancreatitis

Gopakumar Hariharan
Fellow
Neonatal and Pediatric Intensive Care
Royal Hobart Hospital
Lecturer, University of Tasmania
Hobart, Tasmania, Australia
Ch 8: Transient Pseudohypoaldosteronism

Vandana Jain
Professor
Department of Endocrinology and Diabetes, AIIMS
New Delhi, India
Ch 6: Diabetes Ketoacidosis
Ch 7: Central Diabetes Insipidus

V Nancy Jeniffer
Assistant Professor
Department of Pediatrics
MS Ramaiah Medical College and Teaching Hospital
Bangalore, Karnataka, India
Ch 15: Status Eplepticus

Ch 35: Acute Gastroenteritis
Ch 41: Bleeding Child

BP Karunakara
Professor and Intensivist
Department of Pediatrics
MS Ramaiah Medical College and
Teaching Hospital
Bangalore, Karnataka, India
Ch 1: Anaphylaxis
Ch 15: Status Eplepticus
Ch 22: Respiratory Distress
Ch 34: Snakebite
Ch 35: Acute Gastroenteritis
Ch 36: Acute Dysentery
Ch 40: Severe Acute Malnutrition
Ch 41: Bleeding Child

K Prarthana Karumbaiah
Assistant Professor
Department of Pediatrics
MS Ramaiah Medical College and
Teaching Hospital
Bangalore, Karnataka, India
Ch 34: Snakebite

Jayashankar Kaushik
Associate Professor
Department of Pediatrics
Pt B D Sharma Postgraduate
Institute of Medical Sciences
Rohtak, Haryana, India
Ch 14: Acute Seizures

TM Ananda Kesavan
Professor
Department of Pediatrics
Government Medical College
Thrissur, Kerala, India
Ch 33: Scorpion Sting

Khaleel Khan
Pediatric Intensivist
Continental Children's Center
Continental Hospitals
Hyderabad, Telangana, India
Ch 13: Traumatic Brain Injury

Shagufta Khan
Fellow in Infectious Diseases
Institute of Child and
Adolescent Health
London, UK
Ch 25: Pneumonia

Shahid Khan
Fellow in Infectious Diseases
Institute of Child and
Adolescent Health
London, UK
Ch 25: Pneumonia

Rajeev Khanna
Associate Professor in Pediatric
Hepatology
Institute of Liver and
Biliary Sciences
New Delhi, India
Ch 37: Variceal Bleed
Ch 38: Acute Hepatitis

Ramesh Konanki
Consultant Pediatric Neurologist
Rainbow Children's Hospital
Hyderabad, Telangana, India
Ch 16: Super-refractory Status
Epilepticus

Alla Bharath Kumar
Assistant Professor (Ex)
Postgraduate Department of
Pediatrics
Mamata Medical College and
General and Superspecialty
Hospitals
Khammam, Telangana, India
Ch 5: Hematuria

R Kumar
Senior Consultant in Infectious
Diseases
Advanced Medical Center
Liverpool, UK
Ch 32: Influenza

Lokesh Lingappa
Consultant Pediatric Neurologist
Rainbow Children's Hospital
Hyderabad, Telangana, India
Ch 16: Super-refractory Status
Epilepticus

Ranjith K Manokaran
Senior Resident in Child
Neurology
Department of Pediatrics, AIIMS
New Delhi, India
Ch 20: Metabolic Crisis

Shina Menon
Senior Consultant in
Pediatric Nephrology
Apollo Center for Advanced
Pediatrics
Indraprastha Apollo Hospital
New Delhi, India
Ch 3: Hemolytic-uremic
Syndrome
Ch 4: Acute Glomerulonephritis

Doaman Mittal
Resident
Department of Pediatrics
Punjab Institute of Medical
Sciences
Jalandhar, Punjab, India
Ch 12: Annular Pancreas

Nalini Nagalla
Consultant in Pulmonary and
Sleep Disorders
Continental Hospitals
Hyderabad, Telangana, India
Ch 45: Obstructive Sleep Apnea

Pavithra Nagaraj
Assistant Professor
Department of Pediatrics
MS Ramaiah Medical College and
Teaching Hospital
Bangalore, Karnataka, India
Ch 1: Anaphylaxis

Sumitha Nayak
Consultant Pediatrician
The Children's Clinic
Bangalore, Karnataka, India
Ch 22: Respiratory Distress

Sidharth Nayyar
Senior Resident
Department of Pediatrics
Dayanand Medical College
Ludhiana, Punjab, India
Ch 12: Annular Pancreas

Sahil Pandita
Senior Fellow in Pediatrics
Harvard Medical School
Boston, Massachusetts, USA
Ch 24: Acute Bronchiolitis

Contributors

Harsh Patel
Consultant Pediatric Neurologist
Zydus Hospital
Ahmedabad, Gujarat, India
Ch 18: Acute Febrile Encephalopathy

Reesham Pattan
Pediatric Registrar
Neonatal and Pediatric Intensive Care Unit
Royal Hobart Hospital
Hobart, Tasmania, Australia
Ch 8: Transient Pseudohypoaldosteronism

Satya Prasad
Pediatric Nephrologist
Rainbow Hospital for Women and Children
Vijaywada, Andhra Pradesh, India
Ch 28: Acute Severe Hypertension

Hemchand K Prasad
Senior Consultant and Head
Department of Pediatric Endocrinology and Diabetes
Mehta Children's Hospital
Chennai, Tamil Nadu, India
Ch 10: Hypoglycemia
Ch 11: Pheochromocytoma

PK Pruthi
Senior Pediatric Nephrologist
Institute of Child Health
Sir Ganga Ram Hospital
New Delhi, India
Ch 2: Acute Renal Injury
Ch 43: Fluid and Electrolyte Imbalance

Sirisha Rani
Consultant in Pediatric Hematology and Oncology
Rainbow Children's Hospital
Hyderabad, Telangana, India
Ch 42: Tumor Lysis Syndrome

Aathira Ravindranath
Senior Resident in Pediatric Gastroenterology
Sanjay Gandhi Postgraduate Institute of Medical Sciences
Lucknow, Uttar Pradesh, India
Ch 7: Central Diabetes Insipidus

J Leenatha Reddy
Consultant
Pediatric Endocrinology and Diabetes
Rainbow Children's Hospital
Hyderabad, Telangana, India
Ch 9: Acute Adrenal Crisis

Sarah Sege
Intensive Care Consultant
King's Hospital
Hong Kong
Ch 39: Acute Pancreatitis

Rakshay Shetty
Consultant Pediatric Intensivist
Rainbow Children's Hospital
Bangalore, Karnataka, India
Ch 17: Raised Intracranial Pressure
Ch 27: Malignant Hypertension

L Francine Shirley
Pediatrics Trainee
Mehta Children's Hospital
Chennai, Tamil Nadu, India
Ch 10: Hypoglycemia
Ch 11: Pheochromocytoma

Abhilasha Singh
Pediatric Intensivist
Continental Children's Center
Continental Hospitals
Hyderabad, Telangana, India
Ch 13: Traumatic Brain Injury
Ch 23: Acute Respiratory Distress Syndrome
Ch 26: Acute Severe Asthma
Ch 29: Congestive Heart Failure
Ch 31: Cerebral Malaria
Ch 44: Vasculitis Syndrome

Utpal Kant Singh
Professor and Head (Ex)
Department of Pediatrics
Nalanda Medical College
Patna, Bihar, India
Ch 39: Acute Pancreatitis

Gaurav Singla
Senior Resident
Department of Pediatrics
Dayanand Medical College
Ludhiana, Punjab, India
Ch 12: Annular Pancreas

RN Srivastava
Senior Consultant in Pediatric Nephrology
Indraprastha Apollo Hospital
New Delhi, India
Ch 3: Hemolytic-uremic Syndrome
Ch 4: Acute Glomerulonephritis

VR Veeturi
Consultant Pediatric Nephrologist
Rainbow Children's Hospital
Hyderabad, Telangana, India
Ch 28: Acute Severe Hypertension

SN Vishwas
Assistant Professor
Department of Pediatrics
MS Ramaiah Medical College and Teaching Hospital
Bangalore, Karnataka, India
Ch 36: Acute Dysentery

Foreword

Notwithstanding huge advancement in the West in Emergency pediatrics, it still remains an emerging field in the South-East Asia. Mercifully, in India, it has begun to receive increasing attention. Nevertheless, in spite of the World Health Organization having repeatedly drawn attention to the excellence of case-based teaching and learning, there remains a paucity of such literature in dealing with emergencies and intensive care in pediatrics.

It is in this context that the *Case-based Reviews in Pediatric Emergencies* by Dr Suraj Gupte, an icon in pediatrics at national and international level, assumes a special significance.

Empowered by over 50 experts as contributors, the book stands out as a unique and innovative treatise dealing with a wide spectrum of pediatric emergencies. These have been dealt with in a comprehensive, lucid, and easy-to-follow manner.

As a norm, each case scenario is followed by a "Critical Case Review in a Nutshell". The subsequent "Interactive Topic Review" in the form of questions and answers is very pertinent, providing clarity of the subject. The contents, presentation, format, and language are simple, to-the-point, and profusely illustrated using tables, boxes, clinical photographs and other figures, including flowcharts/algorithms. At the end of each chapter, "Key Learning Points" are given to drive home the take-home messages. Each and every chapter is a testimony to the clear and precise thought process of the authors and the editors.

All in all, Dr Suraj Gupte's excellent book, *Case-based Reviews in Pediatric Emergencies*, in my opinion, is a strongly recommended treatise for all pediatricians, more so for those actively involved in emergency and intensive care pediatrics.

Elizabeth Smith MRCP FRCP PhD
Chief of Emergency Pediatrics
Hong Kong Medical Center
Hong Kong

Preface

The new book, *Case-based Reviews in Pediatric Emergencies*, draws its inspiration from the philosophy that enhancing emphasis on clinical scenarios is crucial to the learning of management of pediatric emergencies. The errors committed and the strong positives attained become a stepping stone in improved clinical delivery of optimal care.

Each of the 45 chapters authored by 53 experts in the field kickstarts with one or more case scenarios, focusing on presentation, diagnosis, and management of the problem. It is followed by a short critical review of the case and developments in its management. The error, if any, and important therapeutic points are particularly brought to light. Finally, there appears an extensive interactive discussion in the form of frequently asked questions (FAQs) on the topic as such. In this discussion, such important points that remain elusive in the textbooks receive special attention.

Clinical orientation and practical applicability receive a central stage in each and every chapter. Contents are rationally listed in various sections. In order to enhance the impact of the narration, a large number of illustrations (including algorithms), tables and boxes stand incorporated. In addition to the core matter, "Key Learning Points" are given at the end. "Suggested Reading" have also been incorporated providing some key references for more probing readers. A comprehensive index is also provided to facilitate easy access to requisite issues.

The *Case-based Reviews in Pediatric Emergencies* should turn out to be a welcome and significant educational tool for the target readers, especially the postgraduates, residents and upcoming intensivists, and emergency pediatricians.

Suraj Gupte
Novy Gupte

Acknowledgments

We would like to acknowledge:
- The expert contributors, both from India and abroad, for providing excellent state-of-the-art chapters on various topical issues in pediatric emergencies. They were gracious enough to repose confidence in our editorship
- The peer reviewers for critically reviewing the contributions, providing us the benefit of their expertise
- Dr Elizabeth Smith for reviewing the drafts and generously commending and recommending the book in her Foreword
- The management of Mamata Medical College and Hospitals for blessing this project
- Dr Gagan Hans, Assistant Professor (Psychiatry), All India Institute of Medical Sciences, New Delhi, for voluntarily helping us in various ways in taking the project to its logical conclusion
- Shamma-Bakshi Gupte, Manu Gupte, and Shivani Mahendru for their help at various stages
- Various periodicals and journals for citing their references under "Suggested Readings"
- Jaypee Brothers Medical Publishers (P) Ltd., New Delhi, India, and their dedicated staff for the commendable production qualities of the book.

Contents

Section 1: Life-threatening Emergency

1. **Anaphylaxis** 1
   BP Karunakara, Pavithra Nagaraj

Section 2: Nephrology

2. **Acute Renal Injury** 8
   PK Pruthi

3. **Hemolytic-uremic Syndrome** 14
   Shina Menon, RN Srivastava

4. **Acute Glomerulonephritis** 18
   RN Srivastava, Shina Menon

5. **Hematuria** 26
   Alla Bharath Kumar

Section 3: Endocrine and Metabolic Disorders

6. **Diabetic Ketoacidosis** 31
   Meenakshi Bothra, Vandana Jain

7. **Central Diabetes Insipidus** 37
   Vandana Jain, Aathira Ravindranath

8. **Transient Pseudohypoaldosteronism** 43
   Reesham Pattan, Gopakumar Hariharan

9. **Acute Adrenal Crisis** 46
   J Leenatha Reddy

10. **Hypoglycemia** 52
    L Francine Shirley, Hemchand K Prasad

11. **Pheochromocytoma** 58
    Hemchand K Prasad, L Francine Shirley

12. **Annular Pancreas** 64
    Harmesh S Bains, Doaman Mittal, Gaurav Singla, Sidharth Nayyar

Section 4: Neurology

13. **Traumatic Brain Injury** — 67
    Khaleel Khan, Anjul Dayal, Abhilasha Singh

14. **Acute Seizures** — 75
    Sheffali Gulati, Jayashankar Kaushik

15. **Status Epilepticus** — 83
    BP Karunakara, V Nancy Jeniffer

16. **Super-refractory Status Epilepticus** — 90
    Ramesh Konanki, Lokesh Lingappa

17. **Raised Intracranial Pressure** — 99
    Rakshay Shetty, Dinesh Chirla

18. **Acute Febrile Encephalopathy** — 110
    Sheffali Gulati, Harsh Patel

19. **Acute Flaccid Paralysis** — 121
    Sheffali Gulati, Biswaroop Chakrabarty

20. **Metabolic Crisis** — 129
    Sheffali Gulati, Ranjith K Manokaran

21. **Bacterial Meningitis** — 135
    Suraj Gupte, Gautami Anand, Robert Brakeman

Section 5: Pulmonology

22. **Respiratory Distress** — 140
    BP Karunakara, Sumitha Nayak

23. **Acute Respiratory Distress Syndrome** — 146
    Anjul Dayal, Abhilasha Singh

24. **Acute Bronchiolitis** — 153
    Suraj Gupte, Sahil Pandita, Rita Carswell

25. **Pneumonia** — 160
    Suraj Gupte, Shagufta Khan, Shahid Khan

26. **Acute Severe Asthma** — 168
    Abhilasha Singh, Anjul Dayal

Section 6: Cardiology

27. **Malignant Hypertension** — 176
    Dinesh Chirla, Rakshay Shetty

28.	**Acute Severe Hypertension** VR Veeturi, Satya Prasad	184
29.	**Congestive Heart Failure** Anjul Dayal, Abhilasha Singh	192

Section 7: Infectious Diseases

30.	**Severe Dengue** Anupam Bahe, Anjul Dayal	199
31.	**Cerebral Malaria** Anjul Dayal, Abhilasha Singh	210
32.	**Influenza** Suraj Gupte, R Kumar, Anthony Block	217

Section 8: Envenomation

33.	**Scorpion Sting** TM Ananda Kesavan	224
34.	**Snakebite** BP Karunakara, K Prarthana Karumbaiah	232

Section 9: Gastroenterology

35.	**Acute Gastroenteritis** BP Karunakara, V Nancy Jeniffer	240
36.	**Acute Dysentery** BP Karunakara, SN Vishwas	248
37.	**Variceal Bleed** Rajeev Khanna	251
38.	**Acute Hepatitis** Rajeev Khanna	260
39.	**Acute Pancreatitis** Utpal Kant Singh, Suraj Gupte, Sarah Sege	266

Section 10: Nutrition

40.	**Severe Acute Malnutrition** BP Karunakara, K Anitha	270

Section 11: Hemato-oncology

41. **Bleeding Child** — 278
    V Nancy Jeniffer, BP Karunakara

42. **Tumor Lysis Syndrome** — 285
    Sirisha Rani

Section 12: Homeostasis

43. **Fluid and Electrolyte Imbalance** — 290
    PK Pruthi

Section 13: Rheumatology

44. **Vasculitis Syndrome** — 301
    Abhilasha Singh, Anjul Dayal

Section 14: Sleep Disorders

45. **Obstructive Sleep Apnea** — 308
    Anjul Dayal, Nalini Nagalla

Index — *313*

PLATE 1

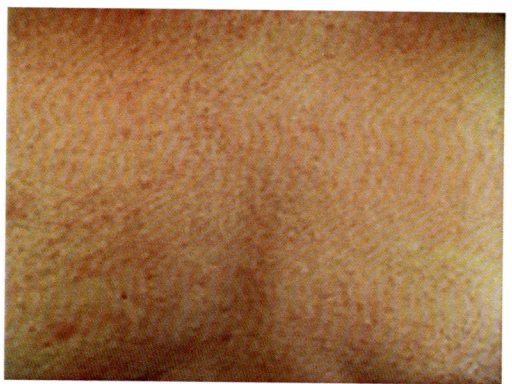

Figure 2: Urticaria and flushing on the back of a subject with anaphylaxis *(Chapter 1)*

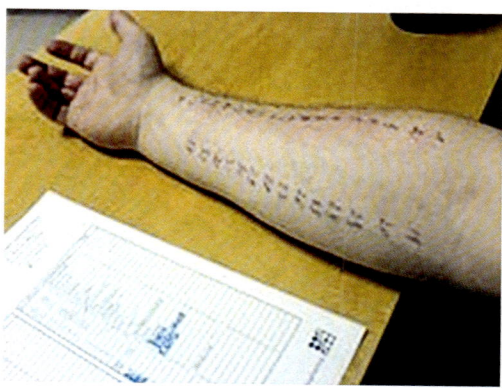

Figure 3: Skin allergy testing being carried out on the right arm *(Chapter 1)*

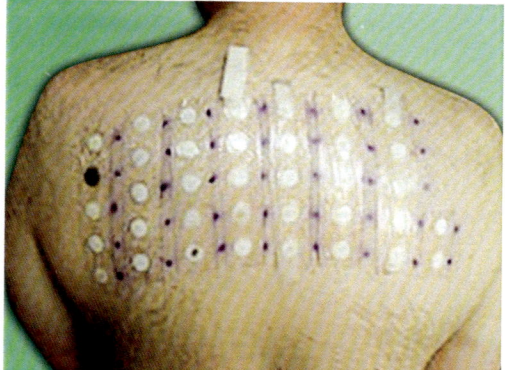

Figure 4: Patch test *(Chapter 1)*

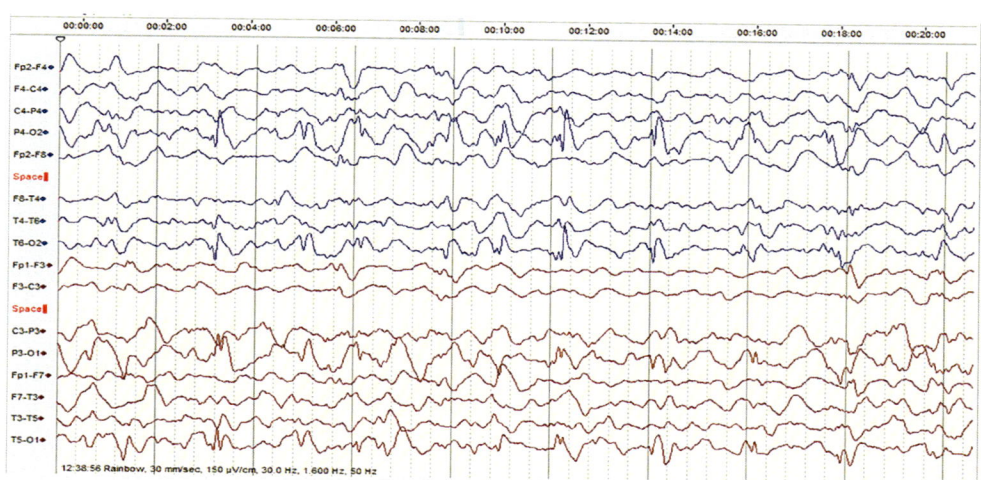

Figure 2: Electroencephalogram showing continuous, generalized sharp-slow wave complexes of 1–2 Hz suggestive of nonconvulsive status epilepticus *(Chapter 16)*

PLATE 2

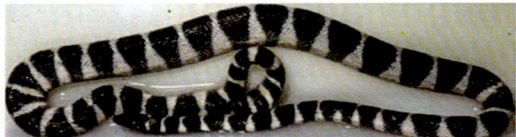

Figure 1: Sea snake *(Chapter 34)*

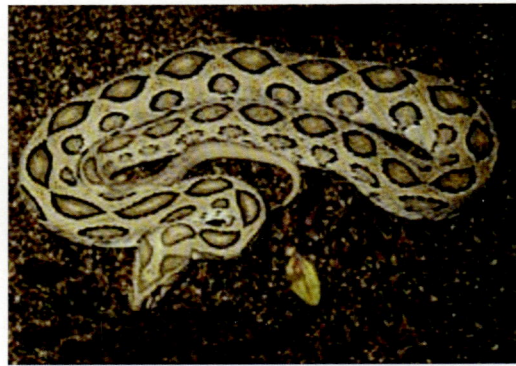

Figure 4: *Daboia russelii* (Russell's viper) *(Chapter 34)*

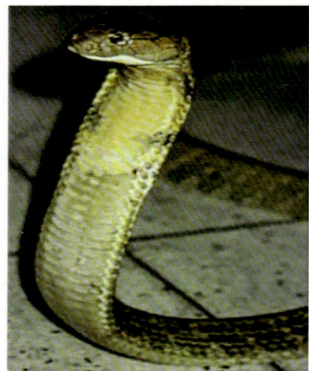

Figure 2: *Ophiophagus hannah* (king cobra) *(Chapter 34)*

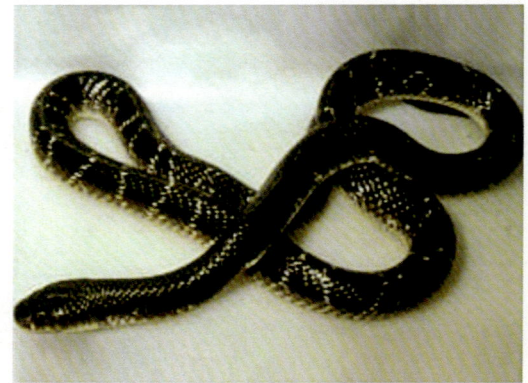

Figure 5: *Bungarus caeruleus* (Krait) *(Chapter 34)*

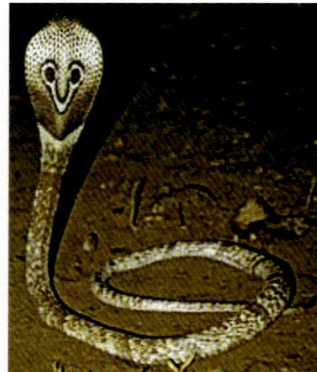

Figure 3: *Naja naja* (common cobra) *(Chapter 34)*

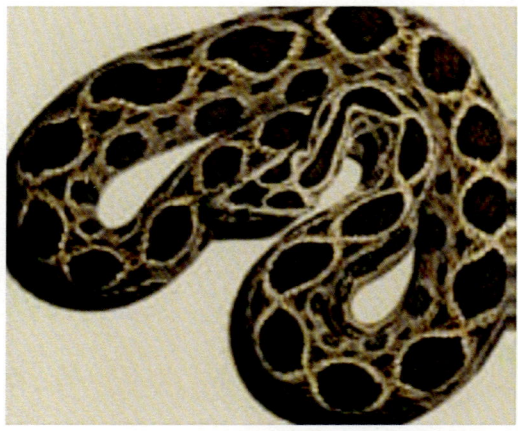

Figure 6: *Echis carinatus* (saw-scaled viper) *(Chapter 34)*

PLATE 3

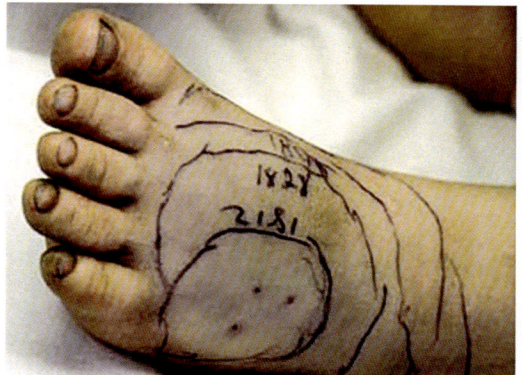

Figure 7: Fang marks *(Chapter 34)*

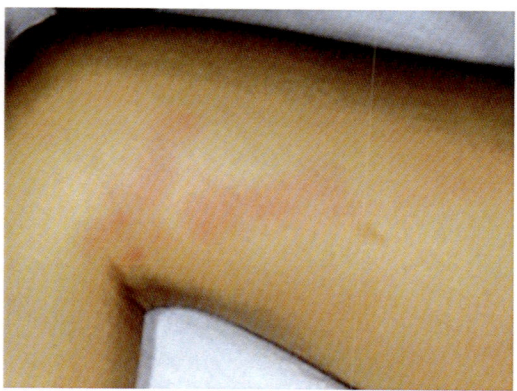

Figure 10: Lymphangitis *(Chapter 34)*

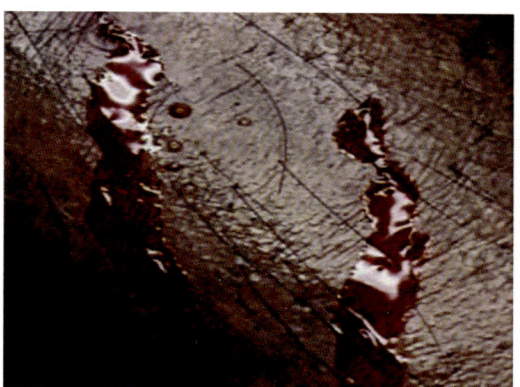

Figure 8: Local bleeding *(Chapter 34)*

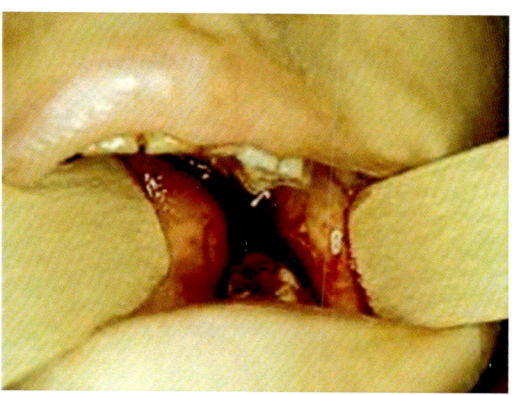

Figure 11: Bleeding from gingival sulci *(Chapter 34)*

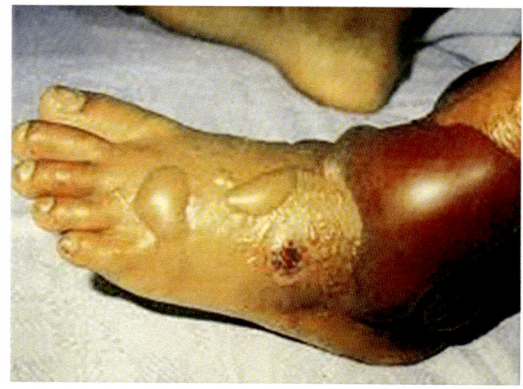

Figure 9: Bruising and blistering *(Chapter 34)*

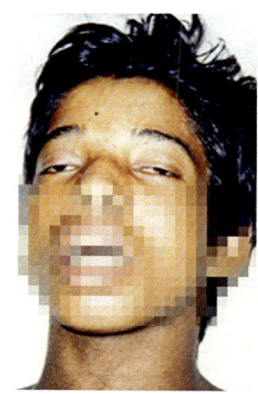

Figure 12: Ptosis *(Chapter 34)*

PLATE 4

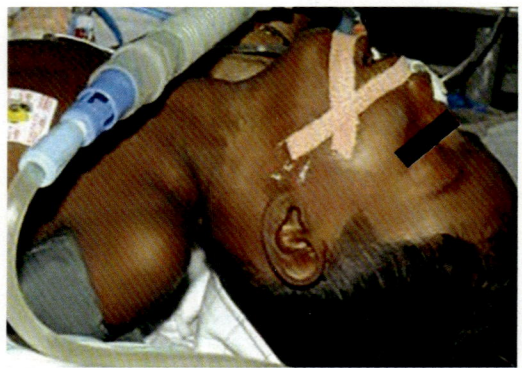

Figure 13: Broken neck sign in a child envenomed by krait *(Chapter 34)*

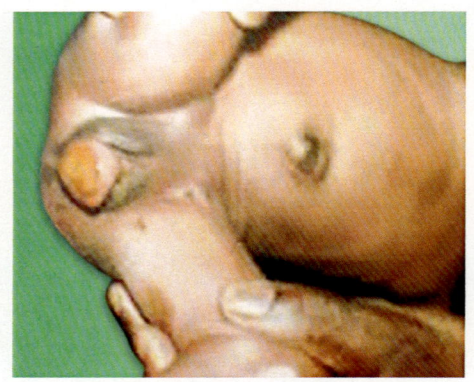

Figure 1: Rectal prolapse in a child with dysentery *(Chapter 36)*

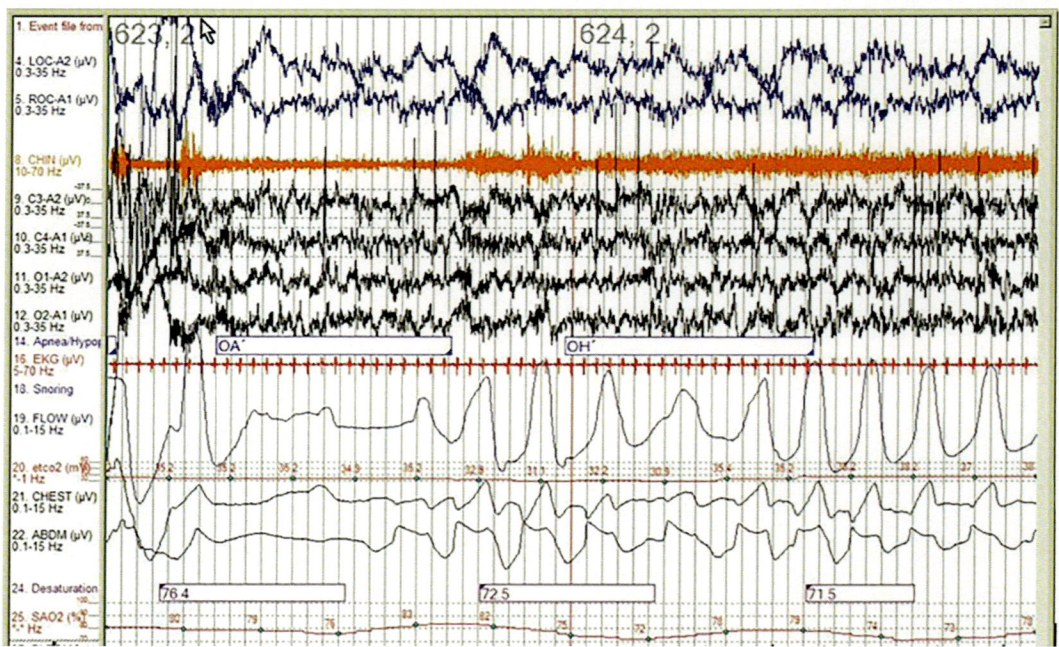

Figure 1: Polysomnographic evaluation for obstructive sleep apnea *(Chapter 45)*

SECTION 1
Life-threatening Emergency

CHAPTER 1

Anaphylaxis

BP Karunakara, Pavithra Nagaraj

INTRODUCTION

Anaphylaxis is an acute, potentially life-threatening immunoglobulin E (IgE)-mediated hypersensitivity reaction, involving the release of mediators from mast cells, basophils, and recruited inflammatory cells. Worldwide, 0.05–2% of the population is estimated to have anaphylaxis at some point in life, and rates appear to be increasing. The term comes from the ancient Greek *ana* "against" and *phylaxis* "protection". The term aphylaxis was coined by Charles Richet in 1902 and later changed to anaphylaxis due to its nicer quality of speech. He was awarded the Nobel Prize in Physiology for his work on anaphylaxis in 1913.

CASE 1

Master X, previously healthy, a 12-year-old boy was brought to the emergency after being stung by a bee on his right forearm. Complained of localized pain and swelling initially followed by shortness of breath after 15 minutes and was observed by his parents to be wheezing. He reported feeling weak and dizzy.
On examination: He is drowsy, pale, but able to answer questions. Temperature 37.1°C; pulse rate (PR) 142/min; respiratory rate (RR) 42/min; blood pressure (BP) 68/44 mmHg (tachycardia, tachypnea and hypotension); and capillary refill time is delayed. Generalized urticaria is present. The bee sting site on his right forearm shows moderate swelling without visualization of a foreign body. Respiratory system: Mild wheezing and subcostal retractions present.
Diagnosis: Anaphylactic shock.
Treatment: Supplemental high flow oxygen was started immediately. Intramuscular adrenaline [1:1,000 (1 mg/mL)] 0.01 mg/kg was given in the anterolateral aspect of thigh. Meanwhile, an intravenous line was established and a fluid bolus of 20 mL/kg with normal saline was started followed by maintenance fluid (normal saline plus potassium chloride). Inhaled β2 agonist (salbutamol) 0.2 mg/kg was started simultaneously. His urticaria resolves, his blood pressure normalizes and his wheezing resolves. After being observed in the emergency department (ED) for 6 hours, he feels "back to normal." He was subsequently discharged from the ED on oral diphenhydramine at 1 mg/kg. His parents were advised of the possibility of a late phase reaction that could result in worsening, so they were advised to monitor his condition carefully and return to the ED if his condition worsens.

CASE 2

An 8-year-old girl presented to the ED with obvious skin rash, puffy face, and loss of consciousness. On arrival to the ED, she could only respond to painful stimulus with the following vitals: temperature of 37.2°C, PR: 44/min, RR: 54/m, BP: 56/20 mmHg, and prolonged clot formation time (CFT). Previous ingestion of groundnut was reported by her mother.
Physical examination disclosed generalized urticaria and dermatographism. Respiratory system

revealed stridor and severe wheezing. The 12-lead electrocardiography (ECG) showed sinus bradycardia with rate of 44/m.

Investigations showed total count: 5,400/µL with neutrophil 66.2%, lymphocyte 20.3%, eosinophil 5.1% and basophil 2.5%, a hemoglobin of 10.9 g/dL, and a platelet count of 313,000/µL.

Diagnosis: Anaphylactic shock.

Treatment: Supplemental high flow oxygen was started immediately. Intramuscular adrenaline [1:1000 (1 mg/mL)] 0.01 mg/kg was given. An intravenous line was established, intravenous atropine 0.02 mg/kg, a fluid bolus of 20 mL/kg with normal saline, and dopamine infusion was administered continuously to maintain heart rate and blood pressure. Inhaled β2 agonist (salbutamol) 0.2 mg/kg is started simultaneously. She was admitted to the intensive care unit (ICU) where she was given intravenous adrenaline, continued with supplemental oxygen and the vitals monitored. Her vital signs were stabilized and dopamine infusion was discontinued 2 days later. Follow-up ECG disclosed normal sinus rhythm with rate of 74/m. She was transferred to regular ward and was discharged 8 days later without any sequelae. Avoidance of groundnuts was advised strongly.

CASE REVIEW IN A NUTSHELL

The clinical profiles of the two cases developing hypotension with respiratory symptoms following bee sting and ingestion of groundnut are consistent with anaphylaxis. Diagnosis of anaphylactic shock rather than just anaphylaxis was made as the child had hypotension and prolonged capillary refill time. This warranted the treatment with supplemental oxygen, intravenous fluid bolus, intramuscular/intravenous adrenaline, and nebulization with salbutamol. However, in the second case the child required prolonged hospital stay in view of severe hypotension and bradycardia (Bezold-Jarisch reflex) requiring inotropic support and ICU care.

INTERACTIVE TOPIC REVIEW

Q. What is anaphylaxis?

Anaphylaxis is an acute, potentially life-threatening IgE-mediated hypersensitivity reaction, involving the release of mediators from mast cells, basophils, and recruited inflammatory cells. Anaphylaxis is defined by a number of signs and symptoms, alone or in combination, which occur within minutes, or up to a few hours, after exposure to a provoking agent.

Q. How about anaphylactic shock?

Interestingly, none of the definitions includes the term "anaphylactic shock". As per current recommendations, the term "anaphylaxis" should also be used in preference to such terms as "allergic reaction", "acute allergic reaction", "systemic allergic reaction", "acute IgE-mediated reaction", "anaphylactoid reaction", or "pseudoanaphylaxis".

Q. What is its pathophysiology?

The term anaphylaxis is often used only for severe allergic reaction affecting the whole body. A second term, nonallergic anaphylaxis, may be used to describe identical reactions that are not caused by allergy, but involve other mechanisms in the body.

In the immunologic mechanism, IgE binds to the antigen (the foreign material that provokes the allergic reaction). Antigen-bound IgE then activates FcεRI receptors on mast cells and basophils. This leads to the release of inflammatory mediators such as histamine, leukotrienes, tumor necrosis factor, and various cytokines. These mediators subsequently increase the contraction of bronchial smooth muscles, trigger vasodilation, increase the leakage of fluid from blood vessels, and cause heart muscle depression. Death may occur from hypoxemia (due to upper airway angioedema, bronchospasm and mucus plugging) and/or shock (due to massive vasodilatation, fluid shift into the extravascular space and depressed myocardial function).

Nonimmunologic mechanisms (other than IgE-mediated reactions) may also be responsible for anaphylaxis. Sometimes termed anaphylactoid reactions (nonallergic anaphylaxis), including direct release of mediators from mast cells by medications and physical factors, nonimmunologic mechanisms involve substances that directly cause the degranulation of mast cells and basophils. These include agents such as contrast medium, opioids, temperature (hot or cold) and vibration.

Q. What are the causes for anaphylaxis in children?

Food allergy is the most common cause in children responsible for about 80% of anaphylactic reactions in which the cause has been identified. The cause remains unknown in 32–50% of cases, referred to as "idiopathic anaphylaxis" (Box 1).

The World Allergy Organization (WAO) guidelines emphasize on risk factors related to age (infancy, adolescence, and advanced age), physiologic state (pregnancy), concomitant diseases including asthma, cardiovascular diseases (CVD) and mastocytosis, and concurrent medications such as β-blockers and angiotensin-converting enzyme inhibitors (ACEIs). The American Academy of Allergy, Asthma and Immunology/the American College of Allergy, Asthma and Immunology (AAAAI/ACAAI) guidelines describe patient-specific risk factors such as asthma, CVD and mastocytosis, and concurrent β-blocker and ACEI use. The European Academy of Allergy and Clinical Immunology (EAACI) guidelines include a major focus on asthma as a patient risk factor.

Q. What are the common clinical features of anaphylaxis in children?

Onset of symptoms varies depending on the cause; reactions from ingested allergens are delayed in onset (minutes to 2 h) compared with injected allergens and tend to have more gastrointestinal symptoms (Fig. 1). The most common areas affected include skin (80–90%), respiratory (70%), gastrointestinal (30–45%), heart and vasculature (10–45%), and central nervous system (10–15%) with usually two or more being involved. Anaphylaxis can follow a biphasic course. Biphasic reactivity was reported with an incidence of 19.4%. The second-phase onset may be 8–10 hours on

BOX 1: Common causes of anaphylaxis in children

- Food: Peanuts, nuts (walnut, hazelnut, cashew), milk, eggs, sea food (fish, shrimp, crab, lobster, oyster), seeds (sesame, cottonseed, pine nuts), wheat
- Drugs: Penicillins, cephalosporins, sulfonamides, nonsteroidal anti-inflammatory agents, opiates, muscle relaxants, vancomycin, dextran, thiamine, vitamin B12, insulin, thiopental, local anesthetics
- Hymenoptera venom: Honeybee, wasp
- Latex
- Allergen immunotherapy
- Exercise: Food-specific exercise, postprandial (nonfood-specific) exercise
- Vaccinations: Tetanus, measles, mumps, influenza
- Miscellaneous: Radiocontrast media, gamma globulin, cold temperature, chemotherapeutic agents, blood products, inhalants (dust and storage mites, grass pollen)
- Idiopathic

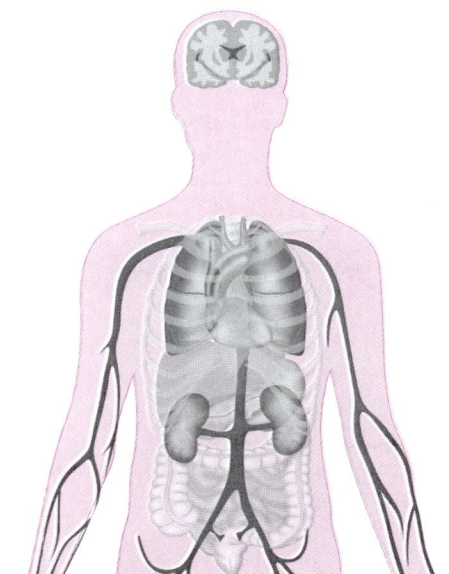

Figure 1: Signs and symptoms of anaphylaxis: Main involvent is of skin (80–90%), respiratory tract (70%), gastrointestinal tract (30–45%), heart and vasculature (10–45%), and central nervous system (10–15%).

average, but it occurred as late as 38 hours. Biphasic anaphylaxis may be related, in part, to undertreatment. Protracted anaphylaxis may occur with symptoms persisting for days.
- Skin reactions—generalized itching, flushing, swelling of the skin and hives (urticaria), a feeling of warmth (Fig. 2). Those with angioedema may describe a burning sensation of the skin rather than itchiness. The skin may also be blue tinged because of lack of oxygen
- Swelling of the eyelids with itchy watery eyes
- Respiratory—include shortness of breath, wheeze or stridor. The wheezing is typically caused by spasms of the bronchial muscles while stridor is related to upper airway obstruction secondary to swelling. Hoarseness, painful swallowing, or a cough may also occur
- Gastrointestinal—abdominal cramps, nausea, vomiting, diarrhea
- Cardiovascular—the coronary spasm is related to the presence of histamine-releasing cells in the heart. While a fast heart rate caused by low blood pressure is more common, a Bezold-Jarisch reflex has been described in 10% of cases where a slow heart rate is associated with low blood pressure. A drop in blood pressure or shock (distributive or cardiogenic) may cause the feeling of light-headedness, dizziness, fainting, or loss of consciousness

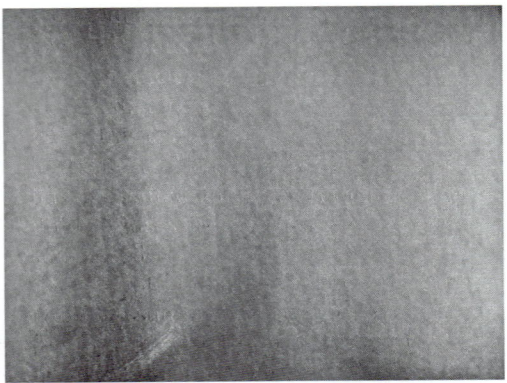

Figure 2: Urticaria and flushing on the back of a subject with anaphylaxis *(For color version, see Plate 1)*

- Others—dilatation of blood vessels around the brain may cause headaches; a feeling of anxiety or impending doom
- Death may occur within minutes, but rarely has been reported to occur days to weeks after the initial anaphylactic event.

Q. What are the mimics of anaphylaxis?

- Vasovagal reactions
- Syncope, panic attacks
- Epiglottitis, status asthmaticus, foreign body aspiration, pulmonary embolism
- Hypoglycemia.

Upper airway obstruction, bronchospasm, abdominal cramps, pruritus, urticaria and angioedema are absent in vasovagal reactions. Pallor, syncope, diaphoresis, and nausea usually indicate a vasovagal reaction but may occur in either condition. Asthma, however, typically does not entail itching or gastrointestinal symptoms, syncope presents with pallor rather than a rash, and a panic attack may have flushing but does not have hives.

Q. What about the diagnosis of anaphylaxis and the role of investigations?

Diagnosis is based on:
- Clinical presentation: Anaphylaxis is diagnosed on the basis of a person's signs and symptoms
- *In vitro* testing for allergen-specific IgE is a useful initial screening test for a variety of allergens. However, it lacks sensitivity and is limited by the range of allergens available (Fig. 3)
- Skin prick tests are more sensitive than in vitro testing (Fig. 4). As these carry a small risk of inducing anaphylaxis, they should only be carried out in an environment in which resources for treating anaphylaxis are available
- Some drug reactions (e.g., nonsteroidal anti-inflammatory drugs, radiographic contrast agents) are independent of IgE, and there are numerous difficulties in assessing

CHAPTER 1: Anaphylaxis

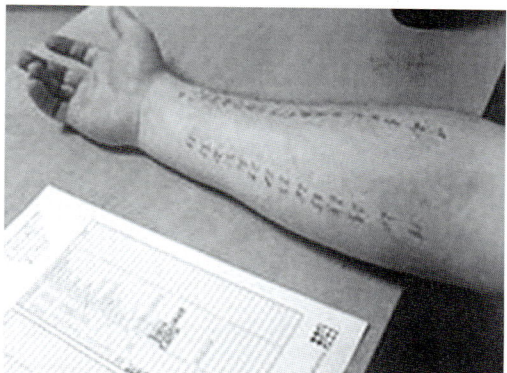

Figure 3: Skin allergy testing being carried out on the right arm *(For color version, see Plate 1)*

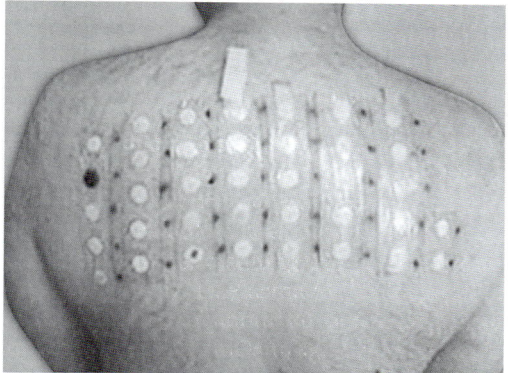

Figure 4: Patch test *(For color version, see Plate 1)*

some cases of antibiotic allergy. In such cases, a challenge testing under controlled conditions may sometimes be required, although a negative challenge test does not always exclude the diagnosis
- During an attack, blood tests for tryptase or histamine (released from mast cells) might be useful in diagnosing anaphylaxis. Serum tryptase takes hours and test results are not available on an emergency basis. Elevation correlates with anaphylaxis severity; however, platelet-activating factor levels appear to correlate better than tryptase or histamine levels do.

Q. How should anaphylaxis be managed at the emergency and after stabilization?

- Anaphylaxis is a medical emergency
- The trigger should be removed if possible. Positioning the patient supine (or semi-reclining in a position of comfort if dyspnoeic or vomiting) with elevation of the lower extremities
- Blood pressure, heart rate, respiratory status, and oxygenation should be monitored at frequent intervals (every 1-5 min), or if possible, continuously
- Airway, breathing, and circulation—measures such as airway management, supplemental high flow oxygen, intubation, and ventilation if required, intravenous fluid resuscitation with a crystalloid such as 0.9% (isotonic) saline. Fluid boluses if required—20 mL/kg of NS. If no improvement in BP start inotropes such as epinephrine, dopamine or vasopressin infusion
- Resuscitation should be started without delay and that H_1-antihistamines, H_2-antihistamines are not initial medications of choice
- Prompt initial treatment of anaphylaxis. Adrenaline [1:1,000 (1 mg/mL)] 0.01 mg/kg, max 0.3 mg (0.5 mg for >12 y), repeated every 5-15 minutes as necessary, intramuscularly in the anterolateral aspect of thigh. The intramuscular route is preferred over subcutaneous administration because the latter may have delayed absorption. Minor adverse effects from epinephrine include tremors, anxiety, and palpitation. Intravenous adrenaline, however, has been associated both with dysrhythmia and myocardial infarction. Adrenaline autoinjectors used for self-administration typically come in two doses, one for adults or children who weigh more than 25 kg and one for children who weigh 10-25 kg
- The WAO guidelines and the AAAAI/ACAAI guidelines do not specifically recommend inhaled epinephrine for patients with stridor during anaphylaxis, although they note that

an inhaled β2 agonist should be considered in patients with bronchospasm that persists despite epinephrine treatment. The EAACI guidelines recommend inhaled epinephrine (adrenaline) in patients with stridor and an inhaled β2 adrenergic agonist in patients with wheezing after, and in addition to, epinephrine injection
- Systemic glucocorticoids—hydrocortisone 1 mg/kg four times a day or methyl-prednisolone, although not helpful in acute phase, will prevent recurrent anaphylaxis
- Second line therapy or adjuncts
    - H1-antihistamines: Diphenhydramine 1–2 mg/kg or 25–50 mg per dose
    - H2-antagonists: Ranitidine 1 mg/kg intravenous
    - Inhaled β2 agonist—salbutamol
    - In severe laryngeal edema—consider adrenaline inhalation
- Observation and monitoring for minimum of 6–8 hours for patients with respiratory symptoms and 12–24 hours for those with hypotension or collapse.

Q. How should anaphylaxis refractory to the initial steps of management be handled?

- People on β-blockers may be resistant to the effects of epinephrine. In this situation if epinephrine is not effective, intravenous glucagons (<25 kg—0.5 mg, over 25 kg—1 mg SC/IM/IV) can be administered which has a mechanism of action independent of β-receptors
- Methylene blue 1–2 mg/kg intravenous 1% solution over 5–10 minutes has been used in those not responsive to other measures due to its presumed effect of relaxing smooth muscle.

Q. What is the prognosis and how to prevent further episodes of anaphylaxis?

- Anaphylaxis emergency action plan: Parents are advised to inform schools of their children's allergies and what to do in case of an anaphylactic emergency
- Prescribe epinephrine intramuscular through autoinjector (EAI)
- Describe allergen avoidance (food, stinging insects, drugs, latex, etc.) and desensitization to drugs
- Immunotherapy is available for certain triggers to prevent future episodes of anaphylaxis
- Yearly review of EAI use, action plan, optimal management of comorbid diseases, adjustment of concurrent medications as needed, allergen avoidance, and immune modulation is required.

Q. Any modern and future strides?

There are ongoing efforts to develop sublingual epinephrine to treat anaphylaxis. Subcutaneous injection of the anti-IgE antibody omalizumab is being studied as a method of preventing recurrence, but it is not yet recommended.

CONCLUSION

Anaphylaxis is a life-threatening condition. Invasive hemodynamic monitoring and stability would elucidate complex hemodynamic status. The importance of the alphabets A, M, and P, denoting allergy, medicines, and past illness, of the "sample" history worth to be emphasized again. Although tachycardia is considered as the early warning sign of shock, a relative bradycardia accompanied with or without hypotension as a benign course leading to delayed resuscitation may contribute to a negative outcome eventually.

KEY LEARNING POINTS

- Anaphylaxis is a life-threatening condition
- Invasive hemodynamic monitoring and stability would elucidate complex hemodynamic status in the patient with anaphylaxis
- The alphabets A, M, and P denoting allergy, medicines and past illness of the "sample" history should be borne in mind
- A relative bradycardia along with or without hypotension may contribute to a negative outcome eventually
- Sublingual epinephrine and subcutaneous injection of the anti-Immunoglobulin E antibody omalizumab may prove breakthrough in its management.

SUGGESTED READINGS

1. Brown SG, Blackman KE, Stenlake V, Heddle RJ. Insect sting anaphylaxis: Prospective evaluation of treatment with intravenous adrenaline and volume resuscitation. *Emerg Med J*. 2004;21:149-154.
2. Campbell RL, Li JT, Nicklas R, Sadosty AT; Members of the Joint Task Force; Practice Parameter Workgroup. Emergency department diagnosis and treatment of anaphylaxis: a practice parameter. *Ann Allergy Asthma Immunol*. 2014;113:599-608.
3. Khan BQ, Kemp SF. Pathophysiology of anaphylaxis. *Curr Opin Allergy Clin Immunol*. 2011;11:319-325.
4. Joint Task Force on Practice Parameters; American Academy of Allergy, Asthma and Immunology; American College of Allergy, Asthma and Immunology; Joint Council of Allergy, Asthma and Immunology. The diagnosis and management of anaphylaxis: an updated practice parameter. *J Allergy Clin Immunol*. 2005;115:S483-523.
5. Sampson HA, Munoz-Furlong A, Campbell RL, Adkinson FN, Bock SA, Branum A, et al. Second symposium on the definition and management of anaphylaxis: Summary report—Second National Institute of Allergy and Infectious Disease/Food Allergy and Anaphylaxis Network symposium. *J Allergy Clin Immunol*. 2006;117:391-397.
6. Simons FE, World Allergy Organization. World Allergy Organization survey on global availability of essentials for the assessment and management of anaphylaxis by allergy-immunology specialists in health care settings. *Ann Allergy Asthma Immunol*. 2010;104:405-412.

SECTION 2
Nephrology

CHAPTER 2

Acute Renal Injury

PK Pruthi

INTRODUCTION

The term acute renal injury (ARI) has now replaced the former nomenclature, i.e., acute renal failure (ARF). It is defined as a sudden loss of renal function, occurring over a period of hour to days, manifested by accumulation of creatinine, urea and other metabolic waste products (azotemia) and often accompanied by reduction in urine volume (oliguria) with associated salt and water retention. The diagnostic criteria for ARI include an abrupt (within 48 h) reduction in renal function, defined as 50% or greater increase in serum creatinine or oliguria (<0.5 mL/kg/h) for more than 6 hours. Children with multisystem failure have a much higher mortality rate. The emphasis has now shifted to diagnose minimal derangements of renal function (not amounting to failure) and prompt treatment.

CASE 1

A 2-year-old boy presented with history of loose stools and vomiting for 2 days. He had not passed urine for the last 12 hours.

Examination: The child was dehydrated, pulse rate 110/min, low volume, blood pressure (BP) 80/55 mmHg, and weight 11 kg. Bladder was not palpable.

Investigations: Hemoglobin 10.2 g/dL, blood urea nitrogen (BUN) 90 mg/dL, serum creatinine 1.8 mg/dL, serum sodium 138 mEq/L, and K 3.8 mEq/L.

Diagnosis: Acute gastroenteritis with dehydration with AKI (preneral).

Treatment given: Intravenous fluids 200 mL of normal saline in 1 hour. As child did not pass urine and was still dehydrated, another bolus of 200 mL normal saline was given in the next 1 hour. At the end of this bolus, the child passed lot of urine and looked better hydrated.

Outcome: At the end of 24 hours, BUN and serum creatinine returned to normal (BUN 18 mg/dL and serum creatinine 0.5 mg/dL), the child looked well hydrated and passed urine 6 times.

CASE REVIEWS IN A NUTSHELL

The 2-year-old child developed oliguria after having loose stools and vomiting. On presentation, he had features of dehydration and peripheral circulatory failure. His renal functions were found to be deranged. With this presentation, a diagnosis of ARI (prerenal) following fluid losses was made.

The child received two boluses of normal saline. Following this, he improved and started passing urine. Prerenal injury is reversible once the blood volume and hemodynamic conditions are restored to normal.

CHAPTER 2: Acute Renal Injury

CASE 2

An 8-year-old boy presented with periorbital puffiness and reduced urine output for last 2 days with history of sore throat 3 weeks back.

On examination: Weight 28 kg; height 125 cm; pulse rate 90/min; respiratory rate 20/min; BP 100/70 mmHg, bladder not palpable, and edema over eyes and feet.

Investigations: Hemoglobin 9.5 g/dL, total leukocyte count 9,800/mm^3, differential leukocyte count—phagocytes 68%, leukocytes 30%, and monocytes 2%. Erythrocyte sedimentation rate 90 mm first hour, serum proteins 6.0 g/dL, albumin 3.0 g/dL, globulin 3.0 g/dL, BUN 100 mg/dL, serum creatinine 3.8 mg/dL, serum C3 78 mg/dL, anti-streptolysin O (ASO) 400 units.

Urine examination: Red blood cells 50/hpf, white blood cells 10–12/hpf and protein 2+.

Throat swab: Normal flora, serum sodium 138 mEq/L, potassium 6.6 mEq/L.

Diagnosis: Acute renal disease with post streptococcal glomerulonephritis with hyperkalemia.

Treatment given:
- Restricted fluids 400 mL/m^2/day plus urine output for last 24 hours, intravenous fluids not needed as child was able to accept orally
- Potassium containing food items were avoided. As electrocardiogram (ECG) did not show any changes of hyperkalemia, the child was not shifted to the pediatric intensive care unit. The child was given salbutamol 5 mg in nebulized form.

CASE REVIEWS IN A NUTSHELL

The 8-year-old child presented with oliguria and mild edema, normal blood pressure, active urine sediment, and deranged renal function with history of sore throat 3 weeks back. The investigations revealed that he had hyperkalemia also. All these findings suggested that he had intrinsic ARI. Intrinsic ARI does not warrant bolus fluid administration rather restriction of fluids immediately. Life-threatening emergencies like fluid overload and pulmonary edema require immediate treatment.

INTERACTIVE TOPIC REVIEW

Q. What is the definition of acute renal injury?

Acute renal injury is considered to be present when there is an abrupt (within 48 h) reduction in renal function defined as an absolute increase in serum creatinine of either more than 0.3 mg/dL (or a percentage increase of >50%) or a reduction in urine output (documented oliguria of <0.5 mL/kg/h for >6 h). These criteria include both an absolute and a percentage change in creatinine to accommodate variations related to age, gender and body mass index, and reduce the need for a baseline level of serum creatinine. It is necessary that the diagnosis be made following estimation of at least two serum creatinine values within 48 hours.

Q. Why has the term acute renal failure been replaced by the term acute renal injury?

The term ARI acknowledges that although there are various causative factors, the acute decline in renal function is secondary to an injury that leads to functional and structural changes in the renal. The word failure reflects only the end of the clinical spectrum.

The definition of ARI suggests that even a marginal increase of 0.3 mg of serum creatinine indicates ARI. For example, if the serum creatinine of a child rises from 0.3 to 0.6 mg/dL, although still in the normal range, indicates some renal injury and alerts the physician to take proper preventive action. Therefore, the term ARI has been proposed to encompass the entire spectrum of the syndrome from minor changes in renal function to requirement for renal replacement therapy (RRT).

Q. What are the criteria for defining and staging acute renal injury?

Recognizing the need for a uniform definition for ARI, the Acute Dialysis Quality Initiative

(ADQI) group proposed a consensus-graded definition called the RIFLE (Risk, Injury, Failure, Loss, End Stage Renal Disease) criteria. A modification of the RIFLE criteria was subsequently proposed by Acute Kidney Injury Network (AKIN), which included the ADQI group as well AKIN criteria.

Another classification called pediatric RIFLE is a modification of RIFLE criteria, and consists of three graded levels of injury (RIF) based on the magnitude of change in estimated glomerular filtration rate (GFR) or urine output. In this classification, estimated creatinine clearance is based on original Schwartz formula to quantitate the change in GFR rather than absolute changes in serum creatinine. This modification takes into account the expected normal changes in serum creatinine concentration that accompany somatic growth, hence more applicable to pediatric patients (Tables 1 and 2).

Q. What are the causes of acute renal injury?

The common causes of ARI are listed in box 1.

Q. How to evaluate a patient of acute renal injury?

The clinical evaluation of a patient begins with assessing whether the patient has renal, postrenal, or intrinsic disease. Postrenal obstruction is suggested by poor urinary stream, voiding dysfunction, palpable bladder, or ultrasonography findings of hydronephrosis with significant postvoid residual urine.

Prerenal azotemia manifests as signs of intravascular volume depletion in the form of hypotension, tachycardia, poor skin turgor, concentrated urine, urine sediment without any casts, or cellular elements.

The ultimate determination of whether a patient has prerenal or intrinsic ARI may require

TABLE 1: RIFLE and Acute Kidney Injury Network criteria

RIFLE stage	AKIN stage	Serum creatinine criteria	Urine output criteria
Risk	1	Rise in serum creatinine >1.5 times the baseline	<0.5 mL/kg/h × 6 h
Injury	2	Rise in serum creatinine >2 times the baseline	<0.5 mL/kg/h × 12 h
Failure	3	Rise in serum creatinine more than 3 times the baseline, or serum creatinine >4 mg/dL with an acute rise ≥0.5 mg/dL	<0.3 mL/kg/h × 24 h or anuria × 12 h
Loss	–	Persistent renal failure >4 weeks	
End-stage renal disease	–	Persistent renal failure >3 months	

AKIN, Acute Kidney Injury Network; RIFLE, risk, injury, failure, loss, end-stage renal disease.

TABLE 2: pRIFLE criteria

	pRIFLE criteria	Estimated CrCl (Schwartz)	Urine output
Early	R (Risk)	Decrease by 25	<0.5 mL/kg/h × 8 h
	I (Injury)	Decrease by 50	<0.5 mL/kg/h × 16 h
	F (Failure)	Decrease by 75 or <35 mL/min/1.73 m²	<0.3 mL/kg/h × 24 h or anuria × 12 h
Late	L (Loss)	Renal failure >4 weeks	
	E (End-stage)	Renal failure >3 months	

CrCl → creatinine clearance by Schwartz formula [k × height (cm)/serum creatinine (mg/dL)], where "k" is a constant. The value of "k" is 0.34 for preterm infants, 0.45 for term infants, 0.55 for children and adolescent girls, and 0.70 for adolescent boys

aRIFLE, pediatric risk, injury, failure, loss, end-stage renal disease.

CHAPTER 2: Acute Renal Injury

BOX 1: Categories of acute renal injury in children

Prerenal
- Intravascular volume depletion
  - Dehydration
  - Gastroenteritis
  - Hemorrhage
  - Burns
  - Diuretics
- Redistribution of fluids/vasodilatation
  - Sepsis
  - Pancreatitis
  - Peritonitis
  - Nephrotic syndrome
  - Hepatic failure
- Decreased cardiac output
  - Congestive heart failure
  - Cardiogenic shock
  - Myocarditis

Intrinsic renal
- Acute tubular necrosis
  - Ischemic injury
    - Prerenal causes
    - Exogenous toxins, nephrotoxic antibiotics, Chemotherapeutic agents, NSAIDs
    - ACEIs and ARBs Radiographic contrast
    - Venoms
    - Heavy metals
    - Ethylene glycol
- Endogenous toxins
  - Myoglobinuria/hemoglobinuria
  - Tumor lysis syndrome
- Acute interstitial nephritis
  - Drug-induced or idiopathic
- Acute glomerulonephritis
  - Postinfectious (Streptococcal)
  - HSP, SLE, Goodpasture syndrome
- Vascular pathology
  - Renal artery/vein thrombosis
  - HUS/TTP
  - Cortical necrosis
- Congenital
  - Renal dysplasia/hypoplasia
  - Polycystic renal disease

Continued

Continued

Postrenal
- Posterior urethral valves
- Obstruction of a solitary renal
- Bilateral ureteral obstruction
- Neurogenic bladder
- Trauma

ACEIs, angiotensin converting enzyme inhibitors; ARB, angiotensin receptor blockers; HSP, Henoch-Schönlein purpura; HUS, hemolytic-uremic syndrome; NSAIDs, nonsteroidal anti-inflammatory drugs; SLE, systemic lupus erythematosus; TTP, thrombotic thrombocytopenic purpura.

a challenge of intravenous fluid administration of isotonic saline 20 mL/kg over 30–60 minutes. Following this infusion, a dehydrated patient generally passes urine within 1–2 hours. If the child is still dehydrated and has not passed urine, another intravenous bolus fluid is given. If the patient becomes euhydrated, and still there in no urine output, injection furosemide can be given slowly in the dose of 2 mg/kg. If still there is no urine output, the child is considered to have intrinsic ARI and further on fluids are restricted.

Table 3 depicts the differentiating features of prerenal and intrinsic ARI.

TABLE 3: The differentiating features of prerenal and intrinsic acute renal injury

	Prerenal acute renal injury	Intrinsic acute renal injury
Urinary Na^+ mEq/L	<20	>40
Fractional excretion of Na^+ (%)	<1	>1
Urinary urea nitrogen/plasma urea nitrogen ratio	>8	<3
Urinary/plasma creatinine ratio	>40	<20
Urine osmolality (mOsm/kg)	>500	<250
Blood urea nitrogen/creatinine ratio	>20	<10 to 15
Renal failure index	<1	>1
Urine sediment	Normal or few RBC or WBC	Granular casts and tubular epithelial cells

RBC, red blood cell; WBC, white blood cell.

> **BOX 2: Investigations in a patient with acute renal injury**
>
> **Blood**
> - Complete blood counts
> - Blood urea and creatinine
> - Electrolytes (sodium, potassium, calcium, phosphate)
> - Blood gas (pH, bicarbonate)
>
> **Urine**
> - Urinalysis
> - Culture (if symptoms of urinary infection are present)
> - Fractional excretion of sodium
> - Osmolality
>
> **Radiology**
> - Chest X-ray (for fluid overload, cardiomegaly)
> - Ultrasonography (to identify any obstruction or dilatation)
> - Renal Doppler (for suspected arterial or venous thrombosis)
> - Micturating cystourethrography (if suspecting urethral obstruction)
> - Diethylenetriaminepentaacetic acid (to rule out obstructive uropathy)
>
> **Electrocardiogram (for hyperkalemia)**
> - Investigations to establish the cause
>   - Peripheral smear examination, platelet count, reticulocyte count, blood lactate dehydrogenase levels, stool culture (in suspected d+ hemolytic-uremic syndrome)
>   - Blood anti-streptolysin O, serum C3 levels, antinuclear antibodies, and antineutrophil cytoplasmic antibodies
>   - Renal biopsy

Some investigations, which can aid in identifying the cause of ARI, are listed in box 2.

Q. What are the indications of renal biopsy?

Indications of renal biopsy are:
- Acute renal injury associated with systemic disease, e.g., systemic lupus erythematosus, Henoch-Schönlein purpura
- Interstitial nephritis
- Significant renal dysfunction persisting beyond 2–3 weeks without obvious etiology
- Rapidly progressive glomerulonephritis
- Prognostication and planning future management.

Q. What is the treatment of acute renal injury?

Management of ARI includes treatment of life-threatening complications, maintenance of fluid and electrolyte balance, and nutritional support. Specific management of underlying disorder is possible in a minority of cases (Table 4). Patients with urinary tract obstruction should be managed urgently.

- Fluid management: Child having prerenal ARI would require one or two fluid boluses. If there is no urine output even after diuretic administration, then fluids need to be restricted as in acute intrinsic ARI, to 400 mL/m^2/day plus the urine output and other losses like from gastrointestinal tract
- Electrolyte management: Sodium levels are usually low in ARI because of fluid overload.

TABLE 4: Management of common conditions causing acute renal injury

Prerenal ARI	Crystalloids and discontinue diuretics, NSAIDs or ACEIs
Acute tubular necrosis	Supportive care, discontinue nephrotoxic drugs, treat cause of circulatory failure
Glomerulonephritis	Supportive care, occasionally antibiotics or immunosuppressive therapy
Hemolytic-uremic syndrome	Supportive care, plasma infusions, plasma exchange
Vasculitis	Immunosuppressive therapy, plasma exchange
Interstitial nephritis	Discontinue offending drug, steroid therapy
Renal artery, vein occlusion	Anticoagulation, thrombolysis or surgery
Urinary tract obstruction	Bladder catheter, nephrostomy, treatment of obstruction

ARI, acute renal injury; ACEIs, angiotensin converting enzyme inhibitors; NSAIDs, nonsteroidal anti-inflammatory drugs.

Sodium intake should be restricted to 2 mEq/kg/day together with fluid restriction to prevent sodium and fluid retention. Symptomatic hyponatremia may need to be corrected with hypertonic saline. Hyperkalemia is common in ARI as the renals handle 90% of daily K excretion. It needs to be treated aggressively as it can be life-threatening and dialysis can be employed in cases not responding to medical treatment

Hyperphosphatemia is treated with restriction of phosphate intake along with binders-like calcium acetate or sevelamer to be given along with food

- Nutrition: The major goals are:
  - Adequate caloric intake
  - Protein 2 g/kg/day with an adequate increase during RRT
  - Minimize potassium and phosphate intake
  - Restrict fluid intake
- Medication: Aminoglycosides, nonsteroidal anti-inflammatory drugs, radiocontrast media, amphotericin B, angiotensin-converting enzyme inhibitors, indomethacin should preferably be avoided, but if necessary the doses should be corrected according to GFR
- Renal replacement therapy: Indications for RRT are oliguria with pulmonary edema, severe metabolic acidosis, hyperkalemia, severe hyponatremia, and uremic symptoms not responding to medical treatment. The modalities available for RRT include peritoneal dialysis, hemodialysis or continuous renal replacement therapy.

Q. What steps should be taken to prevent acute renal injury?

General measures to help prevent ARI include judicious use and close monitoring of serum levels of nephrotoxic drugs, adequate fluid repletion in those with hypovolemia, adequate hydration prior to undergoing diagnostic procedures with radiocontrast media, and aggressive hydration and alkalinization of urine prior to chemotherapy.

CONCLUSION

Acute renal injury is a common and potentially devastating complication encountered in critically ill children. Early diagnosis and prompt treatment is the key to successful treatment.

KEY LEARNING POINTS

- The term acute renal injury (ARI) has replaced the former usage of the term acute renal failure. The word "failure" reflected only the end of the clinical spectrum, while ARI suggests that even a marginal increase of serum creatinine (from 0.3 to 0.6 mg/dL) reflects some renal injury and should alert the physician to take appropriate preventive steps
- Different criteria have been laid down to define or stage ARI. Pediatric Risk, Injury, Failure, Loss, End Stage Renal Disease criteria are based on the change in estimated glomerular filtration rate (GFR) or urine output and the estimated creatinine clearance is based on the original Schwartz formula
- To evaluate a patient of ARI, it is essential to categorize in either prerenal, intrinsic renal, or postrenal groups
- The major goal of treatment is to prevent further damage and to provide renal replacement therapy promptly when indicated
- Prompt correction of hypovolemia prevents intrinsic ARI and saves many lives
- Doses of antibiotics and other nephrotoxic drugs should be modified in ARI, when indicated according to GFR value

SUGGESTED READINGS

1. Andreoli SP. Acute kidney injury in children. *Pediatr Nephrol.* 2009;24:253-263.
2. Bagga A, Bakkaloglu A, Devarajan P, Mehta RL, Kellum JA, Shah SV, et al. Improving outcomes from acute kidney injury: report of an initiative. *Pediar Nephrol.* 2007;22:1655-1658.
3. Devarajan P. Pediatric acute kidney injury: Different from acute renal failure, but how and why? *Curr Pediatr Rep.* 2013;1:34-40.
4. Ricci Z, Cruz D, Ronco C. The RIFLE criteria and mortality in AKI: a systematic review. *Kidney Int.* 2008;73:538-546.
5. Walters S, Porter C, Brophy PD. Dialysis and pediatric acute kidney injury: choice of renal support modality. *Pediatr Nephrol.* 2009;24:37-38.

Hemolytic-uremic Syndrome

CHAPTER 3

Shina Menon, RN Srivastava

INTRODUCTION

Hemolytic-uremic syndrome (HUS) is characterized by the triad of nonimmune hemolytic anemia, thrombocytopenia and acute kidney injury (AKI). It occurs predominantly in children younger than 5 years of age, and is amongst the commonest causes of AKI in that group. The typical form of the disorder, also called diarrhea positive HUS (D+ HUS), is preceded by watery diarrhea, which often progresses to hemorrhagic colitis. The diarrhea precedes the hemolysis and thrombocytopenia by 5–7 days; AKI follows several days later. This type is closely linked to infection with Shiga-like toxin (Stx) producing *Escherichia coli* (most commonly serotype O157:H7), and several bacteria, such as *Shigella* or *Streptococcus pneumoniae*. The outcome for most patients who have D+ HUS is favorable with the majority showing complete recovery.

Approximately 10–15% of cases of HUS are not caused by either Stx-producing bacteria or streptococci, and are classified as atypical HUS (aHUS). Atypical HUS has a poor prognosis with death rates as high as 25% and progression to end-stage renal disease in half the patients. Research has shown that aHUS is related to uncontrolled activation of the complement system.

CASE 1

A previously normal 3-year-old boy presented with progressive pallor for 5 days and gradually decreasing urine out for 2 days with anuria since morning. He had bloody diarrhea for 2 days, 1 week back. There was no history of fever, altered sensorium, rash, or joint complaints. His birth and family history were uneventful and he was immunized for age.

On examination, he had tachycardia, normal respiratory rate and blood pressure that was higher than 95th percentile for his age and height. His anthropometric parameters were within age appropriate limits. He was alert but fussy. He looked pale, oral mucosa was moist with no palatal petechiae. Cardiovascular examination revealed tachycardia and a grade II/VI vibratory systolic ejection murmur at the left sternal border without radiation. Gallop rhythm was also noted. His abdomen was soft and nontender with the liver edge palpable 3 cm below the right costal margin. The spleen was nonpalpable. He had good perfusion with no edema, rash or petechiae.

Diagnosis: Anaphylactic shock.

Investigations: A complete blood count showed leukocytosis (white blood cell 26,000 with 72% neutrophils), hemoglobin 8 mg/dL, platelet count 65,000; peripheral smear showed schistocytes and poly-chromasia. Sodium 133 mEq/L, potassium 6.9 mEq/L, chlorine 96, bicarbonate 16, urea 95 mg/dL, creatinine 3.3 mg/dL, calcium 7.8, PO4 7.1, uric acid 7.3. Lactate dehydrogenase was 680. Urinalysis showed 2+ protein, 10–15 red blood cells/high power field and few casts.

Treatment: He was admitted for observation and supportive management. Due to anuria, fluid overload, hyperkalemia, and acute kidney injury, he was started on peritoneal dialysis. Over the next 2 days, his hemoglobin dropped to 5.8 and platelets to 28,000. He was given a packed red cell transfusion. Platelets were not transfused as he was not bleeding. By day 5 of admission, his urine output started improving and his anemia and thrombocytopenia also showed some improvement. At discharge, on day 10, he was off dialysis; his urea was 45, creatinine 1.1, hemoglobin 9.2, and platelets 125,000. He was discharged on an antihypertensive medication.

Outcome: Over the following 2 weeks, his blood pressure and renal function normalized. His complete blood count was also normal.

CASE REVIEW IN NUTSHELL

Any child with pallor and progressive oligo-anuria presenting to the hospital should undergo a comprehensive evaluation to determine the cause. A good history and physical examination helps in narrowing the differential diagnosis and allowing in focusing on diagnostic testing. All patients with AKI should have a urinalysis with microscopic examination, serum chemistries, and a complete blood count. Based on the history, examination, and laboratory features that fulfilled the triad of anemia, thrombocytopenia, and AKI, a diagnosis of HUS was considered in this patient.

The differential diagnosis of D+ HUS includes inflammatory bowel diseases, intussusception, septicemia with disseminated intravascular coagulation, systemic lupus erythematosus, malignant hypertension, and bilateral renal vein thrombosis. Up to 25% cases with typical HUS may not report a diarrheal prodrome.

Non-Stx-related HUS or atypical HUS can be sporadic or familial. The sporadic form is usually secondary to other infections like *Streptococcus pneumonia*, or drugs like chemotherapeutic agents (mitomycin, cisplatin, bleomycin), immunosuppressants (cyclosporine, tacrolimus) and antiplatelet agents (ticlopidine and clopidogrel). Fewer than 20% cases of aHUS are familial, and these are usually related to abnormalities in the complement pathways.

Treatment for typical HUS is supportive. This includes careful monitoring of fluid balance and correction of electrolyte abnormalities. Packed red blood cell transfusion is indicated for symptomatic anemia or if hemoglobin falls below 6 g/dL. Platelet transfusions are indicated only if there is significant bleeding or of the child has to undergo an invasive procedure. Dialysis (peritoneal or hemodialysis) should be considered when medical management cannot correct fluid and electrolyte imbalances.

There is no evidence to suggest that anti-coagulants, antiplatelet agents, fibrinolytic therapy, immune globulin, plasmapheresis, steroids, and Stx binding agents arrest the disease process in HUS. Antibiotics are also not encouraged for D+ HUS due to the potential risk of increasing toxin release from lysed bacteria. They should, however, be used for pneumococcal-associated HUS cases.

In atypical, plasmapheresis has been found to be beneficial. These patients often have a poorer outcome with significant mortality, and high rate of progression to chronic kidney disease (CKD) among survivors.

INTERACTIVE TOPIC REVIEW

Q. What are the key differences between typical and atypical hemolytic uremic syndrome?

The key differences between typical and atypical HUS are given in table 1.

Q. What are the salient steps in the initial management of a child with hemolytic uremic syndrome?

Once the diagnosis of HUS is suspected, all such cases should undergo complete evaluation including complete blood count, renal profile and urinalysis. In patients where atypical HUS is suspected, complement 3 (C3) level should be checked. These patients should be admitted for monitoring fluid-electrolyte status and renal function. The management is mainly supportive. The key components are maintenance of renal perfusion and fluid and electrolyte balance,

TABLE 1: Differences between typical and atypical hemolytic-uremic syndrome

Clinical feature	D+ HUS	D- or atypical HUS
Pathogenesis	Shiga-like toxin, usually associated with *Escherichia coli* (0157:H7)	• *Streptococcus pneumoniae* infection • Drugs (cyclosporine, tacrolimus) • Familial complement pathway disorders
Prodrome	Watery, then bloody diarrhea	None or respiratory
Morbidity	<5%	25%
End-stage renal disease	Unusual, ~ 10%	Common, ~ 30%
Recurrence	Rare	~ 50%
Management	Supportive, dialysis	Dialysis, plasmapheresis

D+, diarrhea positive; HUS, hemolytic-uremic syndrome; D–, diarrhea negative.

blood pressure control, provision of adequate nutrition, and timely initiation of dialysis as indicated.
- Management of fluid status: This depends on whether the patient is dehydrated or fluid overloaded. A dehydrated patient should receive appropriate fluid resuscitation. This should be followed by balancing the patient's ongoing fluid needs (blood products, medications, nutrition). This should be balanced with the output (urine and insensible losses). Fluid restriction may be needed to avoid worsening fluid overload. If fluid restriction does not work, dialysis may be needed to remove the extra fluid
- Monitoring renal function and electrolytes: Medical management should be started for correction of hyperkalemia and acidosis. Dialysis is indicated for refractory fluid overload, refractory acidosis, severe hyperkalemia and uremic symptoms (e.g., pericarditis, lethargy, bleeding diathesis)
- Monitoring: Packed red blood cell transfusion should be considered for hemoglobin less than 6 or symptomatic anemia. Platelet/FFP transfusions are rarely indicated
- Hypertension control.

CONCLUSION

Hemolytic-uremic syndrome is a common cause of renal failure across the world. Most patients with D+ HUS recover with supportive care. Mortality in the acute phase is 5–10% and is often secondary to infection or neurological complications. Long-term follow up is essential post-discharge as 5–25% patients may have sequelae like hypertension, proteinuria, and low glomerular filtration rate. Atypical HUS tends to have a more guarded prognosis. The remission rates are low and many of them have multiple relapses. A large majority also develops CKD and may have recurrence post-transplant.

KEY LEARNING POINTS

☞ Hemolytic-uremic syndrome (HUS), a common cause of renal failure, is characterized by the triad of microangiopathic hemolytic anemia, thrombocytopenia and acute kidney injury

☞ Two broad subcategories are:
1. Associated with a diarrheal prodrome and is more common in infants and children (D+ HUS)
2. Associated with diarrhea (D- HUS), includes atypical and sporadic forms

☞ Most subjects with D+ HUS recover with supportive care though mortality in the acute phase is 5–10%

☞ Sequelae include hypertension, proteinuria, and low glomerular filtration rate

☞ Atypical HUS tends to have a more guarded prognosis with low remission rates, multiple relapses, chronic kidney disease, and post-transplant recurrence.

SUGGESTED READINGS

1. Gagnadoux MF, Habib R, Gubler MC, Bacri JL, Broyer M. Long-term (15–25 years) outcome of childhood hemolytic-uremic syndrome. *Clin Nephrol*. 1996;46:39-41.
2. Gordjani N, Sutor AH, Zimmerhackl LB, Brandis M. Hemolytic uremic syndromes in childhood. *Semin Thrombo Hemost*. 1997;23:281-293.
3. Michael M, Elliott EJ, Ridley GF, Hodson EM, Craig JC. Interventions for haemolytic-uraemic syndrome and thrombotic thrombocytopenic purpura. *Cochrane Database Syst Rev*. 2009:CD003595.
4. Noris M, Remuzzi G. Atypical hemolytic-uremic syndrome. *N Engl J Med*. 2009;361:1676-1687.
5. Siegler RL. The hemolytic-uremic syndrome. *Pediatr Clin North Am*. 1995;42:1505-1529.
6. Tarr PI, Gordon CA, Chandler WL. Shiga-toxin-producing *Escherichia coli* and *haemolytic uraemic* syndrome. *Lancet*. 2005;365:1073-1086.

Acute Glomerulonephritis

CHAPTER 4

RN Srivastava, Shina Menon

INTRODUCTION

Clinical features of gross hematuria, edema, and hypertension constitute the acute nephritic syndrome or acute nephritis. Varying degrees of oliguria and impairment of renal function are usually associated. In most cases, postinfectious acute glomerulonephritis (AGN), usually poststreptococcal, is the underlying etiology. Other, much less common, causative conditions include renal vasculitis (e.g., Henoch-Schönlein purpura), collagen vascular disorders, immunoglobulin A (IgA) nephropathy, and acute interstitial nephritis. Systemic features are often present in these disorders. Extensive laboratory investigations are usually not required in case of postinfectious AGN, which rapidly resolves with supportive management. In most other conditions and in patients with increasing renal dysfunction, detailed laboratory evaluation and a renal biopsy are performed and appropriate treatment carried out.

CASE 1

A 9-year-old girl was referred to pediatric renal clinic. She was perfectly well until 2 days back when she passed "light brownish red urine". There was no dysuria, flank pain, or fever. On the following day, she had complained of headache and was noted to have mild swelling on the face. She appeared to be passing lesser amounts of urine.

Her pediatrician had found her blood pressure (BP) to be raised to 140/90 mmHg. Urinalysis showed 2+ protein and microscopy revealed numerous red cells, red cell casts, and granular casts. Blood tests showed urea 90 mg/dL, creatinine 1.6 mg/dL, and potassium 5.2 mEq/L.

On inquiry, there was a history of mild sore throat about 10 days earlier that resolved over 3–4 days. No antibiotic was taken. There was no family history of a renal disorder. The parents were well educated.

Physical examination confirmed mild facial edema and hypertension. There was no other abnormality.

A chest X-ray film was normal. Blood samples were obtained for hemogram, total protein and albumin, cholesterol, antistreptolysin O (ASO) titer and C'3. The hemoglobin was 11.5 g/dL, leukocytes 11,056/mm^3, neutrophils 60%, protein 6.2 g/dL, and albumin 3.2 g/dL. Subsequent reports showed ASO titer 512 U and C'3 32 mg/dL.

A diagnosis of AGN was made. The parents were explained about the condition, the nature of kidney disease and the outcome and its treatment. She was managed on outpatient basis with close observation by the parents and her pediatrician.

She was advised rest at home, restriction of fluid- and-salt and protein, and control of hypertension with enalapril.

The urine output gradually increased, gross hematuria disappeared over the next 3 days and the weight declined by 1 kg. The levels of blood urea and creatinine were normal on day 7. Urine contained 1+ protein and red blood cells.

Normal diet and activity was gradually resumed.

CHAPTER 4: Acute Glomerulonephritis

The poststreptococcal etiology was confirmed by the findings of raised ASO titer and low C'3. These tests were repeated after a period of 3 months when ASO titer had declined and the C'3 level was within the normal range.

Box 1: Etiology of acute nephritis
- Postinfectious
  - Bacteria: Group A b-hemolytic *Streptococcus* (most frequent cause), *Staphylococcus*, *pneumococcus*, *Salmonella typhi*. Specific conditions: Shunt nephritis,
  - bacterial endocarditis
  - Viruses: Hepatitis B, HIV, cytomegalovirus, rubella
  - Parasites: Malaria, filaria
- Systemic vasculitis
  - Henoch-Schönlein purpura, systemic lupus erythematosus, renal angiitis
- Primary glomerulonephritis
  - Immunoglobulin A nephropathy, membranoproliferative glomerulonephritis.
- Acute interstitial nephritis

HIV, human immunodeficiency virus.

CASE REVIEW IN A NUTSHELL

This patient had presenting features typical of poststreptococcal AGN. It is important to make the correct assessment and avoid unnecessary laboratory investigations. Such patients do not need antibiotics or any specific medications. She was managed symptomatically and observed at home, as the parents were educated and understood the management with imposition of only the necessary restrictions. The condition improved quickly. It is important to be aware of the unusual presenting features. Patients with marked oliguria and profoundly deranged renal functions, severe hypertension need inpatient supportive care.

TOPIC REVIEW

Q. What is the etiology of the "syndrome" of acute nephritis?

Acute glomerulonephritis is mostly follows β-hemolytic streptococcal pharyngitis or pyoderma. It may, however, be caused by other organisms and be a part of systemic disorders affect the kidney (Box 1). Some of them (e.g., IgA nephropathy, acute interstitial nephritis) may have gross hematuria as the sole indicator of renal involvement.

Q. What is its course and outcome?

Acute poststreptococcal glomerulonephritis carries an excellent prognosis. Renal biopsy is no longer carried out in these cases. Earlier studies have shown that even severe histological abnormalities resolve over a period of time with full recovery of renal function. The only exception is a particularly severe renal injury where glomeruli show extensive crescent formation (the histological lesion is termed as "crescentic glomerulonephritis"). These patients usually show mixed features of nephritis with massive edema, hypoalbuminemia, and severe derangement of renal function, which rapidly progresses. Therefore, patients who do not improve within a week are subjected to renal biopsy. Crescentic glomerulonephritis is managed with aggressive immunosuppressive therapy.

Q. How common is poststreptococcal acute glomerulonephritis?

In some parts of India PSAGN still remains common, whereas in northern regions its incidence has declined, and AGN is more often due to a condition other than streptococcal infection.

Q. What precisely is the cause of poststreptococcal acute glomerulonephritis?

Poststreptococcal AGN occurs following pharyngitis or skin infections caused by group A β-hemolytic streptococci. Strains of streptococci capable of producing AGN are called nephritogenic streptococci. Serotype M49 is most commonly associated with skin infections and 1, 4 and 25 with throat infections.

Poststreptococcal AGN related to pyoderma often occurs in epidemics or clusters, being more common in hot and humid climates, whereas that following pharyngitis is predominantly observed in colder regions.

Q. What is its pathogenesis?

Glomerular injury in PSAGN results from deposition of immune complexes in the glomerular capillaries. Circulating immune complexes may get trapped in glomerular capillaries, or such complexes may form in situ from antibodies reacting with streptococcal antigens deposited in glomeruli or with some component of glomerular wall. The antigen responsible for PSAGN is not definitely known. Streptococcal M protein or/and endostreptosin (derived from streptococcal cell cytoplasm) have been suggested to play a role. Complement 3 (C3) activation in PSAGN is via the alternative pathway. The immune deposits consist of IgG, C3, properdin, and C5 and do not contain C1q and C4 (the classical pathway components). Serum C3 levels are decreased.

Q. What is its pathology?

The glomerular abnormalities are very characteristic. Glomeruli are enlarged and the lobular pattern is accentuated. Proliferative and exudative changes are uniformly distributed. There is proliferation of both endothelial and mesangial cells with obliteration of capillary lumen giving the glomeruli a "bloodless" appearance. Neutrophil infiltration is striking in early stages. The capillary basement membrane and the arterioles do not show significant abnormality, and tubular and interstitial abnormalities are absent or insignificant. In a very small proportion of cases, extensive crescentic changes are present. Immunofluorescence examination shows granular deposits of immunoglobulin G (IgG) and C3 along the capillary walls and in the mesangium. Electron microscopy shows electron dense subepithelial deposits or "humps" deposits. The histological abnormalities resolve rapidly and within 6-8 weeks, there is considerable decrease in exudative changes. Mild mesangial hypercellularity may persist for 1-2 years but eventually disappear.

Q. What is its clinical profile?

In most cases, there is a history of sore throat or pyoderma. The latent period is 7-14 days in the former and 2-4 weeks in the latter. Active or healed lesions of impetigo may be present when AGN develops. Poststreptococcal AGN usually affects children between the ages of 5-12 years and is rare below the age of 3 years. Gross hematuria and mild facial edema are the most common presenting features. Urine is typically reddish brown or smoky or cola-colored. Some degree of oliguria is usually associated, but anuria is infrequent and if persistent suggests rapidly progressive glomerulonephritis. If the fluid intake has been unrestricted, edema may increase to involve the hands and legs. Edema is turgid, unlike the flaccid swelling as in nephrotic syndrome. The child often complains of headache due to hypertension, which usually is mild to moderate and results from volume overload.

The severity of PSAGN is variable and mild cases may just have microscopic hematuria with slight proteinuria. Those at the other end of the spectrum may have oligo-anuria and severe hypertension.

Q. How about its atypical presentations?

The child may present with one or more of the complications of AGN. A history of sore throat and gross hematuria may be absent and the edema mild. Occasionally, urinalysis may not show significant abnormality. A correct diagnosis and prompt management are crucial.
- Acute pulmonary edema: Expansion of extracellular volume may lead to congestive heart failure and pulmonary edema. There is dyspnea and restlessness. The blood pressure is high but in later stages when heart failure and shock supervene, there may be hypotension. A chest X-ray film typically shows mild cardiomegaly and features of pulmonary edema. The condition may be

wrongly diagnosed as bronchopneumonia or myocarditis
- Hypertensive encephalopathy: Children with AGN may develop hypertensive encephalopathy at comparatively lower levels of blood pressure. Drowsiness and convulsions may be the presenting features, and the illness resembles encephalitis. Elevated blood pressure and urine abnormalities confirm the diagnosis
- Acute renal failure: In occasional cases, oligoanuria and azotemia are the chief features and gross hematuria and edema may be absent.

Q. What should be the laboratory investigations in a suspected case?

Gross hematuria is present in a majority of moderate-to-severe cases. Proteinuria is usually mild, but occasionally in the nephrotic range. Microscopic examination shows dysmorphic red cells, red cell casts, and neutrophils. In initial stages, urine may contain a large number of neutrophils, which is often mistakenly regarded to indicate urinary tract infection. A fresh, uncentrifuged urine specimen should be examined for casts as these disintegrate on standing and centrifugation. Hyaline and granular casts also may be seen.

The levels of blood urea and creatinine are elevated. In patients with acute renal failure (ARF), there may be hyponatremia, hyperkalemia and acidosis. A chest X-ray film may show cardiomegaly and pulmonary congestion. Anemia and hypoalbuminemia are secondary to renal sodium and water retention with consequent hemodilution. Renal function studies show a decrease in glomerular filtration rate and renal blood flow, increased distal tubular reabsorption of sodium and water leading to hypervolemia and expansion of extracellular volume.

Evidence of preceding streptococcal infection is indicated by a rise in antistreptolysin O (ASO) titer, which is elevated in 60–80% cases. Early antibiotic treatment may attenuate this response. The rise in ASO titer begins 1–3 weeks after the streptococcal infection, reaches a peak in 3–5 weeks and then falls to insignificant levels in 6 months. It is not related to the severity or the prognosis of disease. In pyoderma, ASO titer is less commonly elevated whereas antihyaluronidase and anti-deoxyribonuclease B are more often raised. The streptozyme test detects several streptococcal antibodies but has low sensitivity and specificity and is not necessary for routine use. Streptococci can occasionally be cultured from the throat or skin infection.

Approximately 90% patients have decreased serum C3 levels that return to normal in 6–8 weeks. Serum C5 levels are mildly reduced but those of C4 are normal. Persistent hypocomplementemia is rare in PSAGN and suggests an alternative condition such as membranoproliferative glomerulonephritis, lupus nephritis or glomerulonephritis related to endocarditis or occult abscesses. The levels of ASO titer or C3 are not related to the severity of the disease.

Q. What should be the therapeutic approach?

The treatment is essentially symptomatic. Mild cases may be managed at home. Those with moderate or severe hypertension and oliguria require hospital care. Strict bed rest is not necessary. Circulatory congestion and edema can be treated with restriction of salt and water and judicious use of diuretics. Moderate-to-severe hypertension with or without encephalopathy usually responds to treatment with nifedipine or enalapril and furosemide.

If oliguria is present and the level of blood urea is elevated, dietary protein should be appropriately restricted. Penicillin may be administered for 7 days if active pyoderma or residual pharyngitis is present, but it has no influence on the course of the disease. Daily weight, urine output, and blood levels of urea and electrolytes are monitored. With careful management, the child should lose weight depending upon the degree of edema. In patients having acute pulmonary edema and shock, adequate supportive measures should be promptly instituted preferably in an ICU. Furosemide is given intravenously in a dose of 4–6 mg/kg. Dopamine or dobutamine should be infused and ventilatory support provided.

Q. What is the course and prognosis of the disease?

The symptoms usually begin to resolve in the first week with loss of edema and fall in the elevated blood pressure levels. Gross hematuria rapidly clears but microscopic hematuria may be detected for 6–12 months or longer. Proteinuria subsides earlier but orthostatic or intermittent proteinuria may be observed, which is of no significance. Occasionally, mild-to-moderate hypertension may persist for a few weeks. Patients, who develop ARF, especially if prolonged, may be left with residual impairment of renal function.

Q. What is crescentic glomerulo-nephritis (rapidly progressive glomerulonephritis)?

Crescentic glomerulonephritis refers to a particularly severe form of glomerular injury characterized by extensive crescent formation. Crescentic glomerulonephritis is most commonly associated with a severe acute nephritic syndrome with heavy proteinuria, which may progress to renal failure over a few days to weeks. However, a rapidly progressive course may occur in other forms of glomerulonephritis or interstitial nephritis, whereas crescentic glomerulonephritis may not invariably have a fulminant course.

Q. What is its etiology and classification?

In children, crescentic glomerulonephritis is usually associated with postinfectious glomerulonephritis, collagen vascular diseases and vasculitis, but in many cases, it presents as an isolated disorder. The condition is classified according to immunohistological examination of renal biopsy (Box 2).

> **BOX 2: Disorders associated with crescentic glomerulonephritis**
> - Antiglomerular basement membrane disease:
>   - Goodpasture's syndrome
> - Immune complex disease:
>   - Postinfectious glomerulonephritis
>   - Immunoglobulin A nephropathy
>   - Henoch-Schönlein purpura
>   - Lupus nephritis
>   - Membranoproliferative glomerulonephritis
>   - Idiopathic
> - Pauci-immune disease:
>   - Idiopathic
>   - Microscopic polyarteritis
>   - Wegener's granulomatosis

Q. What about the pathologic changes?

The light microscopic appearance of the affected glomeruli is very striking. The crescents are large, several cell layers thick and initially cellular, and appear to compress and distort the capillary tufts. With passage of time, the crescents become fibrous and eventually the glomerulus gets sclerosed. Renal biopsies in children with pauci-immune glomerulo-nephritis show features of glomerular inflammation and necrosis; varying degrees of vasculitis may also be present. A majority of patients with pauci-immune crescentic glomerulonephritis have antineutrophilic cytoplasmic antibodies (ANCA), and many have systemic features of vasculitis.

Immunofluorescence examination identifies three distinct groups. There may be linear deposition of IgG and C3 along the capillary basement membrane indicating antiglomerular basement membrane (anti-GBM) antibody mediated involvement. Such a pattern is seen in Goodpasture's syndrome, which is rare in children. More commonly discrete granular deposits of IgG and C3 are seen along the capillary walls and in the mesangium indicating immune complex-mediated glomerulonephritis, characteristically found in postinfectious glomerulonephritis (in children usually poststreptococcal). In pauci-immune crescentic GN, there is no deposition of immune reactants in the glomeruli, except for the nonspecific presence of fibrin in the crescents.

Q. How does it present clinically?

Crescentic glomerulonephritis usually manifests with severe acute nephritic features often associated with heavy proteinuria and moderate-to-severe edema. Renal insufficiency may be present at the onset and steadily worsen. Patients with anti-GBM antibody disease, microscopic polyarteritis, and Wegener's granulomatosis may also have pulmonary hemorrhage.

Whereas almost all patients with PSAGN with typical histological features show significant resolution within a week or two, those with crescentic glomerulonephritis do not show much improvement. In occasional cases, the onset may be insidious with features of steroid-resistant nephrotic syndrome.

A renal biopsy should be promptly carried out in children with severe acute glomerulonephritis, in whom a poststreptococcal etiology is not established or those who do not show rapid resolution. Immunofluorescence (or immunohistology) is necessary to categorize different types of crescentic glomerulonephritis. Hemogram, chest X-ray, blood cultures, serum complement, antinuclear antibody, anti-double stranded DNA antibodies and ANCA, hepatitis B and C serology, cryoglobulins, and anti-GBM antibodies are required to clarify the diagnosis.

Q. What is its treatment?

The patients are treated with aggressive immunosuppression. Early diagnosis is essential since later in the course of the disease when the crescents are mostly fibrotic with severe damage to capillary tufts, no therapy will be of any use. Three to six intravenous methylprednisolone pulses followed by long-term treatment with oral prednisolone, together with oral or intravenous cyclophosphamide for the first 3–6 months are usually employed. Plasmapheresis is used in anti-GBM antibody-induced disease and in patients having pauci-immune glomerulonephritis with pulmonary hemorrhage or those not responding to prednisolone and cyclophosphamide.

The long-term prognosis is uncertain. Even patients who seem to recover from acute renal insufficiency may gradually develop increasing renal damage. The outcome is related to the severity of the crescentic changes and the promptness of the institution of therapy.

Q. What is immunoglobulin A nephropathy?

Immunoglobulin A nephropathy is regarded to be the most frequent form of primary glomerulonephritis worldwide, particularly in Asia-Pacific countries. However, it is very uncommon in children in India. Immunoglobulin A nephropathy is diagnosed by demonstration of deposits of IgA in the mesangium on immunofluorescence examination of renal biopsy. Immunoglobulin G and C3 deposits are usually present, but IgA deposition is predominant. Similar abnormalities are seen in Henoch-Schönlein purpura nephritis.

Q. What is its clinical presentation?

Recurrent gross hematuria is the typical presentation. Flank pain may be associated. Episodes of gross hematuria often immediately follow upper respiratory infections, but microscopic hematuria may persist. In an occasional case, the disorder manifests with acute nephritic features or with heavy proteinuria and nephrotic syndrome, and more rarely with ARF and crescentic glomerulonephritis.

Q. How about its pathogenesis?

The underlying abnormality appears to be a defect in glycosylation of IgA1, which leads to formation of immune complexes. Circulating immune complexes get deposited in the mesangium. Environmental factors seem also responsible to account for the high prevalence of IgA nephropathy in South-East Asian countries. Plasma levels of IgA are increased in a variable proportion of patients, but do not correlate with the severity of renal histologic lesions.

Q. What is its renal histology?

On light microscopic examination, focal, segmental proliferative lesions are characteristic. There is proliferation of mesangial cells with increase in mesangial matrix. In more severe cases, segmental fibrinoid necrosis, capsular adhesions, and small crescents may be seen. These proliferative lesions are observed early in the course of the disease and may gradually decrease after a few months, when focal segmental sclerosis or hyalinosis may be more prominent. Diffuse proliferative lesions are uncommon. In the rare patient presenting with rapidly progressive glomerulonephritis, extensive crescent formation is observed. Vascular lesions are usually absent. Deposits in the mesangium are predominantly composed of IgA1.

Q. What is its course and outcome?

The long-term course of the disorder is not clearly defined but the prognosis in children is much better than in adults. A small proportion of patients are reported to develop progressive renal injury and chronic kidney disease on long-term follow-up.

Factors indicating poor outcome include:
- Persistent heavy proteinuria
- Diffuse proliferation with sclerosis
- Extensive crescentic changes on renal biopsy.

Q. How to treat this condition?

Patients with microscopic hematuria with or without mild proteinuria (<1 g/1.73 m²/day) do not require any specific medications. In those having heavy proteinuria and severe histological changes, prednisolone alone or together with azathioprine may be used. Other drugs including cyclophosphamide and mycophenolate have been employed with variable results. Patients with extensive crescentic changes have a poor outcome and need aggressive treatment. Administration of angiotensin converting enzyme inhibitors, enalapril, or lisinopril leads to reduction in proteinuria. Use of omega-3 fatty acids (fish oil, 6–12 g daily) may also retard the decline in renal function.

Q. What is acute interstitial nephritis?

Gross hematuria may occasionally be caused by exposure to drugs (such as ampicillin, ciprofloxacin, methicillin, rifampicin, phenytoin, furosemide, nonsteroidal anti-inflammatory drugs, and several others). Fever, rash, mild arthralgia, and flank pain may be associated. In about 15% cases, acute kidney injury may develop being of the nonoliguric form. Eosinophilia and eosinophiluria may be present. Acute interstitial nephritis is considered to be caused by cell-mediated immune injury. Renal histology shows acute interstitial inflammatory abnormalities with associated damage to tubular cells. Immunofluorescence examination usually does not show immune deposits.

Infiltrative changes can be diffuse but often they are patchy, mostly in the deep cortex and outer medulla. They are composed of T cells, monocytes/macrophages, plasma cells, and eosinophils. Interstitial edema is associated.

Q. How to treat it?

The offending agent should be promptly removed, which often leads to rapid recovery function. A short course of treatment with prednisolone (1–2 mg/kg/day, tapered off over 3–4 weeks) may hasten recovery. In patients with acute kidney injury, 3–5 pulses of intravenous methylprednisolone (30 mg/kg/day) may lead to rapid improvement of renal function.

Q. What is its course?

Patients, who develop renal failure, especially if prolonged, may be left with residual impairment of renal function.

Q. Are there some disorders with acute nephritic features with systemic abnormalities?

A number of conditions may present with one or more features of acute nephritis. Systemic manifestations may be mild or develop subsequently. Presence of purpuric rash or other cutaneous lesions, joint involvement, fever and

CONCLUSION

Acute occurrence of gross hematuria, edema, and hypertension indicates an underlying renal disorder which is referred to as "acute nephritic syndrome". Varying degrees of oliguria and renal functional impairment are associated. The most common etiology is acute postinfectious glomerulonephritis, usually related to group A β-hemolytic streptococcal pharyngitis or pyoderma.

Renal vasculitis, IgA nephropathy, and collagen vascular disorders occasionally present with similar features are usually associated with systemic involvement (fever, arthropathy and rash). Occasionally, PSAGN manifests with atypical features such as pulmonary edema, encephalopathy and ARF. Careful evaluation and supportive management are carried out, and unnecessary tests and hazardous drugs avoided.

The outcome in PSAGN is satisfactory and almost all patients make a complete recovery. However, in unresolving cases renal biopsy is performed to detect crescentic glomerulonephritis, which requires aggressive immunosuppressive therapy and carries a guarded prognosis.

KEY LEARNING POINTS

- Clinical features of gross hematuria, edema, and hypertension constitute the acute nephritic syndrome or acute nephritis
- Varying degrees of oliguria and impairment of renal function are usually associated
- In most cases, postinfectious acute glomerulonephritis (AGN), usually poststreptococcal, is the underlying etiology
- Extensive laboratory investigations are usually not required in case of postinfectious AGN, which rapidly resolves with supportive management.

SUGGESTED READINGS

1. Bagga A, Menon S. Acute and rapidly progressive glomerulonephritis. In: Srivastava RN, Bagga A, (Eds). *Pediatric Nephrology*. New Delhi: Jaypee Brothers Medical Publishers; 2015:136-154.
2. Eison TM, Ault BH, Jones DP, Chesney RW, Wyatt RJ. Poststreptococcal acute glomerulonephritis in children: Clinical features and pathogenesis. *Pediatr Nephrol*. 2011;26:165-180.
3. KDIGO. Clinical Practice guidelines for glomerulonephritis. *Kidney Intern*. 2012;2:139-274.
4. Srivastava RN, Menon S. Acute glomerulonephritis revisited. In: Gupte S, Gupte SB, Gupte M (Eds). *Recent Advances in Pediatrics-23 Hot Topics*. New Delhi: Jaypee Brothers Medical Publishers; 2015:262-273.

Hematuria

CHAPTER 5

Alla Bharath Kumar

INTRODUCTION

Hematuria is defined as the presence of at least five red blood cells (RBCs) per microliter of urine and occurs with a prevalence of 0.5–2.0% among school-age children. Quantitative studies demonstrate that normal children can excrete more than 500,000 RBCs per 12 hour period; this increases with fever and/or exercise. The presence of 10–50 RBCs/µL may suggest underlying pathology, but significant hematuria is generally considered as more than 50 RBCs/µL. False negative results can occur in the presence of formalin (used as a urine preservative) or high urinary concentrations of ascorbic acid (i.e., in patients with vitamin C intake >2,000 mg/day). False-positive results may be seen in a child with an alkaline urine (pH >8), or more commonly following contamination with oxidizing agents such as hydrogen peroxide used to clean the perineum before obtaining a specimen. Microscopic analysis of 10–15 mL of freshly voided and centrifuged urine is essential in confirming the presence of RBCs suggested by more than 10 RBCs/µL, or a 1+ positive urinary dipstick reading.

The detection of microscopic hematuria in a child's urine prompts evaluation for renal and urinary bladder causes. Microscopic hematuria identified during a routine physical examination by the pediatrician is much more common than macroscopic hematuria. Persistent microscopic hematuria is particularly worrisome and may require a percutaneous needle core kidney biopsy to determine whether the etiology is secondary to glomerular disease, tubulointerstitial disease, urinary tract infection, urinary tract structural abnormalities, medications, or toxins.

The physician should ensure that serious conditions are not overlooked, avoid unnecessary and often expensive laboratory studies, reassure the family, and provide guidelines for additional studies if there is a change in the child's course. This article provides an approach to the evaluation and management of hematuria in a child. Many tests have been recommended for the child with hematuria, but no consensus exists on a stepwise evaluation.

CASE REVIEW IN A NUTSHELL

This 10-year-old girl presented in hypertensive urgency because of acute renal failure. For this she was initially started on nitroglycerine drip. BP got controlled over 48 hours. Subsequently, child was started on enalapril. The patient also had hyperkalemia for which she was given intravenous calcium gluconate, 1 mL/kg, and insulin dextrose infusion. As a result, her potassium got normalized. She also had

CASE SCENARIO

A 10-year-old female child presented with passage of cola colored urine for 3 days, decreased urine output for 2 days, and puffiness of eyes for 1 day with preceding history of upper respiratory infection 10 days back.

Examination: Child had hypertension [blood pressure (BP) 145/85 mmHg], periorbital puffiness with ascites.

Investigations: Blood urea: 86 mg/dL, creatinine: 1.4 mg/dL, urine routine examination 10–15 RBC/μL, albumin +++.

Diagnosis: Hypertensive urgency on acute glomerulonephritis.

Treatment: During the hospital stay, child was initially started on nitroglycerine drip in view of hypertensive urgency. Subsequently, BP having got controlled over 48 hours, she was kept on enalapril and a loop diuretic.

Course: She slowly improved. Edema subsided over 1 week, azotemia improved over 10 days and proteinuria got subsided in 5 days.

azotemia with anasarca for which she was started on nasal prong oxygen and loop diuretic. Subsequently, her urine output improved over 4 days, edema subsided over 1 week, azotemia improved over 1 week and proteinuria regressed over 5 days. Her slightly high anion gap metabolic acidosis, detected at the time of first presentation, regressed during hospital stay.

She was also evaluated for active streptococcal infection. However, throat swab, antistreptolysin O antibodies and anti-double stranded deoxyribonucleic acid titers turned out to be negative. Though C3 was low, C4 levels were normal.

INTERACTIVE TOPIC REVIEW

Q. What is Hematuria?

Hematuria is the presence of RBCs in the urine, either visible to the eye (macroscopic hematuria) or as viewed under the microscope (microscopic hematuria) and is usually detected by a dipstick test during a routine examination.

Hematuria is defined as the presence of at least five RBCs per microliter of urine and occurs with a prevalence of 0.5–2.0% among school-age children. The presence of 10–50 RBCs/μL may suggest underlying pathology, but significant hematuria is generally considered as more than 50 RBCs/μL. False negative results can occur in the presence of formalin (used as a urine preservative) or high urinary concentrations of ascorbic acid (i.e., in patients with vitamin C intake >2,000 mg/day). False-positive results may be seen in a child with an alkaline urine (pH >8), or more commonly following contamination with oxidizing agents such as hydrogen peroxide used to clean the perineum before obtaining a specimen. Microscopic analysis of 10–15 mL of freshly voided and centrifuged urine is essential in confirming the presence of RBCs suggested by more than 10 RBCs/μL, or a 1+ positive urinary dipstick reading.

Hematuria is one of the most important signs of renal or bladder disease, but proteinuria is a more important diagnostic and prognostic finding, except in the case of calculi or malignancies. Bright-red urine, visible clots, or crystals with normal-looking RBCs suggests bleeding from the urinary tract. Cola-colored urine, RBC casts, and deformed (dysmorphic) RBCs suggest glomerular bleeding. An absence of RBCs in the urine with a positive dipstick reaction suggests hemoglobinuria or myoglobinuria.

Q. What is the Pathophysiology of Hematuria?

Origin of hematuria may be the glomeruli, renal tubules and interstitium, or urinary tract (including collecting systems, ureters, bladder, and urethra).

In children, the source of bleeding is more often from glomeruli than from the urinary tract.

The RBCs cross the glomerular endothelial-epithelial barrier and enter the capillary lumen through structural discontinuities in the capillary wall. These discontinuities seem to be at the capillary wall-mesangial cell reflections. In most cases, proteinuria, RBC casts, and deformed (dysmorphic) RBCs in the urine accompany hematuria caused by any of the glomerulonephritides.

Renal papillae are vulnerable to necrotic injury from microthrombi and anoxia in patients with a hemoglobinopathy or in those exposed to toxins. Patients with renal parenchymal lesions may have episodes of transient microscopic or macroscopic hematuria during systemic infections or after moderate exercise. This may be the result of renal hemodynamic responses to exercise or fever by undetermined mechanisms.

Q. How do you Evaluate a Child with Hematuria?

Medical History

- A history of dysuria, frequency, urgency, or flank or abdominal pain suggests a diagnosis of urinary tract infection or stone
- A history of recent trauma, strenuous exercise, menstruation, or bladder catheterization may be responsible for transient hematuria
- A sore throat or skin infection within the past 2–4 weeks points to postinfectious glomerulonephritis
- Drugs and toxins may cause either hematuria or hemoglobinuria
- A careful family history includes questions about hematuria, hearing loss, hypertension, renal calculus, renal diseases, renal cystic diseases, hemophilia, sickle cell trait, and dialysis or transplant.

Physical Examination

- Presence or absence of hypertension or proteinuria assists in deciding how extensively to pursue the diagnostic evaluation
- In case the BP is normal and the patient is passing normal amounts of urine, it is unlikely that microscopic hematuria, whatever its cause, warrants immediate treatment
- In case the BP is elevated, the hematuria requires a more intensive diagnostic evaluation
- Presence of fever or costovertebral angle tenderness may indicate a urinary tract infection
- An abdominal mass may suggest a tumor, hydronephrosis, multicystic dysplastic kidney, or polycystic kidney disease
- Macroscopic hematuria with proteinuria suggests glomerulonephritis
- Rashes and arthritis often point to Henoch-Schönlein purpura and systemic lupus erythematosus.

Laboratory Studies

As a rule, usually only two diagnostic tests are required for a child with microscopic hematuria:
1. Demonstration of proteinuria and
2. Microscopic examination of the urine for RBCs and RBC casts.

Macroscopic hematuria needs urine culture and renal imaging by ultrasound.

Proteinuria may be present regardless of the cause of bleeding. However, it usually does not exceed 2þ (100 mg/dL) if the only source of protein is from the blood. This is especially true if the child has microscopic hematuria.

Presence of 1–2þ proteinuria should be evaluated for orthostatic (postural) proteinuria. Over 2þ proteinuria should be investigated for glomerulonephritis and nephrotic syndrome.

Red blood cell casts, when present, are a highly specific marker for glomerulonephritis. Their absence does not rule out glomerular disease and their presence does not prove that glomerular injury has occurred. RBC casts need to be searched for meticulously. Even distorted, misshapen erythrocytes (dysmorphic) also suggest a glomerular origin for bleeding.

Q. How to Differentiate Glomerular from Nonglomerular of Hematuria?

Table 1 highlights the differentiating features of glomerular and nonglomerular hematuria.

Q. What are the Gas Exchange Goals in Acute Respiratory Distress Syndrome?

In terms of determining appropriate gas-exchange goals, it should be stressed that oxygenation and ventilation should have "adequate" rather than "optimal" targets.

TABLE 1: Differentiating features of glomerular and nonglomerular hematuria

Features	Glomerular diseases	Nonglomerular causes
History		
Dysuria	Absent	Present in urethritis and cystitis
Systemic complaints	Edema, fever, pharyngitis, rash, arthralgia	Fever with UTI, pain with calculi
Family history	Deafness, hematuria in Alport's syndrome	May be positive with calculi and hypercalcuria
Physical examination		
Hypertention, edema	Usually present	Less common
Abdominal mass	Absent	Present in Wilm's tumor, obstructive uropathy
Rash, arthritis	Lupus erythematosus. Henoch-Schönlein purpura	Absent unless part of drug-induced interstitial nephritis
Urinalysis		
Color	Brown, tea, cola	Bright red, clots may be present
Proteinuria	2+ or more	Less than 2+
Dysmorphic RBCs	More than 20%	Not common, less than 15%
RBC casts	Common	Absent
Crystals	Absent	Positive in few

UTI, urinary tract infections; RBC, red blood cell.

Permissive hypercapnia and permissive hypoxemia should be employed when clinically indicated, to minimize exposure to toxic ventilatory support. The target PaO_2, SpO_2, and $PaCO_2$ are likely to differ between patients and within an individual patient over time, based on the degree of ventilatory support the patient requires (i.e., risk of ventilator-induced lung injury).

Q. How about an Algorithmic Approach?

Yes, that should be very much in place. Flowchart 1 shows a general suggested approach to the management of hematuria.

CONCLUSION

Hematuria, presence of RBCs in the urine (macroscopic or microscope), is one of the most important signs of renal or bladder disease. It warrants thorough clinical and investigative workup. It should be ensured that serious conditions are not overlooked, unnecessary and expensive laboratory studies are avoided, and the family is reassured. Guidelines for additional studies should be provided as and when required.

KEY LEARNING POINTS

- Hematuria is the presence of red blood cells in the urine which may be gross or microscopic
- It is one of the most important signs of renal or bladder disease though proteinuria is a more important diagnostic and prognostic finding, except in the case of calculi or malignancies
- Hematuria is almost never a cause of anemia
- Though all attempts should be made to ensure that serious conditions are not missed, unnecessary expensive investigations should be avoided in its evaluation.

SECTION 2: Nephrology

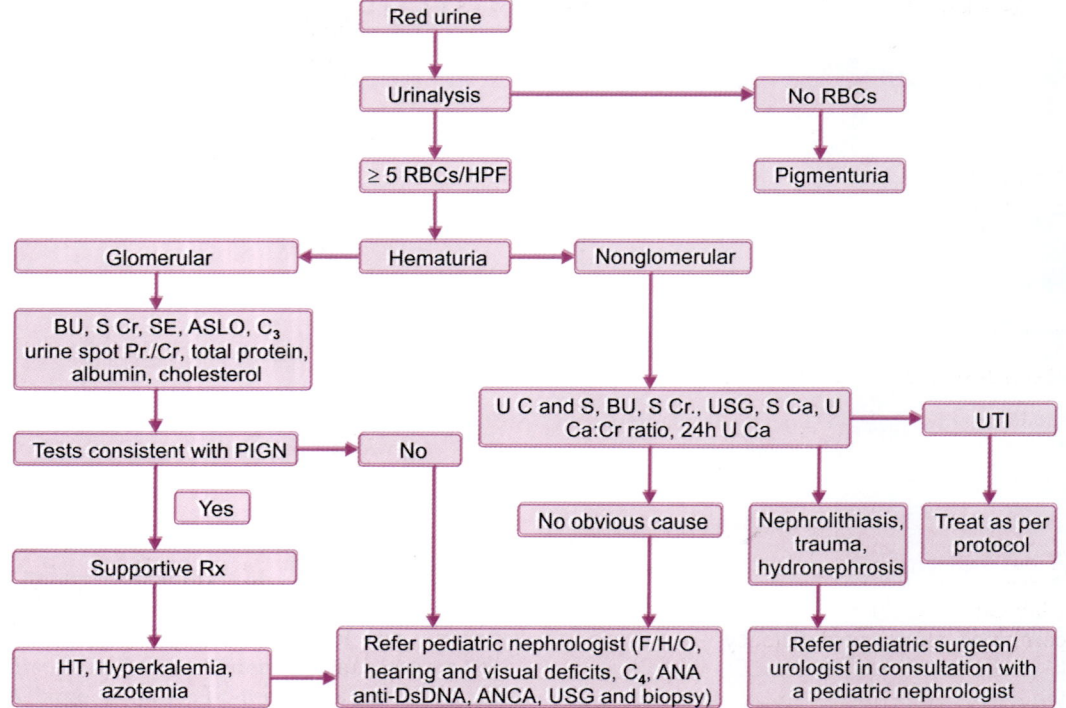

RBC, red blood cell; BU, blood urea; S Cr, serum creatinine; SE, serum electrolytes; ASLO, antistreptolysin O antibodies; C3, complement factor 3; Pr/Cr, protein: creatinine; PIGN, postinfectious glomerulonephritis; Rx: treatment; HT, hematuria; C_4, complement factor 4; ANA, antinuclear antibody; DsDNA, double stranded deoxyribonucleic acid; ANCA, antineutrophil cytoplasmic antibody; USG, ultrasonography; U C and S, urine culture and sensitivity; U Ca: Cr, spot urinary calcium to creatinine ratio; 24h U Ca, 24h urinary calcium excretion; UTI, urinary tract infection.

Flowchart 1: Algorithmic approach to diagnosis and management of hematuria in a child

SUGGESTED READINGS

1. Arpitha G, Gupte S, Shore RM. Pediatric nephrology. In: Gupte S (Ed). *The Short Textbook of Pediatrics*, 12th edn. New Delhi: Jaypee Brothers Medical Publishers; 2016: 612-632.
2. Srivastava RN, Menon S. Acute glomerulonephritis revisited. In: Gupte S, Gupte SB, Gupte M (Eds). *Recent Advances in Pediatrics-23 Hot Topics*. New Delhi: Jaypee Brothers Medical Publishers; 2015:263-272.
3. Srivastava RN, Bagga A. *Pediatric Nephrology*, 4th edn. New Delhi: Jaypee Brothers Medical Publishers; 2005.

SECTION 3
Endocrine and Metabolic Disorders

CHAPTER 6

Diabetic Ketoacidosis

Meenakshi Bothra, Vandana Jain

INTRODUCTION

Diabetic ketoacidosis (DKA) results from the combined effects of deficiency of insulin and high levels of counterregulatory hormones (glucagon, epinephrine, and cortisol), leading to increased production and impaired utilization of glucose (hyperglycemia and hyperosmolality), increased lipolysis and ketone production (ketonemia and metabolic acidosis), and osmotic diuresis (dehydration).

Although DKA is commoner in patients with type 1 diabetes, it is occasionally seen in patients with type 2 diabetes as well, especially those with younger age at onset of diabetes. In type 1 diabetes, DKA may occur either at the onset of diabetes or later, especially in patients with poor compliance to therapy and during intercurrent illness.

Children with mild DKA may be managed on ambulatory basis, but those with moderate-to-severe DKA require hospitalization. Intravenous insulin infusion begun after the initial fluid resuscitation. Close monitoring of clinical and biochemical parameters is required to avert complications like cerebral edema, hypokalemia, and hypoglycemia. Transition is made from intravenous infusion to intermittent premeal subcutaneous insulin with titration of doses to achieve normoglycemia following the resolution of ketoacidosis when the child starts accepting orally.

In order to avoid recurrence of DKA, identification and management of factors precipitating the episode of DKA are of paramount importance.

CASE 1

A 7-year-old girl presented to the pediatric emergency with complaints of abdominal pain and recurrent vomiting for 1 day. She was a known case of type 1 diabetes, diagnosed 1.5 years back. At presentation, she was hemodynamically stable. Her blood glucose was 405 mg/dL and urine ketones were positive (large). A venous blood gas (VBG) showed mild metabolic acidosis (pH = 7.290, HCO_3 = 11 mmol/L).

She had a history of two previous hospitalizations with DKA, first episode was of severe DKA at the time of detection of diabetes mellitus and the second episode was of mild DKA 1 year ago. Blood glucose monitoring was not done regularly at home and the child had not returned for follow-up for the last 1 year. On probing, there were social issues. The child had been living with her maternal grandparents as her father refused to participate in her care. The grandparents could not afford daily blood glucose monitoring.

The child received intravenous normal saline 10 mL/kg in the first hour of treatment and was subsequently started on intravenous fluids (maintenance + 50% dehydration correction) over 48 hours, intravenous regular insulin infusion 0.1 unit/kg/h, which could be tapered off and stopped in 24 hours with resolution of clinical features and improvement in acidosis. She remained hospitalized for another 48 hours for optimization of insulin doses according to blood glucose values.

CASE REVIEW IN A NUTSHELL

- Some of the most common reasons for DKA in a known patient with type 1 diabetes mellitus include:
  - Poor compliance to insulin and dietary therapy
  - Lack of regular blood glucose monitoring at home
  - Omission of insulin doses and poor intake of food and fluids during intercurrent illnesses
  - Adolescent age group
- Clinical features seen in children with DKA include polyuria, polydipsia, dehydration, weight loss, Kussmaul respiration, fruity breath odor, abdominal pain, vomiting, headache, and altered sensorium
- Administration of intravenous fluids is important even before starting insulin infusion
- There is no role of an insulin bolus dose during DKA; continuous intravenous infusion of regular insulin is recommended
- Proper diabetes education to ensure compliance to treatment and regular follow-up is essential to avoid recurrence of DKA and other complications associated with diabetes.

CASE 2

A 2.5-year-old boy presented with recurrent vomiting and fast breathing for 12 hours and altered sensorium (not recognizing parents and not following commands properly) for 8 hours before admission. Six days prior to presenting to us, the child had been admitted in another hospital managed for DKA and discharged in 2 days.

The diagnosis of type 1 diabetes had been made in this child 4 months ago. At that time, he had presented to another hospital with complaints of polyuria and polydipsia for 2 months, and altered sensorium and recurrent vomiting for 2 days. He had been diagnosed to have DKA, was hospitalized for 10 days, and advised insulin therapy. However, the parents had very poor understanding of the child's illness and were not able to comply with the insulin regimen and dietary advice.

In the pediatric emergency room, the child was found to be drowsy, dehydrated with weakly palpable pulses, and having acidotic breathing. He had tachycardia and pallor. Fundus examination did not show papilledema and there were no signs of raised intracranial tension. His blood glucose was "high" and VBG showed severe acidosis (pH = 6.88, pCO_2 = 14.8, pO_2 = 85.3, HCO_3 = 2.3, BE = -30.6), sodium/potassium 130/4.8 urea/creatinine 74/0.7, and urine ketones was positive. His total leukocyte count was 43,200/mm^3 with neutrophils 66% and lymphocytes 32%.

He was diagnosed to have severe DKA with shock, and was given two normal saline boluses of 20 mL/kg each followed by initiation of inotrope therapy along with insulin infusion at 0.1 unit/kg/h and intravenous fluids (maintenance + 70% dehydration correction over 48 h). He was noted to have hepatomegaly and pulmonary crepitations with persistence of altered sensorium. He was intubated and put on mechanical ventilation in view of pulmonary edema and altered sensorium (cerebral edema). Computed tomography head done after initial stabilization confirmed the presence of cerebral edema. His renal functions were subsequently found to be deranged with blood urea/creatinine of 91 and 2.2 mg/dL requiring peritoneal dialysis. The inotropes were gradually tapered off, his sensorium improved and he was extubated after 48 hours. In view of hepatomegaly and generalized lymphadenopathy, the child was worked up and found to have tuberculosis and started on antitubercular treatment (2HRZE + 4HR). The resolution of metabolic acidosis took 3 days. Subsequently, child was shifted to subcutaneous insulin, which was titrated according to blood glucose values.

CASE REVIEW IN A NUTSHELL

- Counseling of parents and ensuring that they are competent with administrating insulin injections, monitoring blood glucose (BG) and understand the actions to be taken for low and high BG values is of utmost importance when a child is diagnosed with diabetes. If the family needs financial assistance for procuring of supplies, the treating physician should be able to guide them appropriately
- Children who present late often have severe DKA with greater risk of complications
- Elevated total leukocyte count with leftward shift is seen in DKA can be due to the effect

of stress hormones epinephrine and cortisol. Thus, leukocytosis during DKA is not a reliable indicator of infection and active screening for possible source of infection (including cultures and chest radiograph) is required
- Cerebral edema is the most common cause of death in children with DKA, and is more likely to occur in patients with newly diagnosed type 1 diabetes, younger age, and greater severity of DKA. Therapy-associated risk factors for cerebral edema include use of bicarbonate, rapid decline in serum osmolality, attenuated rise in sodium during therapy, higher volumes of fluid infused in first 4 hours, and administration of insulin (especially as bolus) within the first hour of treatment.

INTERACTIVE TOPIC REVIEW

Q. How is diabetic ketoacidosis diagnosed?

The biochemical criteria for the diagnosis of DKA are:
- Hyperglycemia (BG >200–300 mg/dL)
- Metabolic acidosis: Venous pH less than 7.3 and/or bicarbonate less than 15 mmol/L
- Ketonemia/ketonuria.

Q. How is diabetic ketoacidosis classified according to severity?

Diabetic ketoacidosis is categorized by the severity of the acidosis:
- Mild: pH 7.25–7.30, HCO_3 10–15 mmol/L
- Moderate: pH 7.10–7.25, HCO_3 5–10 mmol/L
- Severe: pH less than 7.10, HCO_3 less than 5 mmol/L.

Q. What are the indications for admission of a child with diabetic ketoacidosis to intensive care unit?

Intensive care unit admission is recommended for children at the highest risk of cerebral edema.
- Severe DKA (pH < 7.1, HCO_3 <5 mmol/L)
- Decreased level of consciousness
- Age less than 5 years.

Q. What should be the goals of treatment in a child with diabetic ketoacidosis?

Goals of treatment in DKA are:
- Restoration of circulating volume
- Replacement of fluid and electrolyte deficit evenly over 48 hours
- Correction of acidosis and hyperglycemia with continuous insulin infusion
- Avoidance of the complications of DKA and its treatment by frequent monitoring for:
  - Cerebral edema
  - Hypoglycemia
  - Electrolyte abnormalities.

Q. What preliminary investigations are needed in a child with suspected diabetic ketoacidosis?

The preliminary investigations required in a child with suspected DKA include:
- Immediate measurement of blood glucose
- Blood or urine ketones
- Venous blood gas
- Serum electrolytes, urea
- Serum osmolality (if available)
- Electrocardiogram if stat serum potassium is not available
- Complete blood count
- Blood and urine culture, C X-ray in a febrile child.

Q. How should insulin be administered in diabetic ketoacidosis?

- Insulin infusion therapy should be started after an hour of the initiation of intravenous fluids. If the patient has hypokalemia at presentation, potassium supplementation should also be initiated before starting insulin infusion
- Insulin should be administered by continuous intravenous infusion using an electronic infusion pump

- The intravenous tubing should be primed by flushing the insulin solution through the intravenous tubing before connecting to the patient (to saturate the insulin binding sites in the tubing)
- Insulin dose: 0.05–0.1 units/kg/h (children below 3–5 years of age can be managed with the lower dose of 0.05 units/kg/h)
- Insulin infusion is continued even after blood glucose normalization till the acidosis resolves. The dextrose content of the intravenous fluid may be concurrently increased
- If hypoglycemia occurs despite increase of strength of dextrose solution up to 12.5%, the dose of insulin may be reduced in decrements of 0.01– 0.02 units/kg/h up to 0.03 units/kg/h provided that metabolic acidosis continues to resolve.

Q. How much and what fluid should be administered during diabetic ketoacidosis?

- In children with moderate to severe DKA, 10–20 mL/kg of normal saline is infused over 1 hour. In the "rare" patient who presents with shock, up to 2–3 normal saline boluses of 20 mL/kg may need to be given
- A deficit of 30–50 mL/kg is presumed in mild, 50–70 mL/kg in moderate and 70–100 mL/kg in severe DKA
- To this fluid deficit calculated, maintenance fluid requirement for 48 hours is added and all intravenous or oral fluids given in another location including the fluid administered in the first hour are subtracted from this fluid. This is the amount of fluid to be given in the next 47 hours. However, if the patient has presented in shock and has required fluid boluses for resuscitation, this is not subtracted.
- For example, for a 20 kg child with moderate DKA, assuming a dehydration of 5%, (50 mL/kg) and 10 mL/kg normal saline is given in first hour (200 mL)
  - Fluid deficit for this child = 50 mL/kg × 20 kg = 1,000 mL
  - Maintenance requirement for this child weighing 20 kg for 24 hours = 1,500 mL (by Holliday Segar method)
  - Maintenance requirement for 48 hours = 1,500 mL × 2 = 3,000 mL
  - Fluid to be given over next 47 hours = 1,000 mL + 3,000 mL − 200 mL = 3,800 mL
  - Therefore, fluid rate per hour = 3,800/47 = 80 mL/h
- The fluid used initially is normal saline
- After 4–6 hours as the blood glucose approaches 250 mg/dL, fluid containing 5% dextrose with 0.45% (N/2) saline should be used
- The concentration of dextrose in replacement fluid should be increased as required to maintain blood glucose between 150–200 mg/dL
- Potassium is added to intravenous fluids (40 mEq/L) once the child has passed urine and a normal serum K level has been documented, because in DKA, there is an actual deficit in the total body potassium of about 3–6 mEq/kg.
- If the patient is hypokalemic, potassium replacement is begun at the time of initial volume expansion even before starting insulin therapy
- Overzealous fluid resuscitation, indicated by rapid fall in serum Na (>1–2 mEq/L/h) and effective osmolality, is associated with higher risk of cerebral edema.

Q. How should a child with diabetic ketoacidosis be monitored?

Monitoring should include the following:
- Hourly vital signs: Pulse rate, respiratory rate, and blood pressure
- Frequent neurological examination to detect the warning signs of cerebral edema like headache, recurrence of vomiting, changes in sensorium, hypertension, and bradycardia
- Hourly accurate fluid input and output charting
- Hourly blood glucose
- Electrolytes, urea, creatinine, and acid base every 2–4 hours until acidosis has resolved.

Q. How should the patient be transitioned to subcutaneous insulin therapy after resolution of diabetic ketoacidosis?

Transition to subcutaneous insulin therapy:
- Planned when: Metabolic acidosis has been corrected and oral feeds are introduced
- Timing: The ideal time of starting subcutaneous insulin is just before a meal. Regular insulin is started 1-2 hour, while rapid acting insulins (lispro or aspart) are administered subcutaneously 15-30 minutes prior to stopping insulin infusion
- Dose: In patients with known type 1 diabetes, their usual insulin regimen may be restarted. For patients with newly diagnosed diabetes with DKA, the recommended total daily dose (TDD) for toddlers and preschool age children is 0.4-0.7 units/kg, for prepubertal age 0.75-1 units/kg and for pubertal children is 1-1.2 units/kg. If neutral protamine Hagedorn (NPH) and regular insulin are used, two-thirds of TDD before breakfast and one-third of TDD before dinner can be given [one-third as rapid acting (regular) and two-thirds as intermediate acting insulin (NPH)].

Q. What are the complications of diabetic ketoacidosis?

Complications of DKA include:
- Hypoglycemia
- Hypokalemia
- Hyperchloremic metabolic acidosis
- Cerebral edema
- Cerebral venous thrombosis/deep vein thrombosis
- Arrhythmia (due to dyselectrolytemia)
- Pancreatitis
- Renal failure
- Intestinal necrosis
- Rhabdomyolysis
- Pulmonary edema
- Infections (including mucormycosis).

Q. What are the warning signs of cerebral edema?

Warning signs of cerebral edema include headache, recurrent vomiting, change in neurological status, decreased oxygen saturation, fall in serum sodium concentration, hypertension, and bradycardia.

Q. How should a child with features suggestive of cerebral edema be managed?

If cerebral edema is suspected, urgent action is required. The management includes:
- Elevating the head end of the bed
- Reducing the fluid administration rate by one-third
- Securing the airway: Patient may be intubated and mechanically ventilated if Glasgow coma scale is less than 8
- Aggressive hyperventilation ($PCO_2 < 22$ mmHg) should be avoided
- Intravenous 3% saline (5-10 mL/kg over 30 min) or mannitol (0.5-1 g/kg over 20 min) is administered and may be repeated, if required
- Cranial imaging is done to rule out other treatable causes of neurological deterioration like thrombosis or hemorrhage.

CONCLUSION

As DKA is an important cause of morbidity and mortality in children with type 1 diabetes, its prevention, early diagnosis, and appropriate management are very important. Intravenous hydration, insulin infusion and close clinical as well as biochemical monitoring are the mainstay of management. Cerebral edema is the most important cause of mortality in children with DKA and requires a high index of suspicion for timely diagnosis and appropriate management. Proper counseling of the children and their parents, regular follow-up, and ensuring compliance to treatment are necessary to avoid recurrent episodes of DKA.

KEY LEARNING POINTS

- Diabetic ketoacidosis (DKA) is diagnosed when there is hyperglycemia (>200 mg/dL), metabolic acidosis (serum pH <7.3, bicarbonate <15 mEq/L), and ketones in blood or urine
- All children with moderate-to-severe DKA require hospitalization
- Intravenous hydration should be started before starting insulin infusion
- Close monitoring of the clinical condition (including urine output and neurological status) as well as laboratory parameters (hourly blood glucose, 2–4 hourly blood gases and electrolytes) is/are of paramount importance
- Insulin infusion should be continued till the acidosis resolves, with the dose being titrated according to the blood glucose values; following which, transition should be made from intravenous to subcutaneous insulin
- Identification of the precipitating factors for DKA is important to prevent recurrent episodes of DKA.

SUGGESTED READINGS

1. Sivanandan S, Sinha A, Jain V, Lodha R. Management of diabetic ketoacidosis. *Indian J Pediatr.* 2011;78:576-784.
2. Wolfsdorf JI, Allgrove J, Craig ME, Edge J, Glaser N, Jain V, et al. ISPAD Clinical Practice Consensus Guidelines 2014: Diabetic ketoacidosis and hyperglycemic hyperosmolar state. *Pediatr Diabetes.* 2014;15(Suppl 20):154-179.

CHAPTER 7

Central Diabetes Insipidus

Vandana Jain, Aathira Ravindranath

INTRODUCTION

Maintenance of sodium and water homeostasis is an intricately complex process which involves multiple mechanisms. Diabetes insipidus (DI) is a heterogeneous condition that results from a disturbance of this delicate balance. It is characterized by hypernatremic dehydration with inappropriately decreased synthesis, secretion (central DI), or action (nephrogenic DI) of the antidiuretic hormone (ADH), also known as arginine vasopressin (AVP). Central DI is the more common of the two types where there is deficiency of AVP secondary to destruction or degeneration of the neurons originating in the supraoptic and paraventricular nuclei, or due to midline cranial malformations.

CASE 1

A 4-year-old boy was brought to the outpatient department for complaints of noticing a soft rounded swelling in the left temporal region of the skull and excessive thirst and urine output for the past 5–6 months. The child used to pass urine 20 times during the day and 4–5 times during the night with enuresis also, and drank 4–5 L of water per day. There was no history of rash, ear discharge, head injury, intracranial surgeries, meningitis, or visual disturbance. Physical examination revealed a soft swelling around 2 × 2 cm in diameter with underlying bony defect in left temporal skull. There was no other palpable bony defect, no loose teeth, seborrhea, or rash. On evaluation, his fasting blood sugar was 92 mg/dL, blood urea and creatinine were normal, serum sodium was 146 mEq/L, potassium was 3.8 mEq/L, and calcium 9.1 mg/dL. In a paired morning sample, serum osmolality was 300 mOsm/kg and urine osmolality was 188 mOsm/kg, establishing the diagnosis of DI. On administration of injection aqueous vasopressin, urine osmolality escalated to 455 mOsm/kg after 1 hour. Skeletal survey revealed multiple punched out lytic lesions in the skull. Magnetic resonance imaging (MRI) brain showed thickening of the pituitary stalk with absence of posterior pituitary bright spot. Hence, a diagnosis of Langerhans cell histiocytosis (LCH) with central DI was made.

CASE 2

A 6-year-old boy was presented to the emergency room with seizures and dehydration. His serum sodium was 165 mEq/L and serum osmolality was 340 mOsm/kg. The child also had swelling of the left foot and lower leg and Doppler ultrasound confirmed deep vein thrombosis (DVT). This child had been well till 2 months back when he developed diplopia and headache. Computed tomography head had revealed a suprasellar tumor (astrocytoma), for which he underwent extensive neurosurgery. He had developed polyuria and hypernatremia in the postoperative period, diagnosed as DI and initiated on desmopressin nasal spray. However, there was lack of compliance to desmopressin. Parents informed

> that the child did not feel thirst at all and had to be forced to drink water. We made a diagnosis of adipsic central DI with hypernatremic seizures and DVT. Hypernatremia was corrected gradually by increased fluid intake and intravenous vasopressin infusion, and enoxaparin was started for the DVT. The child was subsequently started on a regime of twice daily desmopressin with 2 hourly supervised oral fluid intake, calculated to match the urinary losses.

CASE REVIEW IN NUTSHELL

Case 1 is a vivid description of a classical presentation of DI which is hard to miss. The presence of polyuria with serum osmolality of 300 mOsm/kg and urine osmolality of 188 mOsm/kg clinches the diagnosis of DI. Increase in urine osmolality after administering exogenous vasopressin establishes the central cause of DI. The presence of a calvarial defect immediately points towards LCH as a probable etiology of DI.

Case 2 developed DI after neurosurgical intervention which is not an uncommon association. However, the later presentation with poor thirst, hypernatremic dehydration with seizures, and DVT modifies the diagnosis to the adipsic variant of central DI where the loss of thirst mechanism underlies the severity of the condition.

INTERACTIVE TOPIC REVIEW

Q. How is sodium-water balance maintained?

Thirst and AVP play synergistic roles in maintaining sodium-water homeostasis. The primary stimulants of thirst are increased osmolality of the extracellular fluid (ECF) and hypovolemia. Osmoreceptors (in the anterior hypothalamus) and baroreceptors (in atria and large veins and arteries) respond to the changes in osmolality and volume status, respectively. Changes in osmolality are more potent and sensitive stimulants of thirst than hypovolemia. This may be regarded as an adaptive mechanism to overlook small changes in volume distribution that would occur with assumption of the upright posture in humans. Animal studies have shown that even 1-4% change in osmolality can induce thirst. However, under normal conditions, renal excretion plays a more pivotal role in water balance than thirst. Thirst mechanism rightly takes the backseat as it is influenced by multiple extrinsic factors, including free access to water, developmental status, and age of the child.

Arginine vasopressin is synthesized in the cell bodies of magnocellular neurons located in the supraoptic and paraventricular nuclei of the hypothalamus and transported caudally via the axons of these nuclei. The axons terminate at different levels in the pituitary stalk and posterior pituitary. The AVP-neurophysin II gene is located at 20p13. Arginine vasopressin is synthesized as a preprohormone which sequentially gets cleaved and processed to release AVP, neurophysin II, and copeptin. Neurophysin is believed to stabilize AVP during its transport and storage and copeptin facilitates proteolytic maturation of AVP.

The osmostat located in the hypothalamus anterior to the third ventricle controls AVP release as well as thirst which are closely coupled but can also be regulated independently. Rise in plasma osmolality, AVP secretion, and increase in urine osmolality follow a linear relationship. Low pressure baroreceptors in the left and right atria transmit the stimuli via glossopharyngeal and vagal nerves to nucleus tractus solitarius and then to magnocellular neurons. Although a 10-15% change in volume is necessary to stimulate AVP release compared to 1-2% change in osmolality, the baroreceptor stimuli are much more potent than osmoreceptors as AVP secretion increases exponentially in response to hypotension.

Q. How does arginine vasopressin exert its antidiuretic effect?

The water modulating effect of AVP is mediated by V2 receptors present on basolateral membrane of the principal cells in the renal collecting ducts.

CHAPTER 7: Central Diabetes Insipidus

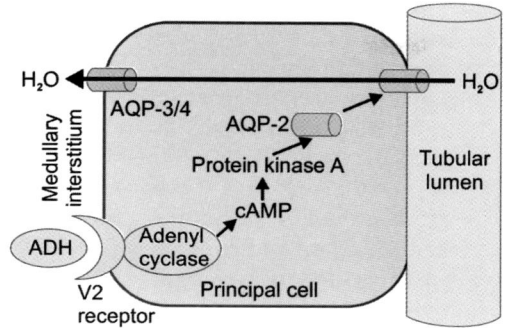

cAMP, cyclic adenosine monophosphate; AQP, aquaporin; ADH, antidiuretic hormone..

Figure 1: Mechanism of action of arginine vasopressin [antidiuretic hormone (ADH)] in the collecting duct. Binding of ADH to V2 receptor results in insertion of aquaporin-2 (AQP-2) channels into the apical membrane. Water enters the principal cells through AQP-2 and exits through the aquaporin-3 and 4 channels into the medullary interstitium

Binding of AVP to these receptors results in generation of cyclic adenosine monophosphate which in turn activates protein kinase A, that promotes insertion of aquaporin-2 (water channels), present in the cytoplasm, into the apical membrane, resulting in increased water reabsorption (Fig. 1). Plasma AVP concentration reaches a peak of about 20 pg/mL at serum osmolality of 320 mOsm/kg, bringing about maximum antidiuresis with urine osmolality of up to 1,000 mOsm/kg. The other receptors on which AVP acts are V1a and V1b. The V1a receptors are located in the vascular smooth muscle cells, hepatocytes, and platelets, and are responsible for mediating the pressor effects of AVP. The V1b receptors are present in the corticotrophs of anterior pituitary and release adrenocorticotropic hormone.

Q. What are the types of diabetes insipidus (DI) and what are the causes of central DI?

Diabetes insipidus can be broadly classified as central and nephrogenic DI. In central DI, which is the commoner of the two types, there is deficiency of AVP and these cases will respond to exogenously administered AVP. In nephrogenic DI, there is resistance to the actions of AVP. Causes of central DI are listed in box 1.

> **BOX 1: Causes of central diabetes insipidus**
> - Congenital anatomic defects
>   - Septo-optic dysplasia, holoprosencephaly
>   - Familial pituitary hypoplasia with absent stalk
> - Neoplasms
>   - Germinomas, pinealomas
>   - Large craniopharyngiomas, optic gliomas
> - Infiltrative, autoimmune, and infectious diseases
>   - Langerhans cell histiocytosis
>   - Lymphocytic hypophysitis
>   - Granulomatous diseases (tuberculoma, sarcoidosis)
>   - Meningitis involving base of the brain
> - Genetic defects in vasopressin synthesis
>   - Familial autosomal dominant type
>   - Autosomal or X-linked recessive
>   - Wolfram syndrome (DIDMOAD)
> - Trauma, septic shock (infarction)
> - Cranial irradiation, neurosurgical intervention
> - Idiopathic
>
> DIDMOAD, diabetes insipidus, diabetes mellitus, optic atrophy, and deafness.

Q. What is the clinical presentation of diabetes insipidus?

Diabetes insipidus is characterized by polyuria (24-h urine production on *ad libitum* fluid intake exceeding 2 L/m²/24 hours or approximately 150 mL/kg/24 hours at birth, 100–110 mL/kg/24 hours till the age of 2 years, and 40–50 mL/kg/24 hours in older children and adults) with hypoosmolar urine. The typical presentation is with passage of large volume of dilute urine, compensated by increased thirst, and hence intake of large volumes of liquids. Many children present with weight loss because of a marked preference for liquid intake to the exclusion of solids. Infants, as well as older children with neurological impairment who are unable to have free access to liquids, often present with failure to thrive, fever, irritability, constipation, and dehydration. Intellectual impairment may occur with repeated episodes of dehydration and hypernatremia. In a small proportion of patients, thirst sensation is impaired due to destruction of the hypothalamic osmoreceptors (adipsic DI) and these present with severe dehydration and hypernatremia and their complications (seizures and thromboembolic events).

Severe dehydration presenting in male infants is highly likely to be due to X-linked nephrogenic DI. Infants with nystagmus and features suggestive of hypopituitarism (jaundice, midline defects, hypoglycemia, and micropenis in boys) are likely to have septo-optic dysplasia. Children (often >5 years of age) presenting with visual symptoms along with polyuria are likely to have intracranial tumors. Children being evaluated for short stature due to congenital or acquired hypopituitarism often give a history of polyuria and nocturia well-compensated by polydipsia. Diabetes insipidus may either be the first manifestation in children with LCH, or may be seen in conjunction with other features such as seborrheic dermatitis, maculopapular rash involving palms and soles, ear discharge, hepatosplenomegaly, and punched out bony defects. Past history of tubercular meningitis is suggestive of basal meningitis or suprasellar tuberculomas as the etiology. Diabetes insipidus in Wolfram syndrome (DIDMOAD, characterized by diabetes insipidus, diabetes mellitus, optic atrophy, and deafness) is partial and its onset is gradual. Diabetes mellitus is usually the first manifestation followed by optic atrophy. Diabetes insipidus develops only in the second or third decade.

Q. How is the diagnosis of diabetes insipidus established?

The diagnostic approach to DI is as follows:
- Quantitate 24-hour urine output/fluid intake
- Measure serum potassium, calcium, glucose, and creatinine to exclude hypokalemia, hypercalcemia, hyperglycemia, and chronic renal insufficiency as the cause for polyuria
- Measure paired early morning serum sodium and osmolality and urine osmolality
    - If serum osmolality more than 300 mOsm/kg, with urine osmolality less than 300 mOsm/kg, DI is confirmed
    - If urine osmolality more than 600 mOsm/kg, or serum osmolality less than 270 mOsm/kg, DI is ruled out
    - For serum osmolality between 270 and 300 mOsm/kg, proceed to water deprivation test
    - Low serum ADH level indicate toward central DI but an isolated ADH level without correlation with plasma osmolality is a futile test and moreover, requires strict sampling technique with rapid centrifugation and immediate freezing
- Keep the child nil per orally and collect samples for serum sodium and osmolality and urine osmolality 2 hourly for up to 10 hours. The endpoints are any of the following: serum sodium more than 150 mEq/L, weight loss more than 5%, intolerable thirst, or less than 30 mOsm/kg variation in osmolality of consecutive urine samples after 5 hours of water deprivation
    - Serum osmolality more than 300 mOsm/kg confirms DI. Urine osmolality less than 300 mOsm/kg indicates complete DI, whereas between 300 and 750 mOsm/kg indicates partial DI. In infants and younger children, urine osmolality more than 450 mOsm/kg after water deprivation, or a urine-to-serum osmolality ratio of 1.5 or higher is also indicative of adequate urine concentrating ability
- Give injection aqueous vasopressin 5 U/m^2 subcutaneously. Greater than twofold rise in urine osmolality after 1 hour confirms central DI, while lack of urinary concentration indicates nephrogenic DI.

Anterior pituitary hormone deficiencies may coexist with central DI and should be actively looked for by performing hormone assays. An MRI brain should be performed to ascertain the cause of central DI. Even without gross structural lesions on MRI, posterior pituitary bright spot which is reflective of vasopressin content may be conspicuous by its absence in cases of central DI. In cases of "idiopathic" central DI, MRI should be repeated periodically (6 monthly or annually) as findings suggestive of germinomas, LCH, or autoimmune hypophysitis may evolve over time.

Q. Case 2 had presented to the emergency room with severe hypernatremia with seizures. How is hypernatremia managed?

The therapeutic goals are to correct both the serum sodium level and the circulatory volume. In children with hypernatremia, water losses are mostly intracellular; the ECF volume being relatively preserved. Hence, clinically the dehydration is underestimated. A simple formula for calculating the minimal amount of fluid necessary to correct the serum sodium is:

$$\text{Water deficit (L)} = \frac{0.6 \times \text{body weight} \times (\text{serum sodium} - 140)}{140 \text{ (L)}}$$

For example, for a 20 kg child with serum sodium of 160 mEq/L, the free water deficit is $0.6 \times 20 \times (160-140)/140 = 1.71$ L. The volume of replacement fluid to be administered will depend on the sodium content, and can be determined as:

$$\text{Replacement fluid volume (L)} = \frac{\text{Water deficit (L)}}{[1 - (\text{sodium concentration in replacement fluid} \div 154 \text{ mEq/L})]}$$

In the above example, if N/5 (0.2%) saline is used (sodium concentration of 34 mEq/L), the replacement volume (L) = $1.8/[1 - (34 \div 154)]$ = 2.3 L. This should be administered over at least 36 hours.

In addition to replacing the calculated water deficit, the normal maintenance fluids should be given and ongoing losses should be replaced. If there is circulatory collapse, normal saline boluses should be administered prior to administering the calculated fluids.

The rate of correction of hypernatremia is guided by its severity, duration, and underlying cause. Due to the relative inability of the brain to extrude idiogenic osmoles, rapid correction of hypernatremia can lead to cerebral edema. It is suggested that unless symptoms of hypernatremic encephalopathy are present, plasma sodium concentration should not be lowered by more than 0.5-1 mEq/L per hour and by no more than 12-15 mEq/L over the first 24 hours. Whenever possible, the safest route is administration of water by mouth or via feeding tube. Child's clinical status and serum sodium should be closely monitored during correction of hypernatremia, so that any neurological worsening can be prevented by slowing the rate of correction or administering a small volume of hypertonic saline.

Q. How is central diabetes insipidus managed?

The treatment of choice for central DI is intranasal or oral desamino-D-arginine vasopressin (DDAVP) which is a synthetic analog of AVP with about 3,000-fold lower pressor effects. The intranasal dose is 5-20 mcg daily, while the oral dose is 20-fold greater (100-400 µg daily) as two doses. The half-life of DDAVP is 3.5 hours and the peak concentration is reached in 50 minutes. Urine output decreases in 1-2 hours and the duration of action of DDAVP lasts for 6-18 hours. As the urine osmolality is fixed at about 1,000 mOsm/kg on chronic DDAVP therapy, there is risk of developing hyponatremia if fluid intake is excessive. This is the situation with infants as they have an obligatory high water intake, all nutrition being liquid. Therefore, central DI in infancy is preferably managed by giving higher volume of feeds with low renal solute load. This is difficult to manage but is preferable to facing the risk of life-threatening hyponatremia. Breastmilk is the recommended fluid as it has low sodium content and renal solute load. Adverse effects reported with intranasal DDAVP include eye irritation, headache, dizziness, rhinitis, epistaxis, nausea, vomiting, chest pain, and palpitations.

Thiazide diuretics increase sodium loss by inhibiting its reabsorption in the distal tubule. The ensuing contraction of ECF results in increased water reabsorption in the proximal tubules. Thiazides decrease polyuria by up to 50% when accompanied by salt restriction, and are effective in both central and nephrogenic DI. Chlorpropamide, clofibrate, and carbamazepine have also been used to treat pediatric cases of partial central DI as they improve sensitivity of the V2 receptors to the residual ADH.

Q. What is adipsic diabetes insipidus?

Children with adipsic DI cannot compensate for the excess free water loss by drinking fluids as there is concomitant destruction of the osmoreceptors as well, secondary to germinomas, congenital malformations, extensive surgeries for brain tumors, and postmeningitis sequelae. Osmoreceptors are circumventricular (to operator: break at ventricular if needed) structures that relay osmolar information to the magnocellular neurons and the thirst center. Destruction of these osmoreceptors abolishes the thirst mechanism which protects against severe hypernatremia. The absence of polydipsia may delay the diagnosis of DI and also predispose the affected children to chronic hyperosmolar state.

Q. What is therapeutic approach for adipsic diabetes insipidus?

Management of adipsic DI is essentially similar to central DI. There is need to address the additional features of chronic hypernatremia and higher risk of developing thromboembolic manifestations with dehydration.

Euvolemia and eunatremia ought to be achieved gradually with fluids and DDAVP after which fixed dose of DDAVP and fluid intake should be continued. Daily fluid intake and weight measurements along with weekly sodium estimation form the cornerstone of management in adipsic DI. Fluid intake needs to be increased during periods of fever, diarrhea, exercise, and climatic changes. Insensible water losses also should be accounted for while calculating the fluid intake.

Education of the family is the bedrock in the management of these children.

In case of repeated episodes of hypernatremia, DVT prophylaxis with low molecular weight heparin can be given.

CONCLUSION

Diabetes insipidus can present not only with typical symptoms of polyuria and polydipsia but also with severe dehydration, coma, and DVT, if it is the adipsic variant. After establishing the diagnosis of central DI, the underlying cause needs to be established. Management of central DI involves intricate regulation of fluid intake and desmopressin administration.

KEY LEARNING POINTS

- Diabetes insipidus (DI) is characterized by polyuria (urine output >2 L/m²/24 h) with low urine osmolality (<300 mOsm/kg) in the presence of high serum osmolality
- If serum osmolality is more than 300 mOsm/kg, with urine osmolality less than 300 mOsm/kg in paired early morning samples, the diagnosis is established. If serum osmolality is between 270 and 300 mOsm/kg, water deprivation test needs to be performed to establish the diagnosis. Response to vasopressin challenge confirms the DI to be central
- Central diabetes is managed with oral or intranasal desmopressin along with fine-tuned fluid regimen. In young infants, desamino-D-arginine vasopressin (DDAVP) therapy carries a higher risk of hyponatremia, and therefore, it is preferable to manage them with increased fluid intake, with addition of thiazide diuretic, if needed
- Adipsic DI poses a special challenge in diagnosis and management because of lack of polydipsia

SUGGESTED READINGS

1. Di Lorgi N, Napoli F, Allegri AE, Olivieri I, Bertelli E, Gallizia A, et al. Diabetes insipidus—diagnosis and management. *Horm Res Paediatr.* 2012;77:69-84.
2. Ooi HL, Maguire AM, Ambler GR. Desmopressin administration in children with central diabetes insipidus: a retrospective review. *J Pediatr Endocrinol Metab.* 2013;26:1047-1052.
3. Rivkees SA, Dunbar N, Wilson TA. The management of central diabetes insipidus in infancy: desmopressin, low renal solute load formula, thiazide diuretics. *J Pediatr Endocrinol Metab.* 2007;20:459-469.
4. Yadav J, Satapathy A, Jain V. Endocrine causes of disturbed water and sodium homeostasis. In: Jain V, Menon RK (Eds). *Case Based Reviews in Pediatric Endocrinology.* New Delhi: Jaypee Brothers Medical Publishers; 2015:157-168.

CHAPTER 8

Transient Pseudohypoaldosteronism

Reeshma Pattan, Gopakumar Hariharan

INTRODUCTION

Vomiting, lethargy, and poor weight gain in neonatal and early infancy could be due to a variety of causes. Sepsis remains a major cause that needs to be ruled out in the first instance. Electrolytes are also done as corroborative evidence for dehydration wherein sodium is expected to be elevated due to hemoconcentration.

Transient pseudohypoaldosteronism is a rare association with severe urinary tract infection and may mimic congenital adrenal hyperplasia (CAH) clinically and on initial baseline electrolyte profile. Considering this entity as a differential diagnosis is important in addition to considering the diagnosis of CAH.

CASE 1

A 5-week-old baby born at term following an uneventful delivery and postnatal period presented with worsening vomiting and inadequate weight gain. Baby was described to have vomiting from birth although considered to be secondary esophageal reflux at that stage. Vomiting was projectile and nonbilious. On examination, he was listless, lethargic, moderately dehydrated with sunken eyes, depressed fontanel, prolonged capillary refill time, and tachycardia. Weight at presentation was 3,840 g, which was below birth weight.

CASE REVIEW IN A NUTSHELL

In clinical practice, it is a dictum that any electrolyte abnormality not in keeping with the clinical picture should raise suspicion of other medical conditions. In this case, the blood tests revealed hyponatremia and hyperkalemia raising possibility of CAH. This led to detailed hormonal testing. In retrospect, the electrolyte abnormalities were attributed to pseudohypoaldosteronism which is a rare accompaniment of urinary tract infection especially noted in early infancy.

INTERACTIVE TOPIC REVIEW

Q. What are the differential diagnoses in this case scenario?

The differential diagnoses in this case scenario are as follows:
- Gastroesophageal reflux
- Pyloric stenosis
- Intestinal obstruction
- Food allergy
- Sepsis
- Metabolic disorders.

Q. List the first line of investigation in this case.

From the clinical picture, the baby is significantly dehydrated and checking the electrolytes and renal function along with investigation to rule out blood or urosepsis would be the first priority. To diagnose metabolic disorder, a baseline venous gas, especially looking at ammonia, acid-base status, and lactate levels, would be appropriate. An ultrasound to rule out pyloric stenosis is also reasonable in case of clinical suspicion.

In this case, hyponatremia and hyperkalemia were noted. In a case of pseudohypoaldosteronism, urinary sodium is generally high with a low potassium excretion. However, normokalemia may be seen in older children in a setting of pseudohypoaldosteronism.

Q. What are the essential hormonal tests in such situations?

- Serum aldosterone
- 17-hydroxyprogesterone (17-OHP)
- Serum cortisol
- Plasma renin activity
- Adrenocorticotropic hormone.

In this case, 17-OHP levels were within normal limits ruling out the most common hormonal abnormality associated with CAH.

Q. Electrolytes are remarkable with a very low sodium and high potassium level. What could be the causes for this?

This can be due to following conditions:
- Congenital adrenal hyperplasia
- Primary adrenal insufficiency
- Inadequate mineralocorticoid secretion or action.

Q. What is the proposed pathophysiology of pseudohypoaldosteronism associated with urinary tract infection?

Pseudohypoaldosteronism following urinary tract infection is especially seen in the first 3 months of life and the risk of salt wasting is seen to diminish as age advances. It is proposed that the bacterial endotoxins transiently damage aldosterone receptors resulting in interstitial inflammation causing loss of sodium and accompanying increase in aldosterone levels. The nephrotoxic effect of urinary tract infection in addition causes renal tubular resistance that could lead to hyperkalemia. The decreased blood volume secondary to dehydration could explain the hyperreninemia.

A possible genetic etiology inherited as autosomal dominant/sporadic is also described which results from a mutation of the mineralocorticoid receptor gene, which prevents normal receptor function causing salt wasting.

Q. Describe the features of pseudohypoaldosteronism.

Features of pseudohypoaldosteronism are as follows:
- Hyponatremia
- Hyperkalemia
- Decreased aldosterone levels.

Q. How is pseudohypoaldosteronism managed?

- Appropriate antibiotics for urinary tract infection
- Hyponatremia generally responds to fluid resuscitation for dehydration and antibiotic therapy for urinary tract infection. In certain situations, 3% sodium chloride correction may be required
- Hyperkalemia: An ECG is taken to look for any cardiac effects of high potassium levels and managed with sodium bicarbonate, calcium gluconate, glucose infusion, and potassium binders as the situation warrants.

Q. What is the usual course of illness?

With successful treatment of urinary tract infection with antibiotics, the electrolyte abnormalities resolved. Baby was managed with fluids, antibiotics, and glucose insulin infusion for hyperkalemia. The electrolyte abnormalities returned to normal by second day of illness. Ultrasound of kidneys done was reported normal.

CONCLUSION

Transient pseudohypoaldosteronism in severe urinary tract infection could mimic CAH. In a child with urinary tract infection, this condition should be considered as a differential diagnosis, especially in cases where there is a dramatic response to fluid resuscitation and antibiotics.

KEY LEARNING POINTS

☞ Transient pseudohypoaldosteronism is an entity seen in very young children with severe urinary tract infection and could mimic congenital adrenal hyperplasia

☞ Considering this differential diagnosis in the context of a urinary infection is important, especially in cases where there is a dramatic response to fluid resuscitation and antibiotics.

SUGGESTED READINGS

1. Bogdanovic R, Stajic N, Putnik J, Paripovic A. Transient type 1 pseudohypoaldosteronism: report on an eight patient series and literature review. *Pediatr Nephrol.* 2009;24:2167-2175.
2. Rodriguez-Soriano J, Vallo A, Quintela MJ, Oliveros R, Ubetagoyena M. Normokalemic pseudohypoaldosteronism is present in children with acute pyelonephritis. *Acta Paediatr.* 1992;81:402-406.
3. Melzi ML, Guez S, Sersale G, Terzi F, Secco E, Marra G, et al. Acute pyelonephritis as a cause of hyponatremia/hyperkalemia in young infants with urinary tract malformations. *Pediatr Infect Dis J.* 1995;14:56-59.
4. Pujo L, Fagart J, Gary F, Papadimitriou DT, Claës A, Jeunemaître X, et al. Mineralocorticoid receptor mutations are the principal cause of renal type 1 pseudohypoaldosteronism. *Hum Mutat.* 2007;28:33-40.

CHAPTER 9

Acute Adrenal Crisis

J Leenatha Reddy

INTRODUCTION

In the year 1855, Thomas Addison described the clinical syndrome of adrenal insufficiency characterized by wasting and hyperpigmentation. This description remains relevant even today. It is a potentially lethal disease.

The adrenal cortex produces more than 50 steroid hormones of which cortisol and aldosterone are by far the most abundant and physiologically active steroids. Adrenal insufficiency is caused by destruction or dysfunction of the adrenal gland, which results in impaired secretion of cortisol and aldosterone essential for maintaining circulating blood volume and homeostasis and combating stress. When there is sudden severe worsening of adrenal insufficiency symptoms, it is called "adrenal crisis". As signs and symptoms are nonspecific, this can cause delay in diagnosis and treatment. Management of this condition includes replacement therapy with the life-saving glucocorticoid hydrocortisone, which has been available from 1949.

CASE 1
A 20-day-old male infant was referred for a surgical opinion for progressing history of vomiting, poor feeding, irritability, and weight loss. He was born at term by normal vaginal delivery to consanguineous parents. His birth weight was 2.8 kg.

Examination: He was noted to be clinically dehydrated with reduced skin turgor, dry lips, sunken anterior fontanel, listlessness, and poor respiratory effort. His weight was 1.9 kg.

Investigations: Blood sugar was 26 mg/dL and blood gas showed metabolic acidosis. Serum sodium was 118 mmol/L, potassium of 7.2 mmol/L, chloride of 90 mmol/L, and calcium of 8.4 mmol/L. Further blood tests showed 17-hydroxyprogesterone (17-OHP) was 340 ng/mL, adrenocorticotropic hormone (ACTH) was 220 pg/mL, and cortisol was 6.2 µg/dL.

Diagnosis: Congenital adrenal hyperplasia (CAH) due to 21-hydroxylase deficiency.

Treatment: Intravenous bolus of 2 mL/kg of 10% dextrose given for hypoglycemia, bolus of 0.9% of saline for dehydration, followed by intravenous maintenance fluids of 0.9% normal saline and 10% dextrose. He was started on 50 mg/m² stat dose of hydrocortisone succinate followed by 50 mg/m²/day in four divided doses.

Outcome: Electrolytes and blood sugar were stabilized with intravenous fluids.

CASE REVIEW IN A NUTSHELL

This 20-day-old male infant was referred for a probable surgical problem because of the history of vomiting, poor feeding, and weight loss. Acute surgical emergencies are common in this age group, while adrenal crisis though rare, present with a similar history and should

CHAPTER 9: Acute Adrenal Crisis

be suspected especially in male infants because of salt losing crisis secondary to CAH. Acute surgical emergencies can present with a similar clinical and biochemical picture. The notable difference is that hypokalemic alkalosis is more often associated with surgical emergencies rather than hyperkalemic acidosis as in adrenal insufficiency and crisis.

Once the adrenal crisis was suspected because of metabolic acidosis, hypoglycemia, hyperkalemia, and hyponatremia, fluid replacement and correction of hypoglycemia and electrolyte disturbances was done which is the key to managing the adrenal crisis. Samples for serum cortisol, ACTH (which needs to be sent to laboratory urgently on ice) and 17-OHP levels were sent before starting on intravenous hydrocortisone. The results supported the diagnosis of adrenal insufficiency secondary to CAH that presented in acute adrenal crisis. Hydrocortisone replacement therapy was continued and later changed to oral hydrocortisone and fludrocortisone.

CASE 2

A 7-year-old girl presented with a few days history of profuse vomiting and abdominal pain. She had suffered from two similar episodes in the previous 2 weeks. During both the previous episodes, she had been noted to have low serum sodium levels attributed to vomiting. Her serum potassium levels had been within the normal range and she had been treated with intravenous fluids briefly and discharged.

Examination: She was severely dehydrated, tachycardic, and hypotensive with systolic blood pressure of 80 mmHg.

Investigations: Serum sodium 122 mmol/L, serum potassium level of 5 mmol/L, and metabolic acidosis (pH 7.26).

Additional History: Mother revealed that she had not been well for the past several weeks with general malaise, lethargy, weight loss, and darkening of her skin noted over her face, extremities, and trunk.

Additional Investigations: Short synacthen test revealed base line cortisol of 1.2 µg/dL with an elevated ACTH of 653 pg/mL. Post synacthen, the serum cortisol level drawn at 30 minutes was 6.2 µg/dL (normal is >18 µg/dL).

Treatment: Intravenous bolus of 20 mL/kg of normal saline was given followed by intravenous maintenance fluids. After the diagnosis was confirmed, she was started on hydrocortisone at the dose of 15 mg/m^2/day in 2–3 divided doses and fludrocortisone 100 µg once a day.

CASE REVIEW IN A NUTSHELL

As adrenal crisis is rare in the pediatric age group, one should have a high suspicion of this emergency. The presenting features are very similar to that seen in common gastroenteritis, as it was probably suspected in this young girl on her two previous presentations with similar features. Eliciting key pointers in the history is vital (mentioned later) to suspect the diagnosis. Hyperkalemia is not a consistent presenting sign in adrenal insufficiency in childhood; its absence cannot rule out this condition. If the diagnosis was not suspected, and samples for cortisol and ACTH were not sent at the time of adrenal crisis, the diagnosis could be confirmed by doing a synacthen test. In this patient, the synacthen test confirmed the diagnosis of adrenal insufficiency, most likely secondary to an autoimmune cause.

One should have a low threshold for suspecting other associated autoimmune endocrine problems in children presenting with adrenal insufficiency and investigate as needed. It is well-known that adrenal insufficiency can occur as a part of autoimmune polyendocrine syndrome.

INTERACTIVE TOPIC REVIEW

Q. What is adrenal insufficiency?

Adrenal insufficiency is a condition which results in impaired secretion of cortisol and/or aldosterone essential for maintaining circulating blood volume and homeostasis and combating stress. Management of this condition includes replacement therapy with the life-saving glucocorticoid hydrocortisone, which has been available from 1949. There are two types of adrenal insufficiency:
1. Primary
2. Secondary.

Q. What is adrenal crisis?

Adrenal crisis is a physiological event caused by an acute insufficiency of adrenal hormones. If this condition is not recognized and treated, the crisis can cause death.

Q. What are the causes of primary adrenal insufficiency?

Primary adrenal insufficiency is characterized by deficiency of both cortisol and aldosterone. Congenital adrenal hyperplasia is the most common cause of primary adrenal insufficiency followed by autoimmune causes of adrenal insufficiency. In CAH, newborn females are identified at birth because of ambiguous genitalia due to increased production of adrenal androgens, whereas males are usually diagnosed at 2–3 weeks of age when they present with salt wasting crisis.

Autoimmune adrenal insufficiency can occur alone or as part of a polyendocrine syndrome. Autoimmune polyendocrinopathy syndrome type 1 is characterized by adrenal insufficiency, hypoparathyroidism, and mucocutaneous candidiasis with onset in childhood. Autoimmune polyendocrinopathy syndrome type 2 comprises of adrenal insufficiency, thyroid disease, diabetes, and other autoimmune disorders. Other rare causes of adrenal insufficiency and crisis in the pediatric age group include infarction; infection; adrenoleukodystrophy; Wolman, triple A, and Zellweger syndromes..

Q. What are the causes of secondary adrenal insufficiency?

Secondary adrenal insufficiency is characterized by deficiency of cortisol alone, as aldosterone secretion is normal and is regulated by the renin angiotensin system.

Secondary adrenal insufficiency is the result of ACTH deficiency caused by dysfunction of the hypothalamic-pituitary axis. Etiologies include primary hypopituitarism, pituitary hypothalamic pathology including cranial irradiation.

However, the most common cause is suppression of hypothalamic-pituitary-adrenal axis by exogenous glucocorticoid administration (oral, inhaled, intravenous, creams, or ophthalmic drops). In this iatrogenic form of secondary adrenal insufficiency, the abrupt discontinuation of exogenous glucocorticoids or relative insufficiency in stress related situations while on suppressive doses could lead to adrenal crisis.

Q. When to suspect adrenal crisis?

As adrenal crisis is relatively rare in the pediatric age group, pediatricians need to be aware and should suspect this in the following clinical scenarios, and any child with:
- Refractory hemodynamic shock
- Unexplained hypoglycemia
- Nonsurgical acute abdomen
- Child who is disproportionately ill for clinical history provided
- Developing pigmentation
- Child with known adrenal insufficiency with an intercurrent illness
- Child who is currently on or recently discontinued exogenous glucocorticoid therapy.

Q. What are the clinical features that point toward adrenal crisis?

Patients can present with any of the following clinical features:
- Vomiting
- Dehydration
- Acidosis
- Hypotension
- Hypoglycemia
- Hyponatremia
- Hyperkalemia (not always present).

Q. What are the key points that need to be obtained from the history?

The important elements that should be elicited from the history of patients with adrenal crisis are:
- Weakness (99%)
- Pigmentation of the skin (98%) in primary causes

CHAPTER 9: Acute Adrenal Crisis

- Weight loss (97%)
- Abdominal pain (34%)
- Salt craving (22%)
- Diarrhea (20%)
- Constipation (19%)
- Syncope (16%)
- Vitiligo (9%).

Q. What investigations to be considered in adrenal crisis?

Once the diagnosis of adrenal crisis is suspected, the following investigations should be considered:
- Complete blood count
- Serum electrolytes
- Blood urea nitrogen level
- Serum creatinine level
- Serum cortisol level
- Serum ACTH (required to be sent to the laboratory urgently on ice)
- 17-hydroxyprogesterone if suspecting CAH
- Serum calcium level
- Thyroid function tests (although will not influence immediate management).

Q. How to confirm the diagnosis of adrenal insufficiency?

It may not always be possible to reliably confirm the diagnosis during management of an acute adrenal crisis, but measurement of serum ACTH and serum cortisol levels before treatment is often sufficient to make a preliminary diagnosis. Of note, a random serum cortisol level of less than 18 µg/dL in a sick and stressed patient is suggestive of adrenal insufficiency.

The diagnosis of adrenal defiiency is adequately established in most patients bydoing a synacthen test, employing the synacthen doses as per Table 1. This includes a baseline assessment of serum cortisol and ACTH levels, followed by administration of synacthen (ACTH) intravenously or intramuscularly, followed by drawing a serum cortisol level 30 minutes after the injection.

TABLE 1: Synacthen doses

Age	Synacthen dose
0–6 months	62.5 µg
6 months–2 years	125 µg
>2 years	250 µg

A normal response is indicated when serum cortisol following the ACTH administration exceeds 18 µg/dL.

However, in emergency situations, the diagnosis can be made on clinical grounds and it is advisable not to delay treatment of possible adrenal crisis, as the diagnosis can be confirmed once the crisis is over.

Q. How to manage the immediate acute crisis?

In patients presenting with symptoms and signs of adrenal crisis, it is critical to support and maintain:
- Airway, breathing, and adequate oxygenation
- Circulation, blood pressure, and hemodynamic with appropriate fluids.

Maintenance fluids for pediatric patients are estimated as given in table 2.

Fluid volume deficit is estimated clinically as a percentage of weight loss as:
  - 100 mL/kg for 10% dehydration
  - 50 mL/kg for 5% dehydration
  - 30 mL/kg for 3% dehydration.
- If a child presents in acute shock or severe dehydration, 10–20 mL/kg bolus of isotonic solution (ringer lactate or normal saline) should be given in the first hour of treatment. This can be repeated if needed

TABLE 2: Estimation of maintenance fluids for pediatric patients

Body weight	mL/kg/day	mL/kg/h
First 10 kg	100	4
Second 10 kg	50	2
Subsequent kg	20	1

- It is essential to replace the fluid deficit and maintenance intravenous fluids over 24 hours with either 5 or 10% dextrose and 0.9% saline
- Once the serum sodium level is corrected to more than 130 mmol/L, consider changing to 0.45% saline and 5 or 10% dextrose
- Mild or no dehydration, intravenous bolus fluid is not required.

Q. How to manage hypoglycemia?

Hypoglycemia (blood glucose <46 mg/dL) should be treated with rapid intravenous bolus of 2–5 mL/kg of 10% dextrose. Blood glucose should be rechecked the blood after 30 minutes to ensure blood sugar is above 72 mg/dL or 4 mmol/L.

> Note: Maintenance fluids may need up to 10% dextrose to keep sugars stable during adrenal crisis. Blood sugars should be monitored 2–4 hourly.

Q. How to treat hyperkalemia?

Hyperkalemia is not always seen in children presenting in adrenal crisis. Hyperkalemia is usually normalized with intravenous fluid replacement and corticosteroids. However, if the serum potassium level is more than 6 mmol/L, then the patient should be on a cardiac monitor with electrocardiogram (ECG) monitoring. If the serum potassium level is more than 7 mmol/L with ECG changes, the patient should be treated urgently with:
- 0.5 mL/kg of 10% calcium gluconate can be given slowly intravenous over 10 minutes through a central line.

  or
- Intravenous insulin infusion at the rate of 0.1 unit/kg/h together with an infusion of 10% dextrose at the rate of 5–10 mL/kg/h. Serum potassium gradually decreases over 30–60 minutes.

Q. What are recommended stress doses of parental hydrocortisone for adrenal crisis?

Steroid replacement: Give intravenous bolus of hydrocortisone succinate. The same dose can be given intramuscularly if intravenous access is not available.

Intravenous hydrocortisone succinate as a stat dose of 50–75 mg/m^2 should be given immediately, followed by 50–75 mg/m^2/day intravenously divided in four doses (body surface area estimations can be made using Broselow tape in the emergency room or using body surface nomograms). It is important to note that intravenous hydrocortisone has some beneficial mineralocorticoid effect.

Q. When to change to oral hydrocortisone replacement?

When the patient has stabilized hemodynamically, intravenous fluids can be reduced, and the patient can be now placed on triple the recommended oral dose of hydrocortisone and then gradually reduced to usual maintenance dose of corticosteroid.

Q. When to consider oral fludrocortisones?

Mineralocorticoid replacement can be started with oral fludrocortisone at the dose of 0.05–0.1 mg/day; once the patient is hemodynamically stable and tolerating oral fluids.

CONCLUSION

Adrenal insufficiency is rare in the pediatric age group, pediatricians should be aware of the presenting symptomatology, know when to suspect this condition, and institute early investigative and supportive measures with aggressive and rapid fluid resuscitation and steroid replacement as indicated. A combination of chronic or subacute clinical symptoms, hypotension, and hyponatremia should alert and raise the suspicion of adrenal insufficiency or adrenal crisis.

KEY LEARNING POINTS

- Though adrenal crisis is rare in children, pediatricians should be aware of the clinical signs to suspect adrenal crisis in sick children
- Of note, hyperkalemia is not always seen in children in adrenal crisis
- Preliminary diagnosis can be made with low cortisol, raised adrenocorticotropic hormone, and clinical features
- Synacthen test can be done to confirm the diagnosis when the child is not in adrenal crisis
- When considering doing a synacthen test, the child should be off hydrocortisone for at least 12 hours.

SUGGESTED READINGS

1. Arlt W, Allolio B. Adrenal insufficiency. *Lancet*. 2003;361: 1881-1893.
2. Fleseriu M, Loriaux DL. "Relative" adrenal insufficiency in critical illness. *Endoc Pract*. 2009;15:632-640.
3. Perry R, Kecha O, Paquette J, Huot C, Van Vliet G, Deal C. Primary adrenal insufficiency in children: twenty years experience at Sainte-Justine Hospital, Montreal. *J Clin Endocrinol Metab*. 2005;90:3240-3250.
4. Shulman DI, Palmert MR, Kemp SF; Lawson Wilkins Drug and Therapeutics Committee. Adrenal insufficiency: still a cause of morbidity and death in childhood. *Pediatrics*. 2007;119:e484-e494.
5. Walter LM. The adrenal cortex and its disorders. In: Brook C, Clayton P, Brown R (Eds). *Brook's Clinical Pediatric Endocrinology*, 6th edn. London: Wiley-Blackwell; 2009:283-325.

Hypoglycemia

CHAPTER 10

L Francine Shirley, Hemchand K Prasad

INTRODUCTION

Hypoglycemia, characterized by a reduction in plasma glucose concentration to a level that may induce symptoms or signs such as altered mental status and/or sympathetic nervous system stimulation, is a common pediatric emergency. Typically, it follows abnormalities in the mechanisms involved in glucose homeostasis.

Hypoglycemia has diverse causes in which low levels of plasma glucose eventually lead to neuroglycopenia. The most common cause of hypoglycemia in patients with diabetes is injecting a shot of insulin and skipping a meal or overdosing insulin.

CASE 1

A 3-year-old female child, developmentally normal, presented to the emergency department with active generalized tonic-clonic seizures. On further probing the history, the mother revealed history of recurrent early morning convulsions. The girl was short for her age. Otherwise systemic examination was normal.

Her capillary blood glucose (CBG) was 21 mg/dL. Ketones were strongly positive and serum lactate was normal.

CASE REVIEW IN A NUTSHELL

Hypoglycemia should be corrected with intravenous dextrose. In the setting of hypoglycemia with short stature, hypopituitarism needs to be suspected. If the critical sample shows low growth hormone (<10 ng/mL) and low cortisol (<5 µg/dL), panhypopituitarism is considered. Magnetic resonance imaging of brain is mandatory to look for pituitary abnormalities.

Hormone replacement prevents the next episode of hypoglycemia.

CASE 2

A 2-year-old boy was brought with lethargy since morning to the emergency room. There was a history of poor oral intake secondary to fever. On examination, the child was poorly built and nourished. Height was on the 75th percentile and body mass index (BMI) was less than 3rd percentile. The child did not have any facial dysmorphism. Systemic examination was normal and external genitalia were also normal.

His CBG was 35 mg/dL. Blood ketones were strongly positive.

CASE REVIEW IN A NUTSHELL

The most likely diagnosis in this child, aged 2 years, is ketotic hypoglycemia. This is a reactive response in extremely thin children with poor muscle stores. The critical sample must be taken and a suppressed insulin and normal growth hormone and cortisol response must be documented to make this diagnosis. These children outgrow the disease in due course. The parents need to ensure regular food intake at times of illnesses to prevent next episode.

CASE 3

A 10-month-old male infant was brought to the emergency room after having a seizure episode at home. Parents gave history of recurrent similar episodes in the past. He was born at term, lower segment cesarean section, a large baby, and weight 4.4 kg. On examination, child was drowsy, responsive to pain, large baby, and height and weight were above the 97th percentile.

His CBG was 17 mg/dL. Blood ketones were negative.

CASE REVIEW IN A NUTSHELL

There is a high index of suspicion of hyperinsulinemia in the child. It is worth remembering that hypoglycemia with absent ketones indicates only two diagnosis—fatty acid oxidation defect and hyperinsulinemia. Parallel to a hypoglycemia, a critical sample must be taken. A glucagon challenge may be given (without dextrose correction). An increment in CBG more than 30 mg/dL proves hyperinsulinemia. Elevated serum insulin more than 2 µU/mL, normal growth hormone response more than 10 ng/mL, cortisol response more than 10 µg/dL, and normal plasma fatty acid levels support the diagnosis. A genetic test for inherited hyperinsulinemia is mandatory.

CASE 4

An 11-month-old female child was brought with hypoglycemia. She had history of one early morning seizure which was not evaluated. On examination, the child had doll-like faces and massive hepatomegaly.

Her CBG was 15 mg/dL.

CASE REVIEW IN A NUTSHELL

Hypoglycemia should be corrected with a dextrose bolus. Glycogen storage disease must be considered and further workup planned. A pediatric gastroenterologist needs to be consulted and further management planned. Night feeding with corn starch must be advised to prevent the recurrence of the hypoglycemia episode.

CASE 5

A 2-week-old male baby was rushed to the neonatal intensive care unit with poor feeding and convulsions. On examination, baby was very dark. Other findings were bilateral undescended testes and severe hypospadias.

His CBG was 20 mg/dL.

CASE REVIEW IN A NUTSHELL

Critical sample should be drawn. About 4 mL/kg of 10% dextrose must be administered. In view of the strong suspicion of adrenal insufficiency, bolus stress dose intravenous hydrocortisone should be administered in the emergency room.

Subsequent reports showed: the serum sodium was 120 mEq/L, potassium 7.5 mEq/L. Ketones were strongly positive; serum lactate was normal; insulin was undetectable; growth hormone was normal (>20 ng/mL); serum cortisol was low (2.5 µg/dL, value <5 µg/dL is suggestive of cortisol deficiency). Further evaluation of the cause of cortisol deficiency was done: ultrasound showed mullerian structures, karyotype was 46,XX and 17-hydroxyprogesterone (17-OHP) was more than 100 ng/mL. A diagnosis of congenital adrenal hyperplasia (CAH) was made.

Remember, there is a suspicion of adrenal insufficiency, to take samples for 17-OHP, adrenocorticotropic hormone, total testosterone, and electrolytes in the emergency room itself. Intravenous hydrocortisone stress dose should be given as follows:
- Less than 3 years: 25 mg hydrocortisone
- 3–12 years: 50 mg hydrocortisone
- More than 12 years: 100 mg hydrocortisone.

CASE 6

A 10-year-old boy, a known case of type 1 diabetes mellitus (T1DM) on insulin over the past 2 years, came to the emergency room in status epilepticus of 1-hour duration. An injection of lorazepam followed by another of diazepam after 15 minutes by a practitioner had failed to control seizures.

In the emergency room, his CBG was found to be 55 mg/dL. He responded to dextrose bolus.

SECTION 3: Endocrine and Metabolic Disorders

CASE REVIEW IN A NUTSHELL

Hypoglycemia is the most important cause of seizures in a child suffering from diabetes and on insulin therapy. A CBG less than 70 mg/dL establishes hypoglycemia. In this child, since CBG had turned out to be just 55 mg/dL, he was given intravenous dextrose bolus with gratifying results. A yet better way of treating severe hypoglycemia in such a child is giving glucagon injection subcutaneously (<12 years: 0.5 mg and >12 years: 1 mg).

Children with T1DM and hypoglycemia without neurological features should be given 15 g of rapid-acting carbohydrates and rechecked in 15 minutes to ensure euglycemia. They need not be hospitalized in the emergency room.

> **CASE 7**
> A 3-year-old toddler was brought to the emergency room in hypoglycemia and altered sensorium. His grandmother was a diabetic and was on glimepiride. A bottle of empty medicines was found near the child.

CASE REVIEW IN A NUTSHELL

In this 3-year-old child, the most likely diagnosis is hypoglycemia due to oral hypoglycemic agent (OHA) poisoning. Routine management of airway, breathing, and circulation (ABC) and dextrose bolus must be administered. A sample must be taken for toxicological analysis also. Activated charcoal may be used. Octreotide may be used if the hypoglycemia is refractory. The child needs to be hospitalized and observed for 24 hours.

INTERACTIVE TOPIC REVIEW

Q. When to suspect hypoglycemia in a child in the emergency room?

All children entering the emergency room must have their CBG checked. It is better to suspect and not find it, rather than not suspect it and find it.

Q. What is the operational definition for hypoglycemia?

There is no cutoff that is universally applicable for all children. Cutoff for hypoglycemia depends on whether the children are prone for hypoglycemia or not.

Children prone for hypoglycemia:
- Diabetes: Blood glucose less than 70 mg/dL
- Suspected OHA poisoning: CBG less than 60 mg/dL
- Newborn: Term baby less than 45 mg/dL.

Children not prone for hypoglycemia:
- Well child with adequate nourishment: 45 mg/dL
- Sick malnourished child: 54 mg/dL
- Common cutoff for practice: 55 mg/dL.

Any child in the emergency room with CBG less than 60 mg/dL is considered to be in hypoglycemia.

Q. Is capillary blood glucose reliable in a sick child? Why?

The values are not reliable in a sick child due to confounding factors like hypotension, hypoperfusion, acidosis, or peripheral edema. Hypotension results in decrease in perfusion and increase in glucose utilization resulting in false results in capillary blood glucose. Hence, any abnormal CBG value should be confirmed by a venous blood glucose estimation.

Q. What are the transitions that occur during hypoglycemia to maintain sugars?

A summary of the transitions occurring is presented in box 1.

Remember that ketones are the most important fuel for the body in the absence of

> **BOX 1: Transitions that occur during hypoglycemia to maintain sugars**
> - Hormonal
>   - Increased catechilamines
>   - Increased glucagon
>   - Increased growth hormone
>   - Increased cortisol
>   - Fall in insulin
> - Enzymes
>   - Fall in glycogen synthase
>   - Rise in glycogen phosphorylase
>   - Rise in phosphoenolpyruvate carboxykinase
> - Receptors
>   - Adaptive changes in the hormonal receptors

sugar. Alternatively, lactate and alanine will act as a fuel too.

Q. What are the counterregulatory hormones that are elevated in hypoglycemia to maintain sugars?

Counterregulatory hormones that are elevated in hypoglycemia to maintain sugars are given in table 1.

Hence, remember that absence of growth hormone and cortisol or excess of insulin can lead to recurrent hypoglycemia.

Q. What are the clinical manifestations of hypoglycemia?

The clinical manifestations of hypoglycemia are given in box 2.

Q. What are the causes for hypoglycemia?

The causes for hypoglycemia could be transient or persistent. These are given in boxes 3 and 4.

TABLE 1: Counterregulatory hormones that are elevated in hypoglycemia

Hypoglycemic state	Counterregulatory hormone
Activating glycogenolytic enzymes	Glucagon, epinephrine
Inducing gluconeogenic enzymes	Glucagon, cortisol
Inhibiting glucose uptake by muscle	Epinephrine, growth hormone, cortisol
Mobilizing amino acids from muscle for gluconeogenesis	Cortisol
Activating lipolysis and thereby providing glycerol for gluconeogenesis and fatty acids for ketogenesis	Epinephrine, cortisol, growth hormone, glucagon
Inhibiting insulin release and promoting growth hormone and glucagon secretion	Epinephrine

BOX 2: Clinical manifestations of hypoglycemia
- Activation of autonomic nervous system and epinephrine release
  - Anxiety
  - Perspiration
  - Palpitation (tachycardia)
  - Pallor
  - Tremulousness
  - Weakness
  - Hunger
  - Nausea
  - Emesis
- Cerebral glucopenia
  - Headache
  - Mental confusion
  - Visual disturbances (↓ acuity, diplopia)
  - Organic personality changes
  - Inability to concentrate
  - Dysarthria, staring
  - Paresthesias
  - Dizziness, amnesia
  - Ataxia, incoordination
  - Refusal to feed
  - Somnolence, lethargy
  - Seizure, coma, stroke, hemiplegia, aphasia
  - Decerebrate or decorticate posture

BOX 3: Causes for transient hypoglycemia
- Inadequate substrate
  - Normal newborn
  - Prematurity
  - Small for gestational age
  - Intrauterine growth retardation
- Transient hyperinsulinism
  - Infant of a diabetic mother
  - Infant of toxemic mother
  - Birth asphyxia
  - Small for gestational age

Q. What are the drugs causing hypoglycemia?

The drugs causing hypoglycemia are:
- Sulfonylureas
- Salicylates
- Beta-blockers
- Quinine
- Disopyramide
- Alcohol.

> **BOX 4: Causes for persistent hypoglycemia**
> - Hyperinsulinism
>   - Diffuse β-cell hyperplasia
>   - Focal β-cell microadenoma
>   - Persistent hyperinsulinemic hypoglycemia of infancy
>   - Inactivating mutation of SUR gene
>   - Activating mutation of glucokinase
> - Deficiency of counterregulatory hormones
>   - Panhypopituitarism
>   - Growth hormone deficiency
>   - Addison's disease
>   - Congenital adrenal hyperplasia
> - Substrate limited
>   - Ketotic hypoglycemia
>   - Glucose-6-phosphate dehydrogenase deficiency
>   - Phosphoenolpyruvate carboxykinase deficiency
>   - Fatty acid oxidation disorders
> - Systemic illness
>   - Liver cell failure
>   - Reye's syndrome
>   - Drug induced

- Accidental exposure to OHA—OHA poisoning
- Previous salt wasting crises/early neonatal death—adrenal insufficiency, CAH
- Increasing pigmentation—CAH
- Consanguineous parentage—metabolic disorders
- Poor growth (height or BMI)—ketotic hypoglycemia, growth hormone deficiency.

Q. What do you look for in a child presenting with hypoglycemia?

- Macrosomic baby/overgrowth—Persistent hyperinsulinemic hypoglycemia of infancy
- Microphallus, cleft palate, undescended testes, cholestatic jaundice—hypopituitarism
- Skin pigmentation, genital abnormalities—adrenal disorders
- Dysmorphism, hypotonia, cardiomegaly—fatty acid oxidation defects
- Hepatomegaly—metabolic diseases
- Features of Beckwith-Wiedemann syndrome.

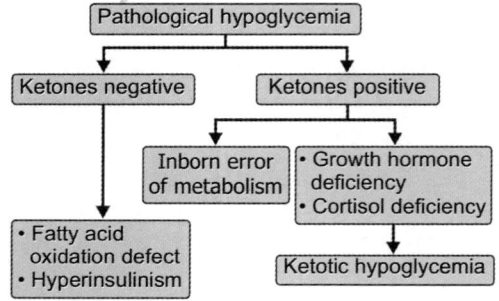

Flowchart 1: Algorithmic approach to pathological hypoglycemia in the emergency room

Q. How to approach pathological hypoglycemia in the emergency room?

Flowchart 1 presents an algorithmic approach to pathological hypoglycemia in the emergency room.

Q. What are the important histories to be taken when a child presents with hypoglycemia to the emergency room?

- Previous hypoglycemia—hypopituitarism, inborn errors of metabolism

Q. What should an emergency room pediatrician do on seeing a child with hypoglycemia?

- Venous blood sugar
- Blood and urine ketones.

At the time of hypoglycemia:
- Insulin, growth hormone, and cortisol
- Lactate, pyruvate
- Free fatty acid, uric acid
- Preserve sample for genetic study.
  Catheterize—for collection of next voided urine for ketones and organic acids.

Q. What is a critical sample?

A critical sample is a sample taken during an acute episode of hypoglycemia (Box 5).

Q. What is the quantity of sample to be taken?

- Plain bulb 6 mL
- Ethylenediamine tetraacetic acid sample 2 mL

CHAPTER 10: Hypoglycemia

> **BOX 5: Types of sample taken during an acute episode of hypoglycemia**
> - Substrates
>   - Glucose
>   - Free fatty acids
>   - Ketones
>   - Lactate
>   - Uric acid
>   - Ammonia
> - Hormones
>   - Insulin
>   - Cortisol
>   - Growth hormone
>   - Thyroxine, thyroid stimulating hormone
>   - Insulin-like growth factor binding protein-1

Q. What is alternate supervised fast test?

This test is used to confirm the diagnosis of ketotic hypoglycemia. Children are put on a 24-hour supervised fast test. Normal children can tolerate fasting up to 24 hours without developing hypoglycemia. Children with ketotic hypoglycemia develop hypoglycemia with elevated fatty acids and ketones within 12–14 hours. It is contraindicated in children with fatty acid oxidation defects.

CONCLUSION

Pediatric hypoglycemia follows abnormalities in the mechanisms involved in glucose homeostasis.

It has diverse causes in which low levels of plasma glucose eventually lead to neuroglycopenia. The most common cause of hypoglycemia in patients with diabetes is injecting a shot of insulin and skipping a meal or overdosing insulin. The cutoff line for blood glucose level to be considered hypoglycemic varies. High index of suspicion is central to its detection. Every pediatrician's office must be equipped with a glucagon vial and point of care testing for blood ketones.

> **KEY LEARNING POINTS**
> ☞ Every pediatrician's office must be equipped with a glucagon vial and point of care testing for blood ketones

☞ Hypoglycemia + short stature + strong ketone response + low growth hormone suggest diagnosis of hypopituitarism

☞ Hypoglycemia + body mass index less than 3rd percentile + strong ketone response + normal growth hormone and suppressed insulin suggest diagnosis of ketotic hypoglycemia

☞ Hypoglycemia + absent ketone response—hyperinsulinemia (after fatty acid oxidation defect is ruled out). An indication for performing glucagon challenge in the emergency room

☞ Pathological hypoglycemia + ketones + low cortisol + normal growth hormone + suppressed insulin suggest diagnosis of adrenal insufficiency. Estimation of 17-hydroxyprogesterone, adrenocorticotropic hormone, and total testosterone in the critical sample should be done and appropriate stress dose of hydrocortisone in the emergency room itself administered

☞ In a diabetic child with mild and moderate hypoglycemia, treatment is as per "rule of 15"

☞ In hypoglycemia with neurological features like convulsions, injection glucagon or dextrose bolus should be given immediately.

SUGGESTED READINGS

1. Clarke W, Jones T, Rewers A, Dunger D, Klingensmith GJ. Assessment and management of hypoglycemia in children and adolescents with diabetes. *Pediatr Diab.* 2009;10(Suppl 12):134-144.
2. Hussain K. Diagnosis and management of hyperinsulinemic hypoglycaemia of infancy. *Horm Res.* 2008;69:2-13.
3. Joint LWPES/ESPE CAH Working Group. Consensus statement on 21-hydroxylase deficiency from the Lawson Wilkins Pediatric Endocrine Society and the European Society for Paediatric Endocrinology. *J Clin Endocrinol Metab.* 2002;87: 4048-4053.
4. Pelavin PI, Abramson E, Pon S, Vogiatzi M. Extended-release glipizide overdose presenting with delayed hypoglycemia and treated with subcutaneous octreotide. *J Pediatr Endocrinol Metab.* 2009;22:171-175.
5. Wilker RE. Hypoglycemia and hyperglycemia. In: Cloherty JP, Eichenwald EC, Hansen AR, Stark AR (Eds). *Manual of Neonatal Care*, 7th edn. Philadelphia: Wolters Kluwer; 2012: 285.

CHAPTER 11

Pheochromocytoma

Hemchand K Prasad, L Francine Shirley

INTRODUCTION

Though most common in adults, around 10% of pheochromocytomas are encountered in childhood. These are neuroendocrine tumors that arise from cells of neural crest origin. About 80–85% pheochromocytomas arise from adrenal medulla. Remaining 10–15% tumors are extra-adrenal in origin.

Clinical presentation of both extra-adrenal and adrenal pheochromocytomas is identical. Clinical manifestations include hypertension, headache, palpitation, and excessive sweating. Notwithstanding surgical excision, long-term prognosis is required, since some 10% of pheochromocytomas are malignant.

CASE 1

A 12-year-old boy presented to the emergency room with complaints of sudden onset headache, palpitations, dizziness, and blurring of vision. On examination, the boy had profuse sweating, heart rate of 110 beats/min, blood pressure of 190/110 mmHg, all four limb pulses were well felt. Cardiovascular examination revealed tachycardia with normal heart sounds and no murmurs were heard.

Chest X-ray was normal. Electrocardiogram (ECG) showed sinus tachycardia with normal rhythm. Echocardiogram (echo) showed structurally normal heart and good cardiac contractility. There was no coarctation of aorta. Ultrasound of the abdomen showed a small mass measuring 2.1 × 2 cm between the left kidney and spleen. Renal Doppler study was normal. Computed tomography (CT) abdomen showed a nodular mass of 2.8 × 2 cm arising from the left suprarenal gland. Hemoglobin, renal parameters, and serum electrolytes were within normal limits. Urinary and serum catecholamine levels were elevated.

CASE REVIEW IN A NUTSHELL

This 12-year-old boy suddenly developed headache, palpitations, dizziness, blurring of vision, profuse sweating, tachycardia, and hypertension.

This clinical profile is consistent with hypertensive crisis. Well-felt peripheral and lower limb pulses ruled out coarctation of aorta. A normal echo and ECG rule out a cardiac cause. Doppler study of the renal vessels rules out renal artery stenosis. In the setting of hypertension, nodular mass in the left suprarenal gland and elevated catecholamine levels, the diagnosis is consistent with pheochromocytoma.

INTERACTIVE TOPIC REVIEW

Q. What are pheochromocytomas/paragangliomas?

Pheochromocytomas are rare, catecholamine-secreting, vascular, neuroendocrine tumors arising from chromaffin cells of the adrenal medulla. About 15-20% of such tumors are extra-adrenal in origin and are termed as paraganglioma or extra-adrenal pheochromocytoma.

Q. What are the most common sites of origin?

The most common site of origin is the adrenal medulla (90%). About 15-20% arise from extra-adrenal chromaffin tissue called paragangliomas.

Q. What is the most common age of presentation?

Only 10-20% of the tumors occur in children. They usually present between 6 and 14 years of age with a slight preponderance in males. They may rarely present during infancy.

Q. How do pheochromocytomas present at initial diagnosis?

The presentation of pheochromocytoma is highly variable. Most of the clinical features of pheochromocytoma are attributed to the hypersecretion of catecholamines, namely epinephrine, norepinephrine, and sometimes, dopamine. Hypertension, either paroxysmal or sustained, is the most common manifestation of pheochromocytoma. Sometimes, the children may be asymptomatic and may be detected by surveillance when they are known carriers of mutation in tumor suppressor genes like Von Hippel-Lindau disease. Other rare presentations include: failure to thrive, polydipsia, and polyuria, unexplained fever. It is a great mimic—it is better to suspect it and not find it rather than not suspect it and find it.

Q. How does hypertension present in pheochromocytoma?

Pheochromocytoma is an underlying cause of 1-2% cases of pediatric hypertension. Hypertension can be either paroxysmal or sustained. Compared to adults, it is sustained in nearly 70% of the children. In case of paroxysmal hypertension, the attacks are initially infrequent, but the frequency increases leading on to a continuous hypertensive state. The children may be symptom-free in between the paroxysms. During paroxysms, children experience headache, dizziness, palpitation, abdominal pain, vomiting, pallor, and sweating. They can also present with convulsions or features of hypertensive encephalopathy.

Q. What are the common triggers for paroxysms?

Paroxysms can occur at rest, but are usually triggered by physical activity, trauma, by direct stimulation of tumor (e.g., urinary bladder distension), or after using certain drugs or taking food (e.g., tyramine in chocolate).

Q. What is the classical symptom triad of pheochromocytoma?

It comprises headache, palpitation, and sweating (Fig. 1).

Q. What are the other clinical features of pheochromocytoma?

- Cachexia despite good appetite

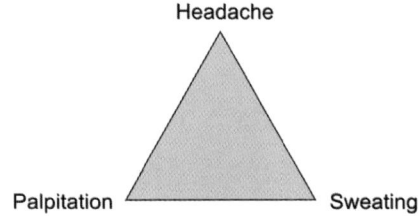

Figure 1: Symptom triad of pheochromocytoma

- Pallor, orthostatic hypotension (secondary to low plasma volume)
- Polyuria, polydipsia, hyperglycemia, growth failure
- Constipation, psychiatric disorders, blurred vision, weight loss, increased erythrocyte sedimentation rate, dilated cardiomyopathy.

Q. What are the important associations with endocrine disturbances and malignancy in a child with pheochromocytoma?

Table 1 lists the important pheochromocytoma associations.

Q. What is the basis for biochemical method of diagnosis?

Biochemical diagnosis of pheochromocytoma is based on demonstration of excessive production of catecholamines. Tumor cells express catechol-o-methyltransferase, hence methylated metabolites are also secreted in excess. Measurement of plasma metanephrines and plasma and urinary catecholamines is the investigation of choice.

Normal values of plasma and urinary metanephrines are shown in table 2.

TABLE 2: Normal values of plasma and urinary metanephrines

Test	Normal range
24-h urinary vanillylmandelic acid	<35 µmol/day
24-h urinary meta-adrenaline	<6.5 µmol/day
Serum adrenaline	30–200 pmol/day
Serum noradrenaline (infants)	<100 pmol/day
Serum noradrenaline (children)	<900 pmol/day

Elevated parameters more than three times, the upper limit is considered as abnormal.

Q. What are the precautions while collecting the sample?

- The sample should be taken in the recumbent posture
- Drugs like acetaminophen, imipramine, and phenothiazines that decrease catecholamine levels should be avoided
- Drugs that increase catecholamines like tetracycline, methyldopa, aminophylline, clonidine, erythromycin, insulin should be avoided
- Abstain from foods like banana, vanilla, caffeine, and nicotine
- A 24-hour sample is always preferred

TABLE 1: Pheochromocytoma associations

Syndrome	Gene involved	Associations
Multiple endocrine neoplasia-2A	• RET proto-oncogene • Chromosome 10	• Medullary carcinoma thyroid • Parathyroid hyperplasia
Multiple endocrine neoplasia-2B	• RET proto-oncogene • Chromosome 10	• Medullary carcinoma thyroid • Mucosal neuromas
Neurofibromatosis type 1	• NF tumor suppressor gene • Chromosome 17	• Retinal angiomas
Von Hippel-Lindau syndrome	• VHL gene • Chromosome 3	• Renal cell carcinoma • Cerebellar and spinal cord hemangioblastomas
Carney triad	• Succinate dehydrogenase deficiency • (SDHB, SDHC, SDHD)	• Mitochondrial disorders
Familial paraganglioma	–	• Gastric leiomyosarcoma • Pulmonary chondroma • Extra-adrenal pheochromocytoma

- The sample should be taken from an indwelling intravenous catheter.

Q. What is the role of imaging in diagnosis?

Most of the tumors are adrenal and can be easily identified by CT or magnetic resonance imaging. Extra-adrenal tumors are often multiple and require a metaiodobenzylguanidine (MIBG) scan for localization (Flowchart 1).

Q. How to treat a child with pheochromocytoma?

The definitive treatment is surgical excision of the tumor in toto. The tumor tissue has to be sent for histopathological examination and 10% of tumors are malignant.

Flowchart 2 presents the algorithmic approach in the treatment of pheochromocytoma.

Q. What are the important steps to be considered in the management of pheochromocytoma?

The important steps to be considered in the management of pheochromocytoma are as follows:
1. Preoperative management (control of hypertension and preparation of surgery)
2. Fitness for surgery
3. Anticipated complications and prepared handedness
4. Postoperative care
5. Follow-up.

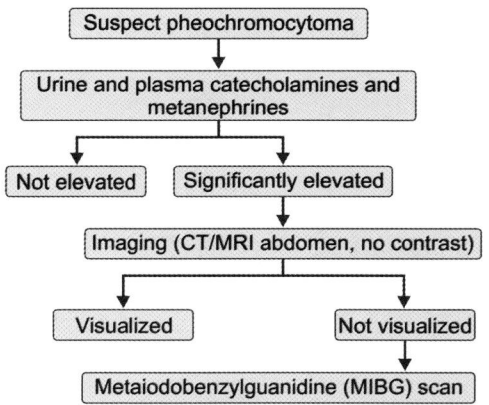

CT, computed tomography; MRI, magnetic resonance imaging.
Flowchart 1: Algorithmic approach to diagnosis of pheochromocytoma

Q. What is the main goal of preoperative evaluation?

- Ensure normal heart rate and blood pressure prior to shifting to operation theater

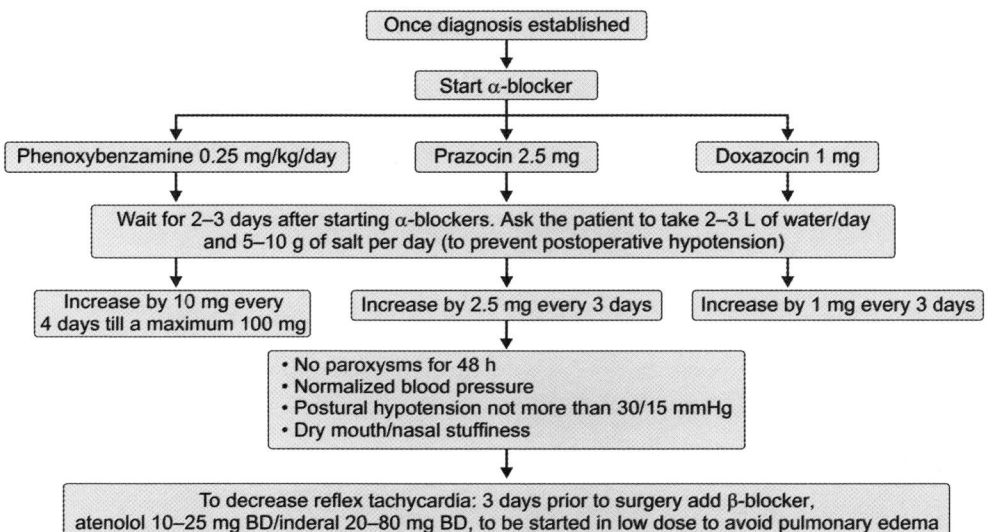

Flowchart 2: Algorithmic approach to treatment of pheochromocytoma

- Normal volume status postoperatively
- Prevent surgery induced catecholamine storm during surgery.

Q. Which is the α-blocker preferred? Why?

Prazocin is preferred to phenoxybenzamine (Table 3).

Q. Can calcium channel blockers be used to treat hypertension?

Calcium channel blockers can be supplemented, if:
- Alpha blockage is inadequate
- Alpha-blockers lead to side effects
- Only intermittent hypertension
- Preferred if coronary spasm (in adults).

Beta-blockers should never be given prior to α-blockers.

Q. Can labetalol be used to treat hypertension?

No. The ratio of α-β blockade is 1:7. Preferred ratio of α-β blockade is 4:1.

Q. When can a child be considered fit for surgery?

No pediatric guidelines exist at present. Hence, we currently follow adult guidelines (Table 4).
- Orthostatic hypotension present
- Normal ECG present.

TABLE 3: Prazocin versus phenoxybenzamine in pheochromocytoma

Factor	Phenoxybenzamine	Prazocin
Availability	Difficult	Easily available
Postoperative fall in blood pressure	More	Less

TABLE 4: Guidelines for surgery in pheochromocytoma

	Standing	Sitting
Heart rate	80/min	70/min
Blood pressure	<160/90 mmHg	>80/45 mmHg

Q. What are the precautions to be taken before surgery?

- Stay in bed/rails
- Start intravenous fluids dextrose normal saline night before surgery
- Calculate mean arterial pressure (MAP) and target MAP, and keep ready all the required medicines
- Shift to operation theater on call
- Skip the morning dose of medicine.

Q. What are the anticipated intraoperative complications and their appropriate management?

- Hypotension: Treat with saline boluses followed by inotropes, preferably vasopressin
- Hypertension: Treat with sodium nitroprusside 0.5 µg/kg/min. Titrate to keep MAP at 50th per centile. Use nonpermeable extension line.
(Alternative: Phentolamine 2.5–5 mg @ 1 mg/min. Repeat every 3–5 min till blood pressure is controlled.)

Q. What is the recommended postoperative care?

A 24-hour elective postoperative pediatric intensive care unit observation and care is warranted.
- Hypoglycemia (β-cell inhibition leads to increased insulin levels)
- Hypovolemia: Fluid boluses may be needed
- Bilateral adrenalectomy should be treated with hydrocortisone
- Cardiomyopathy/pulmonary edema
- If flutter/fibrillation: Intravenous esmolol 0.5 µg/kg over 1 minute.

Q. What should be the follow-up?

As the tumors may recur after a long period at a distant location, a long-term follow-up with imaging and biochemical testing is necessary. Life-long surveillance is warranted because tumors can recur even after several years.

CONCLUSION

Pheochromocytoma, which may be adrenal or extra-adrenal, needs to be kept in mind in any adolescent child presenting with hypertension of obscure etiology. The investigation of choice is measurement of catecholamines and metabolites. Surgical resection followed by life-long follow-up is essential.

KEY LEARNING POINTS

- Pheochromocytoma should be considered in the differential diagnosis in a child presenting with hypertension
- Hypertension is paroxysmal and may not be present at the time of examination
- Other clinical features should be kept in mind to make a diagnosis
- Measurement of plasma and urinary catecholamines and their metabolites is the investigation of choice
- Metaiodobenzylguanidine (MIBG) scan helps in accurate localization and extent of the tumor
- Extensive preoperative care is the cornerstone of management of pheochromocytoma
- Surgical resection and life-long surveillance is necessary

SUGGESTED READINGS

1. Bhansali A, Rajput R, Behra A, Rao KL, Khandelwal N, Radotra BD. Childhood sporadic pheochromocytoma: clinical profile and outcome in 19 patients. *J Pediatr Endocrinol Metab.* 2006;19:749-756.
2. Ganesh HK, Acharya SV, Goerge J, Bandgar TR, Menon PS, Shah NS. Pheochromocytoma in children and adolescents. *Indian J Pediatr.* 2009;76:1151-1153.
3. Lenders JW, Duh QY, Eisenhofer G, Gimenez-Roqueplo AP, Grebe SK, Murad MH, et al. Pheochromocytoma and paraganglioma: an endocrine society clinical practice guideline. *J Clin Endocrinol Metab.* 2014;99:1915-1942.
4. Mishra A, Mehrotra PK, Agarwal G, Agarwal A, Mishra SK. Pediatric and adolescent pheochromocytoma: clinical presentation and outcome of surgery. *Indian Pediatr.* 2014; 51:299-302.
5. Tsirlin A, Oo Y, Sharma R, Kansara A, Gliwa A, Banerji MA. Pheochromocytoma: A review. *Maturitas.* 2014;77:229-238.
6. Waguespack SG, Rich T, Grubbs E, Ying AK, Perrier ND, Ayala-Ramirez M, et al. A current review of the etiology, diagnosis, and treatment of pediatric pheochromocytoma and paraganglioma. *J Clin Endocrinol Metab.* 2010;95: 2023-2037.

CHAPTER

12

Annular Pancreas

Harmesh S Bains, Doaman Mittal, Gaurav Singla, Sidharth Nayyar

INTRODUCTION

Literary meaning of the term annular pancreas is a ring-shaped pancreas. It is a rare embryologic disorder of the pancreas first described by Tedemanin in the year 1818. A large majority of the cases are diagnosed early in life with neonatal obstruction and often prenatally. At times, the condition may remain asymptomatic for many years, presenting with complications such as pancreatitis in adolescence and even adulthood association with other congenital malformations, e.g., cardiovascular anomalies, Down syndrome, Hirschsprung disease, tracheoesophageal and fistula, esophageal atresia.

CASE 1

A 5-month-old male child presented with complaints of recurrent episodes of nonbilious projectile vomiting since early neonatal period, frequency of which increased 3 days prior to admission. The vomiting was nonbilious and projectile in nature containing undigested milk. The child had birth weight of 2,500 g and the pregnancy was uncomplicated. The child was breastfed but not exclusively, it was supplemented with cow's milk (Bottle feeds). The child had recurrent episodes of feed regurgitation which resulted in aspiration. This aspiration leads to recurrent chemical pneumonitis for which the child has been admitted multiple times in the past. The child was lethargic at admission. Physical examination revealed slight upper abdominal distension and signs of dehydration. Possibility of aspiration pneumonia was kept with underlying sepsis. Intravenous fluids and intravenous antibiotics were started. Initial blood counts were normal and C-reactive protein was less than 6. Initial blood gas revealed pH = 7.71, bicarbonate (HCO3) = 60, partial pressure of carbon dioxide (pCO2) = 55, partial pressure of oxygen (pO2) = 50. Electrolytes were sodium/potassium/chlorine = 129/2.77/57 (revealed hypocholoremic metabolic alkalosis). Possibility of underlying intestinal obstruction was considered and a pediatric surgery opinion was taken.

The child underwent a barium meal follow through study (Fig. 1). The study revealed intestinal obstruction at the level of second part of duodenum. Possibilities kept were malrotation and/or annular pancreas. On laparotomy, pancreas was found encircling second part of duodenum. Rest all structures were normal. Duodenojejunal junction was at normal position suggestive of no malrotation. Duodenoduodenostomy was done (first part of duodenum with third part) and annular pancreas was left in situ. The postoperative course was uncomplicated and child was discharged in a stable condition.

CASE REVIEW IN A NUTSHELL

This congenital anomaly affects males more frequently than females, and the majority of cases are observed very early in life. In infants, it is usually characterized by severe duodenal

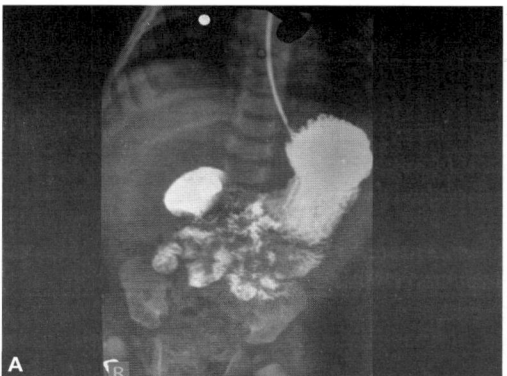
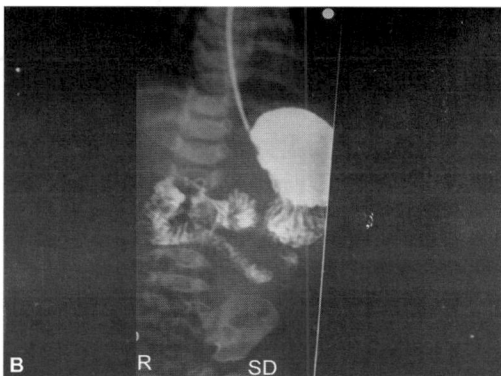

Figure 1: Barium meal follows through sequences of the index case

obstruction requiring immediate surgical intervention. However, in other cases, the obstruction may be of such minimal degree at birth that the patient remains asymptomatic for life. The severity of symptoms and the age at which they occur is presumably determined by the degree of constriction of the duodenum caused by the encircling pancreatic tissue.

In infants, the X-ray films confirm the diagnosis of duodenal obstruction. Wedge resection would be insufficient in newborn babies as it would not cure the underlying duodenal stenosis or atresia. Duodenoduodenostomy around the constricting ring of pancreas appear to be the ideal treatment. Failing this, duodenojejunostomy should be satisfactory. Gastrojejunostomy should be avoided; it will fail to drain the dilated proximal duodenum and incomplete obstruction will result in bile passing backwards into the stomach and the setting up of acute gastritis.

INTERACTIVE TOPIC REVIEW

Q. What is the Embryology of Pancreas?

It is in the 5th gestational week that the development of pancreas takes off as one dorsal and two ventral buds from the primitive foregut. By 7th week, the ventral bud undergoes a rotation, passes behind the duodenum, and fuses with the dorsal bud. In due course, dorsal bud forms the body and tail of the pancreas whereas the ventral bod forms its head, inferior part and uncinate process. Main pancreatic duct is basically formed from the fusion of the buds.

Q. How about the embryology of annular pancreas?

This is an embryological defect of the foregut. According to a hypothesis, the tip of the ventral bud fuses abnormally to the duodenum. As a consequence, incorrect rotation around the duodenum occurs, resulting in a band of fibrous or pancreatic parenchyma tissue around the second part of the duodenum. Another hypothesis stresses on the hypertrophy of the dorsal and ventral buds, resulting in a complete band of pancreatic tissue around the duodenum. Thus, a complete ring is found in around one-fourth of the cases.

Q. How to evaluate character of vomitus: bilious versus nonbilious emesis?

Bilious: Obstruction distal to ampulla of Vater.

Nonbilious: Obstruction proximal to ampulla of Vater or other causes of emesis (infection, metabolic, etc.).

Q. Is that always true?

This is generally true. However, sometimes infants and children do not follow these rules.

Q. What should be done?

Nil per os, 10 Fr nasogastric tube to low continuous suction. Start intravenous fluids: normal saline/lactated ringers bolus and maintenance intravenous fluids, blood gas to assess acid-base status. Additional labs: Complete blood counts, biochem panel, urinalysis, and blood/urine cultures

Q. What should be radiological test?

It depends on what is the index of suspicion. Plain films of the abdomen may provide clues to the level of obstruction and help determine what follow-up fluoroscopic exam is necessary. This should be performed concurrent with fluid resuscitation and decompression. Radiologic work-up should be discussed with the consulting surgical team. A well-appearing child with a low index of suspicion for volvulus may benefit from a barium enema before an upper gastrointestinal (GI). In cases with a high index of suspicion, an upper GI is indicated. However, if a child is ill-appearing, urgent laparotomy may be performed without prior radiologic studies.

Q. What is the surgical intervention of choice?

Surgical bypass of the duodenum is indicated in severe stenosis. Local resection of the annular segment is avoided because of the fear of development of pancreatic fistula and is often difficult because of dense adhesions due to local fibrosis.

Q. What should be the preferred procedure?

Duodenoduodenostomy or duodenojejunostomy are the procedures of choice. Gastrojejunostomy is an alternative option in case of grossly fibrotic duodenal C loop.

CONCLUSION

Acute duodenal obstruction due to annular pancreas is seen more often in infants, presenting with vomiting and dehydration. Vomiting may or may not be bilious and abdominal distension is absent because of the high obstruction. Early diagnosis and definitive treatment is essential to preserve the metabolic status of the already depleted infant. Treatment modality of choice is surgical bypass of the affected segment.

KEY LEARNING POINTS

- Annular pancreas, a ring-shaped pancreas, is a rare embryologic disorder of the pancreas, usually diagnosed early in life with neonatal obstruction and often prenatally
- Association with cardiovascular anomalies, Down syndrome, Hirschsprung disease, tracheo-esophageal fistula, and esophageal atresia are common
- Ultrasound or cross-sectional imaging techniques are required to specifically identify annular pancreas
- Though urgent surgical intervention is required in cases of duodenal obstruction, annular creas without complication(s) requires no treatment
- Overall prognosis is dictated by the severity of associated congenital defects
- Diagnosis may be made prenatally with evidence of duodenal obstruction though more specific markers for prenatal detection of annular pancreas are currently under investigation

SUGGESTED READINGS

1. Dankovcik R, Jirasek J, Kucera E, Feyereisl J, Radonak J, Dudas M. Prenatal diagnosis of annular pancreas: reliability of the double bubble sign with periduodenal hyperechogenic band. *Fetal Diagn Ther.* 2008;24:483-490.
2. Patra DP, Basu A, Chanduka A, Roy A. Annular pancreas: a rare cause of duodenal obstruction in adults. *Indian J Surg.* 2011;73:163-165.
3. Rickham PP. Annular pancreas in the newborn. *Arch Dis Child.* 1954;29:80-83.
4. Zyromski NJ, Sandoval JA, Pitt HA, Ladd AP, Fogel EL, Mattar WE, et al. Annular pancreas: dramatic differences between children and adults. *J Am Coll Surg.* 2008;206:1019-1025.

SECTION 4
Neurology

CHAPTER 13

Traumatic Brain Injury

Khaleel Khan, Anjul Dayal, Abhilasha Singh

INTRODUCTION

The management of severe traumatic brain injury (TBI) centers on meticulous and comprehensive intensive care that includes multimodel, protocolized approach involving careful hemodynamic support, respiratory care, fluid management, and other aspects of therapy, aimed at preventing secondary brain insults, maintaining an adequate cerebral perfusion pressure (CPP), and optimizing cerebral oxygenation. This approach clearly requires the efforts of a multidisciplinary team including neurointensivists, neurosurgeons, bedside nurses and respiratory therapists, and other members of the medical team.

CASE 1

A 10-year-old girl with alleged history of fall from balcony of her first floor, brought to emergency room in unconsciousness state. Her vitals: heart rate: 84/min, respiratory rate: 22/min, blood pressure (BP): 115/60, unarousable, decerebrates on painful stimuli with right pupil 3 mm SL and low-titer 1.5 mm NRL, nasal bleed with raccoon eyes, cold peripheries, and low volume pedal pulses.

A multidisciplinary team approach was adopted in the management of our patient. Neurosurgeons operated on him after stabilization by the pediatric intensive care unit (NICU) team. The child also needed exploratory laparotomy, done by the pediatric surgeons because of a query of collection of fluid or blood in the intra-abdominal cavity. The patient remained hospitalized for further management and observation for one month, after which she was discharged in a good condition.

CASE REVIEW IN A NUTSHELL

Clinical profile of this 10-year-old child with alleged history fall from first floor with altered sensorium and ear, nose, throat bleed with raccoon eyes pointed to severe TBI, which warranted immediate attention including:
- ABC (no head tilt chin left with rapid sequence induction, assessment of Arpu/Ges/NICU) stabilization and primary survey
- In addition, urgent computed tomography (CT) head was performed and it showed a severely comminuted depressed fracture of the right frontal bone extending to orbital roof with an associated frontal scalp hematoma and multiple air pockets (Fig. 1). Petechial, tiny hemorrhagic foci in the right frontal lobe were evident on the brain window images as well as subdural hematoma which was evident as the hyper density of the inter hemispheric fissure anteriorly
- A right frontal intracranial pressure (ICP) monitor was placed on the day of admission. The child was started on hypertonic saline

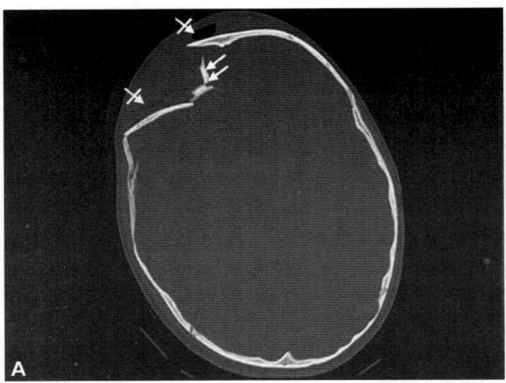
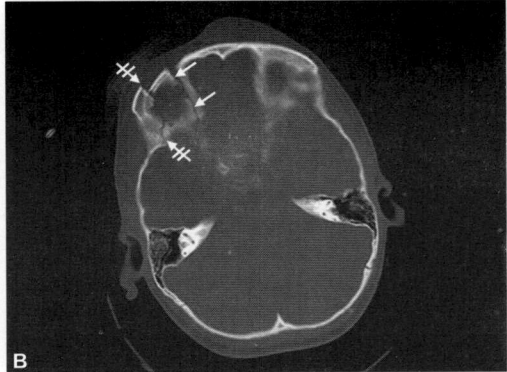

Figure 1: Computed tomography scan (bone window) showing the depressed fracture of the right frontal bone extending to orbital roof

and intravascular volume and blood pressure were maintained to maximize CPP
- The child was also started on prophylactic anticonvulsants and vasoactive agents to maintain BP
- Subsequent CT scan showed mild diffuse cerebral atrophy, complete regression of the subdural effusions on the right side, and considerable regression of the left subdural effusion with only a small subdural collection on the left side
- Management of raised ICP with:
  - Head elevation at 30°
  - Euthermia
  - Sedation
  - Hypertonic saline.

INTERACTIVE TOPIC REVIEW

Q. How to assess severity of head injury?

Assessment of grading of severity of head injury is presented in table 1.

Q. What is primary brain injury?

Immediate or primary brain injury results from the initial forces generated following trauma. Focal injuries such as contusions and hematomas are generated by contact, linear forces when the head is struck by a moving object. Inertial, angular forces produced by acceleration deceleration can lead to immediate physical shearing or tearing of axons termed "primary" axotomy.

Q. What are the reasons for secondary brain injury?

Following primary brain injury, two forms of secondary brain injury can occur. The first form of secondary brain injury, such as hypoxemia, hypotension, intracranial hypertension, hypercarbia, hyper- or hypoglycemia, electrolyte abnormalities, enlarging hematomas, coagulopathy, seizures, and hyperthermia are potentially avoidable or treatable. The primary goal in the acute management of the severely head-injured pediatric patient is to prevent or ameliorate these factors that promote secondary brain injury.

The other form of secondary brain injury involves an endogenous cascade of cellular and biochemical events in the brain that occurs within minutes and continues for months after the primary brain injury that lead to ongoing or "secondary" traumatic axonal injury and neuronal cell damage (delayed brain injury) and ultimately, neuronal cell death. Intense research continues in the ultimate hopes of discovering novel therapies to halt the progression or inhibit these mechanisms for which there is no current therapy.

Secondary brain injury can be minimized by preventing and correcting hypoxemia,

CHAPTER 13: Traumatic Brain Injury

TABLE 1: Assessment and grading of severity of head injury

Minor	• No loss of consciousness • Up to one episode of vomiting • Stable, alert conscious state • May have scalp bruising or laceration • Normal examination otherwise
Moderate	• Brief loss of consciousness at time of injury • Currently alert or responds to voice • May be drowsy • Two or more episodes of vomiting • Persistent headache • Up to one single brief (<2 min) convulsion occurring immediately after the impact • May have a large scalp bruise, hematoma or laceration • Normal examination otherwise

Severe	• Decreased conscious state: Responsive to pain only or unresponsive
	• Localizing neurological signs (unequal pupils, lateralizing motor weakness)
	• Signs of increased intracranial pressure:
	  ○ Uncal herniation: Ipsilateral dilated nonreactive pupil due to compression of the oculomotor nerve
	  ○ Central herniation: Brainstem compression causing bradycardia, hypertension, and widened pulse pressure (Cushing's triad)
	  ○ Irregular respirations (Cheynes-Stokes)
	  ○ Decorticate: Arms flexed, hands clenched into fists, legs extended, feet turned inward
	  ○ Decerebrate: Head arched back, arms extended by the sides, legs extended, feet turned inward
	  ○ Penetrating head injury
	  ○ Cerebrospinal fluid leaks from nose or ears

hypotension, anemia, hypoglycemia, and hyperthermia, and by evacuating certain intracranial masses.

Q. What is the relationship between mean arterial pressure (MAP), cerebral perfusion pressure, and intracranial pressure and its importance?

Cerebral perfusion pressure = (Mean arterial pressure − Intracranial pressure)

It is important to appreciate that cerebral ischemia is the single most important secondary event affecting outcome following severe TBI.

Cerebral perfusion pressure, defined as the MAP minus ICP, (CPP = MAP - ICP), below 50 mmHg must be prevented. A low CPPs likely to damage regions of the brain with preexisting ischemia, enhancement of CPP may help to avoid cerebral ischemia.

It is advisable to maintain the CPP value above the ischemic threshold at a minimum of 60 mmHg. Maintenance of a CPP 60 mmHg is a therapeutic option that may be associated with a substantial reduction in mortality and improvement in quality of survival. It may enhance perfusion to ischemic regions of the brain after the severe TBI.

Incidence of intracranial hypertension, morbidity, or mortality does not increase by the active maintenance of CPP above 60 mmHg with normalizing the intravascular volume or inducing systemic hypertension.

The CPP should be maintained at a minimum of 60 mmHg in the absence of cerebral ischemia, and at a minimum of 70 mmHg in the presence of cerebral ischemia.

Age-appropriate CPP:
- For 2-6 years, greater than equals to 50 mmHg
- For 7-10 years, greater than equals to 55 mmHg

- For 11–15 years, greater than equals to 60 mmHg.

Q. What is osmolarity? What is the role of hyperosmolar therapy in TBI?

Osmolarity = (2Na + Glucose/18 + BUN/2.3), where Na is sodium and BUN is blood urea nitrogen.

Mannitol, which creates a temporary osmotic gradient and increases the serum osmolarity from 310 mOsm/kg to 320 mOsm/kg H_2O, is an effective method to decrease raised ICP after severe TBI. However, its prophylactic administration is not recommended. Mannitol is contraindicated in patients with TBI and renal failure because of the risk of pulmonary edema and heart failure.

Hypertonic saline, typically 3% saline, is an effective therapy for intracranial hypertension. It increases serum osmolality, causing the shift of water from intracellular compartments to the intravascular space, with subsequent decrease in cellular edema. Improved vasoregulation, cardiac output, immune modulation, and plasma volume expansion are its other advantages.

Children with TBI appear to tolerate a high osmolar load with the use of hypertonic saline, reaching serum osmolarities around 360 mOsm/L. Some of these patients may develop reversible renal insufficiency when serum osmolality approaches 320 mOsm/L. Effective dose is 6.5–10 mL/kg; continuous infusion of 3% saline ranges from 0.1 mL/kg/h to 1 mL/kg/h administered on a sliding scale. Minimum dose needed to maintain ICP of less than 20 mmHg should be used. Serum osmolality should be maintained at less than 360 mOsm/L.

Q. What are the indications for doing computed tomography scanning in case of traumatic brain injury?

Computed tomography scanning is required if any of the following features:
- Witnessed loss of consciousness more than 5 minutes
- Amnesia (anterograde or retrograde) more than 5 minutes
- Abnormal drowsiness
- Three or more discrete episodes of vomiting
- Post-traumatic seizure (no history of epilepsy nor history suggestive of reflex anoxic seizure)
- Suspicion of open or depressed skull injury or tense fontanelle
- Any sign of basal skull fracture [hemotympanum, "panda" eyes, cerebrospinal fluid (CSF) leakage from the ear or nose, Battle's sign]
- Focal neurological deficit
- If under 1 year, presence of bruise, swelling or laceration of more than 5 cm on the head
- Dangerous mechanism of injury (high-speed road traffic accident, fall from more than 3 m height, high-speed injury from a projectile or an object).

Q. What is prophylactic hyperthermia?

Moderate systemic hypothermia at 32–34°C reduces cerebral metabolism and cerebral blood volume (CBV), decreases ICP, and increases CPP. Evidence of the impact of moderate hypothermia on the outcome of patients with TBI was controversial. Initially, studies showed that moderate hypothermia, established on admission was associated with significantly improved outcome at 3 months and 6 months after TBI. However, in a large randomized controlled trial (RCT), no effect of moderate hypothermia has been demonstrated on outcome after TBI. However, temperature should be controlled and fever should be aggressively treated in patients with severe TBI. Moderate hypothermia may be used in refractory, uncontrolled ICP.

Q. What are early measures to be taken in emergency room on arrival?

Early airway management involves providing proper airway position, clearance of debris while keeping cervical spine precautions in place, and orotracheal intubation. Hypercarbia and hypoxia must be avoided because they are both potent cerebral vasodilators that result in increased cerebral blood flow and volume and, potentially, increased ICP and intracranial hypertension. Orotracheal intubation allows for airway protection in patients who are severely obtunded and allows for better control of oxygenation and ventilation (Table 2).

In the initial resuscitation period, efforts should be made to maintain eucapnia at the low end of the normal reference range ($PaCO_2$ of 35–39 mmHg) and prevent hypoxia (PaO_2 <60–65 mmHg) to prevent or to limit secondary brain injury.

Achieving normotension and euvolemia is the goal in cardiovascular management unless there is evidence of increased ICP requiring supraphysiologic BP to drive CPP. Adequate volume resuscitation with isotonic solutions is indicated to maintain adequate filling pressures, normal cardiac output, and, ultimately, normotension.

Q. What is the role of intracranial pressure monitoring in traumatic brain injury?

It is recommended that ICP should be monitored in all salvageable patients with a severe TBI and an abnormal CT scan. Based on physiological principles, potential benefits of ICP monitoring include earlier detection of intracranial mass lesion, guidance of therapy and avoidance of indiscriminate use of therapies to control ICP, drainage of CSF with reduction of ICP and improvement of CPP, and determination of prognosis. Currently, available methods for ICP monitoring include epidural, subdural, subarachnoid, parenchymal, and ventricular locations. Historically, ventricular ICP catheter has been used as the reference standard and the preferred technique when possible. It is the most accurate, low-cost, and reliable method of monitoring ICP. It also allows for continuous measurement of ICP and for therapeutic CSF drainage in the event of intracranial hypertension to control raised ICP. Subarachnoid, subdural, and epidural monitors are less accurate. Intracranial hypertension is

TABLE 2: **Assessment and stabilization in emergency room**

Airway	• Consider possible injury to the cervical spine • Maintain head and neck in a neutral position • Immobilization: Sandbags, intravenous solution bags, towel rolls (younger patients) • Age-appropriate rigid cervical collar or manual in-line immobilization (older patients) • Orotracheal intubation if cannot maintain airway adequately with positioning and after suctioning
Breathning	• Intubation if unable to maintain adequate oxygenation and ventilation, despite provision of supplemental oxygen • Use rapid-sequence induction technique • Maintain cervical spine precautions
Circulation	• Hemodynamic instability unlikely to be caused by intracranial injury alone (exception: significant intracranial or scalp bleeding in a young infant) • If present: Investigate extracranial lesions causing hemorrhagic or hypovolemic shock. Insert two large-bore intravenous catheters; fluid bolus of 20 mL/kg of normal saline • Repeat until vital signs improve

Disablity	• Perform rapid assessment, including:
	  ○ Glasgow Coma Scale score adapted to age
	  ○ Pupil size and reactivity to light
	  ○ Tone, reflex and movement of all four limbs
	  ○ Fontanelle (infants)
	  ○ Signs of basal skull fracture: Periorbital ecchymosis ("raccoon eyes"), ecchymosis over the mastoid bone (Battle's sign), obvious leakage of cerebrospinal fluid from the nose or ears, hemotympanum. If one or more of these signs is present, no tube should be placed by the nasal route.

associated with poor neurologic outcome. In the intensive care unit, continuous ICP monitoring is predominantly used to help target therapies to maintain adequate CPP, which is equal to the mean arterial BP minus either the ICP or the central venous pressure, whichever is greater.

Although no RCTs have been conducted to assess the use of ICP monitoring, it is widely accepted as an essential tool in major pediatric centers to guide therapies for the treatment of severe TBI. The exact threshold of pathological ICP or intracranial hypertension for a given age has not been established, but the general consensus is that treatment efforts should, at a minimum, attempt to keep ICP less than 20 mmHg.

Q. What are the role of analgesics, anesthetics, and sedatives'?

Such narcotics as morphine and fentanyl are the first line therapy. They provide analgesia, mild sedation, and depression of airway reflexes (cough) which are required in intubated and mechanically ventilated patients.

Propofol is the hypnotic of choice in an acute neurologic insult. It is easily titratable and rapidly reversible once discontinued. It should be avoided in hypotensive or hypovolemic patients because of its deleterious hemodynamic effects.

Benzodiazepines, like midazolam and lorazepam, are good in the form of a continuous infusion or intermittent boluses. Over and above sedation, they provide amnesia and anticonvulsive effect. However, prolonged infusion, high dose, presence of renal or hepatic failure, and old age are risk factors for accumulation and over-sedation.

Nuromuscular blocking agents to paralyze patients with TBI may be considered as second-line therapy for refractory intracranial hypertension.

Q. How about the role of anti-seizure prophylaxis?

Post-traumatic seizures are often complicated with TBI and can cause secondary injury by increasing metabolic demands and raising ICP, with an incidence varying from 4 to 25% within the first 7 days of injury. Prophylactic anticonvulsants decrease the incidence of early posttraumatic seizures (level II evidence), but have not been shown to decrease mortality, improve neurological dysfunction, or affect late seizures that occur after 7 days postinjury. Valproic acid and phenytoin have been shown to have similar efficacies. Emerging studies have shown that levetiracetam has similar efficacy as phenytoin, which is recommended as an agent for the first line prophylaxis because of its higher availability and lower cost.

Q. Any role of hyperventilation?

Indeed, it is quite significant since hyperventilation tends to reduce intracranial hypertension via reflex vasoconstriction in the presence of hypocapnia, resulting in decreased cerebral blood flow, decreased CBV, and a subsequent decrease in ICP. Its adverse effects include cerebral vasoconstriction and the subsequent risk for cerebral ischemia. Avoidance of prophylactic severe hyperventilation to a $PaCO_2$ of less than 30 mmHg may be considered in the initial 48 hours after injury.

Severe hyperventilation ($PaCO_2$ <30 mmHg) may be necessary in emergencies such as impending herniation (e.g., a patient with the Cushing triad), but it should not be commonly used for prolonged therapy unless there is refractory intracranial hypertension. If aggressive hyperventilation is used for an extended period, advanced neuromonitoring for cerebral ischemia (e.g., cerebral blood flow, brain tissue oxygen monitoring, jugular venous oxygen saturation, transcranial Doppler, near-infrared spectroscopy) is suggested.

Q. What is the role of steroids in traumatic brain injury?

There are theoretical benefits to administering glucocorticoids, but studies show that they might increase mortality and morbidity. In Corticosteroid Randomization After Significant Head Injury (CRASH) study showed a significant increase in number of deaths in patients given steroids compared with patients who received no treatment. The significant increase in deaths with steroids suggests that steroids should no longer be routinely used in children with traumatic head injury.

Q. What intravenous fluids should be used in traumatic brain injury?

Generally, patients should be kept euvolemic. Hypotensive patients should receive isotonic fluids. Normal saline and hypertonic saline are the fluids of choice in the treatment of patients with TBI.

Q. Why is it important to manage hypotension and hypoxemia in children with traumatic brain injury?

Hypoxemia and hypotension are to be avoided or treated to prevent or minimize secondary brain injury from hypoxic-ischemic brain damage, which may promote diffuse cerebral swelling and intracranial hypertension.

Q. What is the correlation of hyperglycemia and outcome in severe traumatic brain injury in children?

The stress response in trauma patients, including those with severe TBI, generates a hypercatabolic state leading to rapid muscle protein breakdown and hyperglycemia. At a cellular level, there are deleterious effects in macrophage and neutrophil function and there is also some evidence suggesting axonal dysfunction.

It is unclear whether hyperglycemia or lack of insulin during the metabolic stress response affects outcome, but it is clear that an adequate level of glucose in plasma is associated with lower morbidity and better outcome.

Q. What is the role of barbiturate coma in traumatic brain injury?

Barbiturate is proven as efficient therapy for refractory intracranial hypertension. Barbiturates reduce cerebral metabolism and CBF, and lower ICP. High-dose barbiturate.

Q. What is the role of surgical decompression in traumatic brain injury?

Surgical decompressive craniectomy and hemicraniectomy are promising therapeutic approaches for patients with acute severe TBI who are at risk to develop severe brain and death edema, especially when medical treatment has failed and death is imminent.

There are only few studies on decompressive craniectomy in TBI in children. However, a recent RCT found that early bifrontal decompressive craniectomy for refractory ICP elevations resulted in lower ICPs, and decreased the length of ICU stay.

Q. Does early nutrition in traumatic brain injury indeed help?

Yes, it does. The usual coexistence of hypermetabolic, hypercatabolic, and hyperglycemic states with altered gastrointestinal function plus malnutrition increases morbidity and mortality rate in TBI. Enteral feeding is superior to parenteral feeding. Hence, early enteral feeding is recommended in patients with severe TBI. It is safe, cheap, cost-effective, and physiologic. Additionally, it promotes stimulation of all gastrointestinal tract functions, preservation of the immunological gut barrier function, intestinal mucosal integrity, and prevention of complications related to superimposed infections.

CONCLUSION

Children are more susceptible to TBI because they have a larger head to body size ratio, thinner cranial bones providing less protection to the intracranial contents, less myelinated neural tissue which makes them more vulnerable to damage, and a greater incidence of diffuse injury and cerebral edema compared to adults. Diffuse TBI is the most common type of injury and results in a range of injury severity. The diagnosis of TBI is primarily made by CT of the brain and is associated with increased ICP. The acute treatment of pediatric TBI is directed at preventing secondary injury from systemic hypotension, hypoxia, hypocarbia, and hyperglycemia.

KEY LEARNING POINTS

- Traumatic brain injury is common and a major cause of morbidity and mortality worldwide
- Severe traumatic brain injury patients should be stabilized and have rapid neurosurgical consultation
- Diagnostic imaging with computed tomography should be performed promptly to quantify the extent of injury and need for intervention
- Aggressive therapy should be started immediately to reduce secondary injury
- Management is based on avoidance of secondary injury, maintenance of cerebral perfusion pressure, and optimization of cerebral oxygenation
- Evidence-based guidelines and management protocols help to guide target-driven care and are associated with better outcome
- Multimodality monitoring of the injured brain enables individualized therapeutic targets to be set to optimize patient management
- Patients with moderate or severe brain injury should be managed in a specialist neurosurgical center

SUGGESTED READINGS

1. Dayan PS, Holmes JF, Hoyle J Jr, Tunik MG, Lichenstein R, Alpern E, et al. Association of traumatic brain injuries (TBI) in children after blunt head trauma with degree of isolated headache or isolated vomiting. *Acad Emerg Med.* 2008;15:S175-176.
2. Kuppermann N, Holmes JF, Dayan PS, Hoyle JD Jr, Atabaki SM, Holubkov R, et al. Identification of children at very low risk of clinically-important brain injuries after head trauma: a prospective cohort study. *Lancet.* 2009;374:1160-1170.
3. Kuppermann N, Holmes JF, Dayan PS, Hoyle J, Atabaki SM, Monroe D N, et al. Does isolated loss of consciousness predict traumatic brain injury in children after blunt head trauma? *Acad Emerg Med.* 2008;15:82-84.
4. Lee LK, Monroe D, Bachman MC, Glass TF, Mahajan PV, Cooper A, et al. Isolated loss of consciousness in children with minor blunt head trauma. *JAMA Pediatr.* 2014;168:837-843.
5. Palchak MJ, Holmes JF, Vance CW, Gelber RE, Schauer BA, Harrison MJ N, et al. Does an isolated history of loss of consciousness or amnesia predict brain injuries after blunt head trauma? *Pediatrics.* 2004;113:e507-513.
6. Quayle KS, Holmes JF, Kuppermann N, Powell EC, Mahajan P, Hoyle JD Jr, et al. Epidemiology of blunt head trauma in children in U.S. emergency departments. *N Engl J Med.* 2014;371:1945-1947.
7. Stocchetti N, Conte V, Ghisoni L, Canavesi K, Zanaboni C. Traumatic brain injury in pediatric patients. *Minerva Anestesiol.* 2010;76:1052-1059.

CHAPTER 14

Acute Seizures

Sheffali Gulati, Jayashankar Kaushik

INTRODUCTION

Acute seizure refers to transient occurrence of signs and/or symptoms due to abnormal excessive or synchronous neuronal activity in brain [International League Against Epilepsy (ILAE), 2005]. In contrast, epilepsy (ILAE, 2014) is defined as disease of the brain defined by any of the following conditions:
- At least two unprovoked (or reflex) seizures occurring more than 24 hours apart
- One unprovoked (or reflex) seizure and a probability of further seizures similar to the general recurrence risk (at least 60%) after two unprovoked seizures, occurring over the next 10 years
- Diagnosis of an epilepsy syndrome.

The overall prevalence of epilepsy in India was estimated to 5.33 (4.25–6.41). There are diverse etiologies for acute seizure in children. Broadly, acute seizure can be divided into provoked and unprovoked seizures. Common cause of provoked seizure includes febrile seizure, head trauma, and dyselectrolytemia including hypoglycemia, hypocalcemia, and hyponatremia. The common causes for unprovoked seizure in children include neurocysticercosis, tuberculoma, and past neurological insult (ischemic infarct, hypoxic ischemic insult).

CASE 1

A 6-year-old boy presented with complaints of one episode of seizure in the evening. He was playing in the playground, when he felt uncomfortable in abdomen followed by vomiting. He was made to sit in the playground bench. Within few minutes, he complained of severe headache and immediately started gazing strangely toward the right side and remained unresponsive. This was followed by resultant fall to floor and jerk involving right upper limb that lasted for almost 30–40 seconds, then remained unresponsive till child was shifted to nearby hospital.

On examination, he was conscious, alert, was recognizing the parents, and was speaking with clarity; heart rate 92/min; respiratory rate 20/min; blood pressure 98/72 mmHg, and temperature 97°F. There were no evident neurocutaneous markers and no dysmorphism. Higher mental function was normal. Fundus examination was normal. Muscle bulk and tone were normal. Muscle power was around 3/5 in right upper limb across proximal and distal joint. Power in rest of limbs was normal. Deep tendon reflexes were normal. There were no meningeal signs. There were no cerebellar signs.

Child was admitted in pediatric casualty.

Investigations: His blood sugar (88 mg/dL) and serum calcium (1.0 mEq/L) were normal. Blood urea was normal (22 mg/dL). Contrast-enhanced computed tomography (CT) scan revealed 0.5 cm by 0.5 cm, ring-enhancing lesion in left temporoparietal lobe with scolex with perilesional edema suggestive of neurocysticercosis.

Treatment: He was administered injection phenytoin 20 mg/kg loading dose and subsequently started on oral phenytoin at the rate of 5 mg/kg/day. Investigations including mantoux test and chest X-ray were normal. Indirect ophthalmoscopy was performed to rule out intraocular cysticerci. He was started on oral albendazole 15 mg/kg/day for 28 days under initial cover of oral dexamethasone (0.6 mg/kg/day for 3 days before to 2 days after albendazole). His muscle power returned to normal within 24 hours.

At follow-up after 6 months, repeat CT scan revealed calcified granuloma. His antiepileptic drug (AED) (phenytoin) was continued for 2 years. Electroencephalography (EEG) had done at the end of 2 years revealed a normal study. His AEDs were tapered over next 2 months and was doing fine.

CASE REVIEW IN A NUTSHELL

The presentation of this 6-year-old boy's manifestations may be analyzed as per table 1.

TABLE 1: Analysis of the index case

Question	Analysis
Is it true seizure, could it paroxysmal nonepileptic event?	Presence of abdominal symptoms (aura) at onset followed by version of eyes to right side with focal clonic jerking of right upper limb with impairment of consciousness with return to normalcy is more likely to be seizure
Is it focal or generalized seizure?	It appears to be right focal seizure
Is it provoked or unprovoked seizure?	In absence of obvious provoking factors like fever, head trauma, obvious dyselectrolytemia, it is more likely to be unprovoked seizure
What is age at onset?	6 years
How is the development of child?	Appropriate for age

Continued

Continued

Question	Analysis
Is there a positive family history of epilepsy?	None
What could have led to transient paresis of right upper limb in this child?	Todd's paralysis
What is etiology of seizure based on investigation?	Neurocysticercosis
Do we need long-term AED	Yes
Is the etiology treatable?	In this case, yes. Cysticidal treatment has proved beneficial role
How long to give AED?	AEDs need to be continued till resolution of lesion or 2-year seizure freedom following calcification

AED, antiepileptic drug.

INTERACTIVE TOPIC REVIEW

Q. What are common causes of acute seizure in children?

Following are the causes of acute seizure in children:
- Infective cause (neurocysticercosis, tuberculoma, meningoencephalitis, brain abscess)
- Traumatic cause (intracranial bleed due to recent or past head trauma)
- Vascular cause (hemorrhage, infarct)
- Metabolic cause like hypoglycemia, dyselectrolytemia, hypoxic ischemic, inborn errors of metabolism
- Structural cause (congenital malformation)
- Toxic (drug or toxin induced).

Q. What history should be elicited among children presenting with acute seizure?

History is often provided by caregiver or parents. In those presenting with acute seizure, it is essential to elicit history from the person who has witnessed the seizure rather than caregiver alone who might not have witnessed the event.
- Age at onset

- How is prior development of child?
- Is there positive family history of seizure or epilepsy?
- Is this first episode of seizure? If not, what is the frequency of seizure?
- Describe the seizure semiology in detail with emphasis on preceding events (awake, sleep, playing, exercise, following cry), presence of aura (somatosensory, auditory, visual, abdominal), ictal manifestations (motor, sensory, autonomic, cognitive, behavioral), postictal period (postictal dizziness, loss of consciousness, immediate return to normal).
- Does the semiology suggest a nonepileptic event rather than epileptic seizure?
- Which seizure type could you classify after analyzing the seizure semiology (generalized or focal)?
- Is it single seizure type or multiple types of seizures are seen?
- Do the seizure semiology, age at onset, and development give a clue to any specific epilepsy syndrome?
- Are there any obvious provocation factors (head trauma, fever, preceding diarrheal illness)?

Q. What are the common provoked seizures in children and when to think of it?

The provoking factors in children include fever, head trauma, previous central nervous system infection or tumor, hypoglycemia, electrolyte imbalance (hyponatremia, hypernatremia, hypocalcemia), or history of toxic or drug ingestion. A Simple approach to a child presenting with fever and seizure is given n flowchart 1. New terminology of simple febrile seizure plus is to emphasize that those children with otherwise simple febrile seizure but more than one episode behaves more like simple febrile seizure rather than complex febrile seizure in terms of risk of recurrence and future evolution to epilepsy. Among the factors that predict future risk of epilepsy, prolonged seizure (duration >15 min) is the most consistent factor.

Developmentally normal infant especially those on bottle/top feeds who present with an episode of generalized seizure, no postictal loss of consciousness with return to normal activity should be evaluated for hypocalcemic seizure. Children who present with seizure in setting of acute diarrhea and vomiting are more likely to have dyselectrolytemia. Children who have a past history of perinatal brain injury (birth asphyxia) or postnatal brain injury (vascular insult, encephalitic sequelae) are more likely to have convulsive seizure in presence of structural deficits on neuroimaging.

Q. How do we classify acute seizure?

International League Against Epilepsy Task Force has classified seizures as generalized onset and focal-onset seizures. Generalized

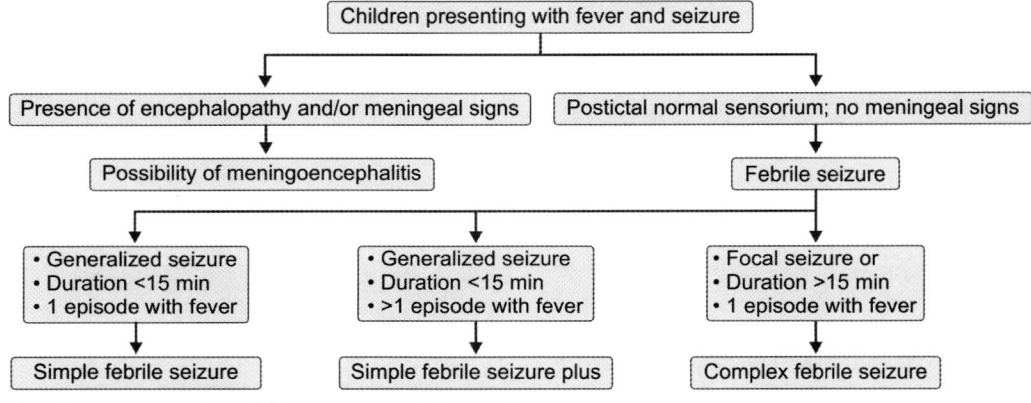

Flowchart 1: Approach to child presenting with fever and seizure

seizure refers to those arising within and rapidly engaging bilateral distributed networks.

Generalized seizures include seizures with tonic, clonic, tonic-clonic, absences (typical, atypical, myoclonic absence, eyelid myoclonia), myoclonic seizures (myoclonic, myoclonic-atonic, myoclonic-tonic), epileptic spasms, and atonic seizures. Focal-onset seizures refer to those that originate within networks limited to one hemisphere characterized by one or more of aura, motor, autonomic, altered awareness (dyscognitive) which may evolve to bilateral convulsive seizure. Earlier terminologies of simple partial seizures (without impairment of consciousness) and complex partial seizures (with impairment of consciousness) have been abandoned by newer ILAE classification.

Epileptic seizure could have variety of clinical symptoms including sensory symptoms, motor symptoms, symptoms of alteration in sensorium, and autonomic symptoms. Hence, based on semiology, seizures have been classified as seizures with aura, autonomic seizures, dialeptic seizures, motor seizures, special seizures (with negative ictal events like atonic, astatic, akinetic, negative myoclonic seizure), and paroxysmal events.

Ictal episodes with alteration in consciousness as the main manifestations are called dialeptic seizures. The consciousness during the seizure is defined in terms of responsiveness (ability to respond to external stimulus during the seizure) and awareness (ability to recall the events occurring during the ictal period). Dialeptic seizures are seen in both generalized and focal-onset epilepsy. However, they are more frequently associated with generalized EEG abnormalities (absence seizures). Dialeptic seizures with less abrupt onset and termination with more prolonged duration (atypical absence) are common among those with Lennox-Gastaut syndrome. In addition, dialeptic seizures can be seen in focal epilepsies like frontal lobe and, temporal lobe epilepsies (associated with automatism).

Motor seizures could have simple or complex motor features. Simple motor seizures include myoclonic, tonic, clonic, versive, and generalized tonic-clonic seizures (Table 2).

TABLE 2: **Types of seizure based on semiology of the event**

Seizure semiology	Seizure type
Muscle jerk of short duration <0.4 s which do not recur in rhythmic fashion	Myoclonic jerks
Sustained contraction of one or more group of muscle lasting >3 s leading to positioning	Tonic seizure
Regular, repeated short contraction of various group of muscles	Clonic seizure
Forced sustained turning of head and eyes to one side	Versive seizure
Sudden reduction of postural tone that result in loss of posture (head drops and falls), often preceded by myoclonic jerk, generalized, affect axial muscle	Atonic seizure
Epileptic falls due to atonic, myoclonic, or tonic seizure	Astatic seizure
Short period of atonia during the muscle contraction	Negative myoclonus
Inability to perform voluntary movement with preserved consciousness	Akinetic seizure
Speech arrest with preserved consciousness	Aphasic seizure

Complex motor features include motor automatism like lip licking, lip smacking, chewing, tooth grinding, swallowing, grimacing, smiling, scratching, and rubbing (temporal or extratemporal lobe). Negative component of seizure could be motor (atonic, astatic, akinetic seizure) or cognition (aphasic seizure). The other seizure type includes gelastic seizure characterized by ictal laughter and hypermotor seizures characterized by bilateral forceful limb movement.

Q. What are the situations when one should think of nonepileptic event rather than a true seizure?

Paroxysmal episode that occurs following an exercise (prolonged QT syndrome or cardiogenic syncope), crying (breath-holding spells), or trivial head trauma (reflex anoxic seizure) are more likely to be nonepileptic. It is essential to know whether these clinical events occur during sleep (nocturnal epilepsy or parasomnias) or awake state.

Paroxysmal events that occur following psychological stressor (school maladjustment, peer bullying, parental quarrels, and separation anxiety) could hint toward psychogenic paroxysmal nonepileptic events. Presence of provoking factors like prolonged standing, crowded place, lack of food, unpleasant circumstances could point to syncope. History of drug ingestion (metoclopramide or prochlorperazine) to rule out a possibility of dystonic reaction, like oculogyric crises, must be elicited.

Q. What are the common seizure mimickers in infants?

The common seizure mimickers in typically developing infants include benign sleep myoclonus, breath-holding spells, shuddering attacks, paroxysmal torticollis, spasmus nutans, gratification, and rhythmic movements of sleep. Rhythmic jerks that affect one or more limbs and facial muscles that occur during early part (nonrapid eye movement) of sleep in otherwise developmentally normal infant is more likely to be benign sleep myoclonus. It is essential to reassure the mother by showing video of another baby with benign sleep myoclonus, as AEDs tend to worsen the condition.

Attacks of generalized muscle stiffness, violent shaking of limbs, apnea, cyanosis, and bradycardia during sleep in infant could be owing to hyperekplexia. A simple bedside test by tapping tip of nose repeatedly will elicit eye blinking and flexor spasm of trunk with no habituation is highly suggestive of hyperekplexia. This attack is often perceived as startle response to parents. This condition often responds dramatically to oral benzodiazepines including clonazepam. Shuddering attacks are paroxysmal movement in which baby trembles with head flexed and arms abducted, it often resembles as if baby is straining on stool or as if cold water has been poured on his back. Gratification consists of dystonic posturing of lower limbs as if trying to stimulate genitals associated with grunting, rocking, and sweating that stops when the child is distracted. Paroxysmal attacks of torticollis with pallor and irritability suggest benign paroxysmal torticollis.

Q. What is the role of developmental and family history in child with acute seizure?

Presence of developmental delay points to the underlying etiology of acute seizure. The possible causes include cerebral palsy, postencephalitic sequelae, neurometabolic disorders, epileptic encephalopathy, neurocutaneous syndromes, and genetic epilepsy. Children with global developmental delay are more likely to have acute seizure when compared to those with isolated motor or language delay. Family history of epilepsy and febrile seizures are essential to understand the genetic basis of epilepsy. Most of early onset epileptic encephalopathy like Dravet syndrome (SCN1A) and West syndrome have genetic basis.

Q. What should we focus on examination in a child with acute seizure?

Initial vital assessment for patency of airway, and adequate breathing should be ensured. Stabilize the peripheral perfusion. General physical examination should focus on presence of neurocutaneous markers like ash leaf macules, shagreen patch (tuberous sclerosis), cutaneous hemangioma (Sturge-Weber syndrome), and café-au-lait macules (neurofibromatosis). It is essential to characterize the facial dysmorphism to depict the possible underlying syndromic diagnosis.

Q. What are steps involved in managing a child with acute seizure?

Flowchart 2 presents the algorithmic approach to acute seizure. Initial stabilization includes maintenance of airway, breathing, and circu-

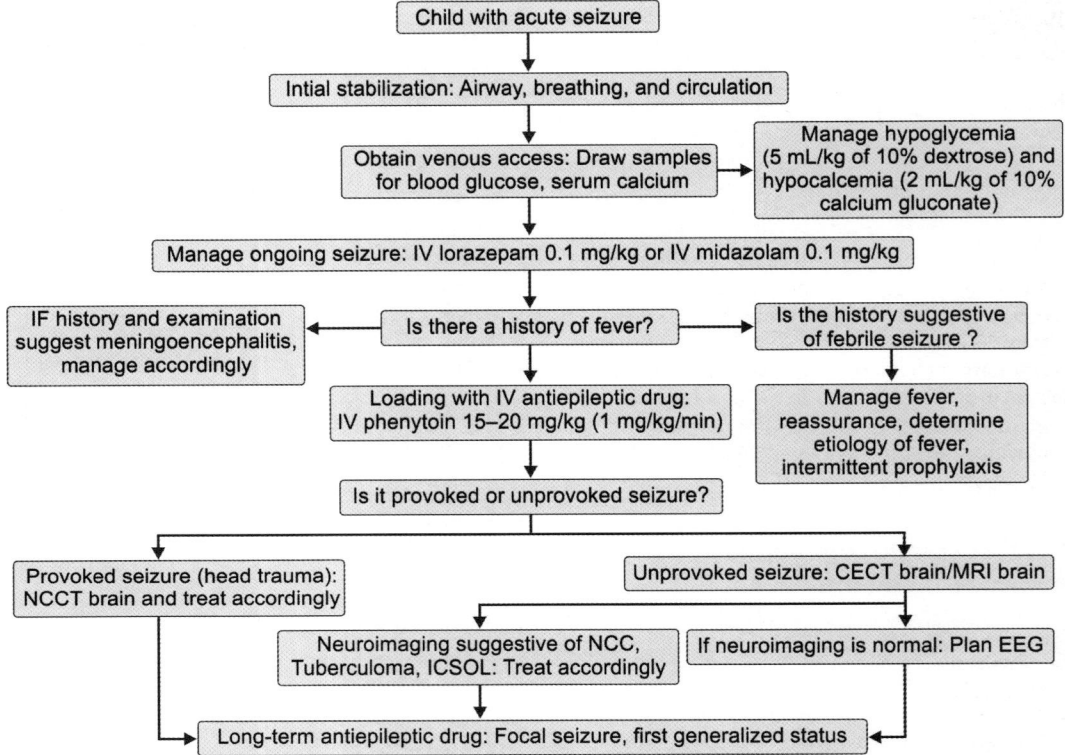

CECT, contrast-enhanced computed tomography; NCCT, noncontrast computed tomography; NCC, neurocysticercosis; ICSOL, intracranial space occupying lesions; EEG, electroencephalography; MRI, magnetic resonance imaging; IV, intravenous.

Flowchart 2: Workup of child with acute seizure

lation. Once the child is hemodynamically stable, abortive measure to stop the ongoing seizure is essential. A venous access needs to be established and samples for blood sugar and serum calcium assessed. Acute abortive drug in hospital setting includes intravenous lorazepam (0.1 mg/kg) or midazolam (0.2 mg/kg). Once the seizures are controlled, detailed history must be elicited to determine provoking factors like fever, head trauma, and dyselectrolytemia. Manage the hypoglycemia, dyselectrolytemia, and febrile seizures as per the protocol. Children with epileptic seizure must be loaded with intravenous AEDs. Indications for neuroimaging and EEG are listed in box 1. Guidelines for AED therapy are given in box 2.

Q. What are essential treatment advice at discharge?

- To continue the prescribed AEDs in doses as explained
- All doses must be measured using a syringe and not to be given by teaspoon
- In case of syrup or suspensions, shake the bottle well before using
- Chrono or sustained-release preparation tablets must not be broken
- To use midazolam nasal spray (0.2 mg/kg) in case of seizure that lasts for more than 3–5 minutes
- To use recovery position while the child is convulsing

BOX 1: Indications of neuroimaging and electroencephalography in acute seizures

Indications for neuroimaging in acute seizure in children
- Children with history of seizure following head trauma
- All children presenting with unprovoked seizure where obvious causes, like febrile seizures, hypoglycemia, and dyselectrolytemia, have been ruled out (perspective of developing country)
- Presence of focal seizure, focal neurological deficit, altered sensorium, status epilepticus, and focal EEG abnormalities

Indications for electroencephalography in acute seizure in children
- All children with unprovoked seizure where obvious causes, like head trauma, febrile seizures, hypoglycemia, and dyselectrolytemia, have been ruled out
- All children with unprovoked seizure with normal neuroimaging where common causes like neurocysticercosis, tuberculoma have been ruled out (perspective of developing country)

Stepwise protocol for investigating a child with acute seizure
- Step 1: Blood glucose and serum calcium
- Step 2: If history of fever and encephalopathy, total leukocyte count and differential leukocyte count, blood culture, and decision for lumbar puncture (manage accordingly)
- Step 3: If there is history of head trauma preceding the acute seizure, noncontrast CT head
- Step 4: In case of unprovoked seizure (focal or generalized), contrast-enhanced CT head to rule out common causes like neurocysticercosis or tuberculoma (manage accordingly)
- Step 5: All unprovoked seizure (focal or generalized) with normal neuroimaging must be subjected to EEG
- Step 6: Magnetic resonance imaging Brain (indications same as step 4) must be planned in nonemergent conditions (can avoid the risk of radiation associated with CT head, but disadvantage includes relatively a long procedure when compared to CT brain and need for sedation/anesthesia)

EEG, electroencephalography; CT, computed tomography.

BOX 2: Guidelines for AED therapy and acute seizures

Indications of loading AEDs among children with acute seizure
- No role of AED in febrile seizure, hypoglycemia, and dyselectrolytemia
- Children with acute seizure following head trauma
- Children with epileptic seizure (focal or generalized)

Indications for long-term AED in children with acute seizure
- Children with acute seizure following head trauma
- Children with first unprovoked generalized seizure need not be started on long-term AED, except in those with status epilepticus or parental anxiety for recurrence
- Children with focal seizure, focal neurological deficit, altered sensorium must be started on long-term AED

Duration of AED among children with acute seizure
- Traumatic brain injury (head trauma): 1 week
- Parenchymal involvement (central nervous system tuberculosis, meningoencephalitis with parenchymal involvement): 3 months
- Neurocysticercosis/tuberculoma: Till resolution of lesion following antihelminthic treatment or 2-year seizure freedom following calcification whichever is applicable
- If semiology, electroencephalography and age at onset suggest epileptic syndrome: Duration of AED will depend on the type of epileptic syndrome

AED, antiepileptic drugs.

- Avoid using spoon, spatula, or wooden objects inside the mouth while the child is convulsing
- Avoid giving anything orally during or after the convulsion
- Do not get panic in case of seizure, bring the child to casualty or emergency room once the seizures have subsided or if ongoing despite use of intranasal midazolam
- If possible, other bystander can record the event in video using a mobile phone; this helps the physician understand the semiology much better than verbal description.

CONCLUSION

Acute seizure, a transient occurrence of signs and/or symptoms due to abnormal excessive or synchronous neuronal activity in brain, may be provoked or unprovoked. Initial stabilization includes maintenance of airway, breathing, and circulation. A venous access needs to be established. Acute abortive drug in hospital setting includes intravenous lorazepam (0.1 mg/kg) or midazolam (0.2 mg/kg). Once the seizures are controlled, detailed history must be elicited to determine provoking factors like fever, head trauma, and dyselectrolytemia. Manage the hypoglycemia, dyselectrolytemia, and febrile seizures as per the protocol.

- After the child is hemodynamically stable, an acute abortive drug (lorazepam or midazolam) needs to be given intravenously
- Management of the hypoglycemia, dyselectrolytemia, and febrile seizures is as per the standard protocol.

LEARNING POINTS

- Acute seizures are defined as transient occurrence of signs and/or symptoms due to abnormal excessive or synchronous neuronal activity in brain
- Provoked seizures include febrile seizure, head trauma, and dyselectrolytemia (hypoglycemia, hypocalcemia, and hyponatremia)
- Unprovoked seizures include neurocysticercosis, tuberculoma, and past neurological insult (ischemic infarct, hypoxic ischemic insult)

SUGGESTED READINGS

1. Duchowny M, Cross JH, Arizimanoglou A. Approach to the child with epilepsy. In: Duchowny M, Cross JH, Arizimanoglou A (Eds). *Pediatric Epilepsy*. New Delhi: Tata McGraw Hill; 2012:1-46.
2. Gulati S, Chakrabarty B, Dubey R, Kaushik JS. Guidelines for diagnosis and management of childhood epilepsy: Expert committee on pediatric epilepsy. Indian Academy of Pediatrics. (Revised and updated) 2014.
3. Panayiotopoulos CP. Epileptic seizure and classification. In: Panayiotopoulos CP (Ed). *A Clinical Guide to Epileptic Syndrome and their Treatment*. London: Springer; 2010:21-61.

Status Epilepticus

CHAPTER 15

BP Karunakara, V Nancy Jeniffer

INTRODUCTION

Status epilepticus (SE) is a medical emergency, requiring an organized and skillful approach to management to minimize the associated mortality and morbidity. A febrile seizure lasting for more than 30 minutes, particularly in a child younger than 3 years of age, is the most common cause of SE. Incidence of childhood convulsive status epilepticus (CSE) in developed countries is approximately 20/1,00,000/year, but will vary depending among others, on socioeconomic and ethnic characteristics of the population. Age is a main determinant of the epidemiology of CSE and even within the pediatric population, there are substantial differences between older and younger children in terms of incidence, etiology, and frequency of prior neurological abnormalities or prior seizures. Incidence is highest during the first year of life, febrile CSE is the single most common cause, around 40% of children will have previous neurological abnormalities and less than 15% will have a prior history of epilepsy.

Children who develop SE are at risk of neuronal injury and consequent morbidities. They are also at risk of respiratory and/or hemodynamic compromise during an attack. Also, most antiepileptic drugs (AEDs) have a cardiac depressive effect. Thus, management includes securing the airway, breathing, circulation (ABC) of the child, termination of the present episode with simultaneous efforts to identify the etiology, prevention of further episodes, and treatment of its complications.

CASE 1

A 2-year-old girl with normal developmental milestones was bought to the emergency room by ambulance during her second seizure of the day. Her first seizure occurred 30 minutes earlier and was described as rhythmic, whole-body jerking with her eyes rolling back in her head and lasting approximately 8 minutes. After the first seizure stopped, she was very sleepy and unarousable. She has now been seizing for 15 minutes. She had history of fever, cough, and cold since 1 day, with no history of vomiting, irritability, or excessive cry. She also has no history of head injury, ear discharge, or rash. However, she had history of previous episode of typical febrile convulsions 6 months back. On examination, child was convulsing, febrile, heart rate (HR) was 160/min, respiratory rate 28/min, blood pressure 100/60 mmHg, plethysmographic pulse oximeter waveform, and general random blood sugar (GRBS) of 80 mg/dL. Pupils were dilated but bilaterally equal and reactive to light. Other systems were within normal limits. She was given intravenous lorazepam which was repeated after 5 minutes again as she continued to convulse following which convulsions stopped. She had irregular respiratory efforts for which she was intubated and given positive pressure ventilation. Electrolytes and serum calcium were within normal limits. Other supportive measures were taken as needed. Intravenous phenytoin sodium 20 mg/kg was given over 20 minutes and child was shifted to intensive care unit. Child was ventilated 12 hours and extubated. She was put on maintenance Intravenous phenytoin sodium 5 mg/kg/day. She had no further convulsions and no neurological deficits. Cerebrospinal fluid analysis was normal.

CASE REVIEW IN A NUTSHELL

Febrile convulsions are the most common cause of SE in children, especially in children less than 3 years old with an incidence of 20/1,00,000 in developed countries.

This child with history of previous episodes of febrile convulsions was now brought with generalized tonic-clonic SE. There has been no gain of consciousness between convulsions for approximately 30 minutes. There is no history suggestive of central nervous system (CNS) infection. General random blood sugar is normal. She is diagnosed to have febrile SE. Her convulsions subsided with two doses of intravenous lorazepam. However, due to respiratory compromise, she was ventilated and started on phenytoin sodium to prevent further convulsions. In febrile children, correction of hyperthermia is also of prime importance to prevent further seizures. Though diagnosis of febrile SE is considered, other causes of symptomatic convulsions and electrolyte abnormalities were ruled out.

Thus, the aims of management are:
- Termination of SE—achieved by giving short-acting benzodiazepines (BZDs)
- Prevention of seizure recurrence by giving long-acting drugs like phenytoin sodium and phenobarbitone
- Management of the precipitating causes—hypoglycemia, treating infection, surgery for space occupying lesions, etc.
- Management of complications—respiratory acidosis, metabolic acidosis, cardiac arrhythmias, electrolyte imbalance, hyperthermia, rhabdomyolysis.

INTERACTIVE TOPIC REVIEW

Q. Define status epilepticus.

Status epilepticus is defined as a continuous convulsion lasting longer than 30 minutes or the occurrence of serial convulsions between which there is no return of baseline consciousness.

A recent defining duration of SE is 5 minutes differing from the classical 30 minutes duration. Animal data suggest that permanent neuronal injury and pharmacoresistance may occur before the traditional definition of 30 minutes of continuous seizure activity have passed, and seizures that last longer than 5 minutes often do not stop spontaneously. Any case bought to the casualty with active convulsions should be considered to be SE and treatment initiated.

This definition is easy to identify CSE, but nonconvulsive status epilepticus (NCSE) requires a high level of suspicion to diagnose and continuous electroencephalographic monitoring. Nonconvulsive status epilepticus is commoner than previously thought.

Status epilepticus lasting more than 60 minutes, despite optimal therapy with first and second line drugs (BZD, phenytoin) are defined as refractory status epilepticus (RSE).

Q. How is status epilepticus classified?

Status epilepticus can be classified by semiology, underlying etiology, and duration.

Classification Based on Semiology

Status epilepticus (CSE) may be classified as generalized (tonic-clonic, absence) or partial (simple, complex, or with secondary generalization) according to semiology. Generalized tonic-clonic seizures predominate in cases of SE.

Types of NCSE include absence SE, simple partial SE, complex partial SE, NCSE with learning difficulties, and NCSE with coma.

Classification Based on Etiology

The etiological classification is helpful in identifying the cause and prognosticating the course of SE.

CHAPTER 15: Status Epilepticus

Acute symptomatic: 26% of SE occurring during an acute illness (an acute CNS insult/acute encephalopathy) such as meningitis, encephalitis, electrolyte disturbance, sepsis, hypoxia, trauma, intoxication.

Remote status epilepticus: 33% of SE occurring without an acute provocation in a patient with a prior history of a CNS insult (chronic encephalopathy), such as CNS malformation, previous traumatic brain injury or insult, chromosomal disorder.

Remote symptomatic with an acute precipitant: 1% of SE occurring with a chronic encephalopathy, but with an acute provocation such as CNS malformation or previous CNS insult with concurrent infection, hypoglycemia, hypocalcemia, or intoxication.

Progressive encephalopathy: 3% of SE occurring with an underlying progressive CNS disorder such as mitochondrial disorders, CNS lipid storage diseases, and amino or organic acidopathies.

Febrile: 22% of SE occurring when only provocation is a febrile illness after excluding a direct CNS infection such as meningitis or encephalitis, in situations with sinusitis, upper respiratory tract infection, and sepsis.

Cryptogenic: 15% (previously idiopathic) of SE occurring in the absence of an acute precipitating CNS insult, systemic metabolic disturbance, or both.

Classification Based on Duration

Stages of status epilepticus:

Stage 1: Early SE—first 30 minutes of SE, treated with BZDs.

Stage 2: Established SE—30 to 120 minutes, treated with phenytoin sodium, phenobarbital, or valproate.

Stage 3: Refractory SE lasting more than 120 minutes and is treated with general anesthesia like propofol, midazolam, or thiopental/pentobarbital.

After 24 hours—super-refractory status epilepticus (SRSE) which has continued or recurred despite therapy with general anesthesia for 24 hours or more.

Q. What is the pathophysiology of status epilepticus in children?

Seizure initiation occur due to imbalance between excitatory and inhibitory neurotransmission as is the case in adults but seizures are more common in the immature brain (children, especially infants) as excitatory synapses mature earlier than inhibitory synapses and stimulation of γ-aminobutyric acid receptors in brain results in depolarization (in young children) rather than hyperpolarization as in adult brain.

Q. What are the principles of antiepileptic drug therapy?

- Drugs with rapid onset of action and that which can be administered rapidly intravenous (like BZDs) should be used initially as first line
- When two or more drugs are required, aim to use drugs with different mechanism of action or those acting at different receptor level
- When combining drugs, additive effect of respiratory depression caused by drugs to be kept in mind, especially combining BZDs and barbiturates. Hence, following BZDs, hydantoins (phenytoin sodium) are used. However, if the child is ventilated, respiratory depression can be tolerated
- Use drugs which cause minimal/no hypotension to maintain cerebral perfusion
- Antiepileptic drug therapy in SE are classified as:
  - First line drugs: Used for immediate control of seizures like BZDs
  - Second line drugs: Prevent recurrences of seizures such as phenytoin sodium, phenobarbitone, and levetiracetam
  - Third line drugs: Used in cases of refractory seizures which are also

neuroprotective agents like midazolam infusion, high dose.
- Add on drugs like topiramate.

Q. What is the first step in the management?

As in any emergency, the ABC approach (Flowchart 1) takes priority.

Q. What are the investigations you would like to prescribe?

- Blood sugars (GRBS), electrolytes (serum sodium, potassium, and chloride), serum calcium (both ionized and total calcium), and serum magnesium
- In febrile children, blood and urine specimens should be obtained for cultures
- Neuroimaging once the patient is stabilized, in appropriate clinical scenario
- Cerebrospinal fluid analysis to be done in patients with suspected CNS infection but raised intracranial pressure/cerebral edema and mass lesion to be excluded
- In children on chronic AED therapy—AED levels to be measured
- Toxic and metabolic screen in suspected cases
- Electroencephalogram to identify NCSE can also be used differentiate seizures from pseudoseizures. The duration of continuous electroencephalographic monitoring should be at least 48 hours in comatose patients to evaluate for nonconvulsive seizures.

Q. Q. What is the protocol for management of status epilepticus?

Flowchart 2 presents such a protocol. Treatment should be initiated along with measures taken to identify the cause of the present episode. Check GRBS; if low, give 2–4 mL/kg of 25% dextrose bolus.

Q. What are the treatments other than antiepileptic drug?

- Correction of precipitating factors: Hypoglycemia, hyponatremia, and hypocalcemia are the first priority. As metabolic disturbances are common in sick children, which can predispose to the seizures, correcting them appropriately not only corrects the abnormalities but also helps in avoiding unnecessary use of AEDs
- Activated charcoal if drug overdosage is considered in a previously epileptic child or in case of accidental consumption of AEDs after stabilization of AEDs
- In febrile children broad spectrum antibiotics, antivirals (acyclovir) to be considered. Injection ceftriaxone 100 mg/kg up to 2 g intravenous if meningitis is suspected (first dose to be given within 1 h). Empiric antimalarials if cerebral malaria suspected.
- Thiamine 100 mg intravenous or intramuscular in a malnourished child to be considered.

Q. What is the management of super-refractory status epilepticus?

The management of SRSE is described in flowchart 3.

Q. What are the drugs used in status epilepticus and their dosages?

The drugs used in status epilepticus and their dosages have been listed in table 1.

```
Airway: Check airway of the child
• If maintainable or not
• Use artificial airway if needed
• Left lateral position the child
• Immobilze cervical spine if trauma suspected
• Start O₂ inhalation
        ↓
Breathing
• Intubate if evidence of ineffective respirations/oxygenation
        ↓
Circulation
• Establish IV access within 30 sec or insert an IO access (all drugs administered through IV can be given IO
• Treat shock if identified
```

Flowchart 1: "ABC (Airway, breathing, and circulation) approach" to initial management in status epilepticus

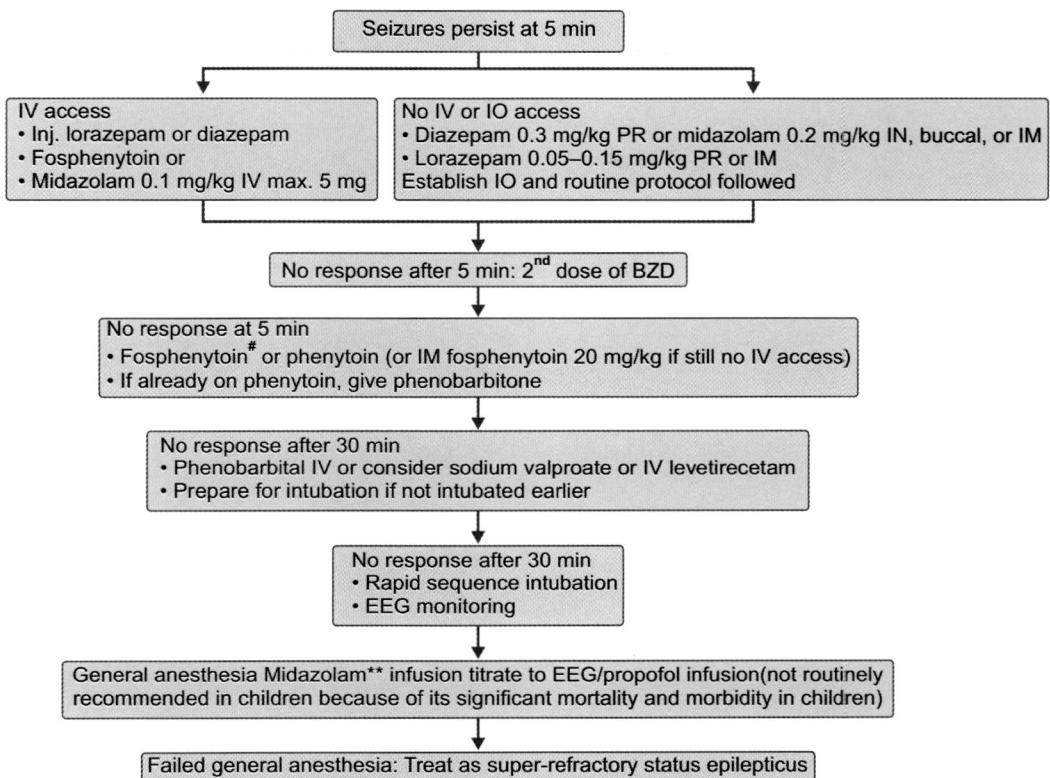

Flowchart 2: Protocol of management

IO, intraosseous; IM, intramuscular; IN, intranasal; BZD, benzodiazepine; EEG, electroencephalogram; SE, status epilepticus; max. maximum.

*(Or sodium valproate 10 mg/kg at 3–5 mg/kg/min if patient is on sodium valproate and subtherapeutic) (IV valproate 1:1 diluted normal saline 20–40 mg/kg over 1–5 min given as continuous infusion at a rate of 5 mg/h).

#Fosphenytoin—20 mg phenytoin equivalents/kg IV at 3 mg/kg/min and intubation should preferably be carried out by using sedative and muscle relaxants (rocuronium is preferred), and an expert caregiver in intubation. The most preferred agent would be thiopental but BZD and narcotic combination are safer.

**Midazolam—titrate Q 15 minutes upwards by 0.05 mg/kg/h till control; max 2 mg/kg/min).

Q. How do we proceed once seizures are controlled? How to wean off from life support systems and continuous infusions?

Once the seizures are controlled and the child remains seizure free for reasonable period of time (at least 24 h), plan to wean off from life support systems and continuous infusions.

In general, maintenance AEDs are given in doses sufficient to maintain therapeutic concentrations during and after weaning of the continuous infusion. Therapeutic concentrations may exceed published target concentrations for many AEDs and dosing should be individualized to achieve seizure control and minimize adverse effects. Gradually taper and stop the infusion medications. Plan the maintenance therapy, further evaluation, and follow-up in consultation with pediatric neurologist.

Ensuring that the child is seizure free, hemodynamically stable, lungs are clear, blood gases and chest X-ray are normal or within acceptable limits, wean off from mechanical

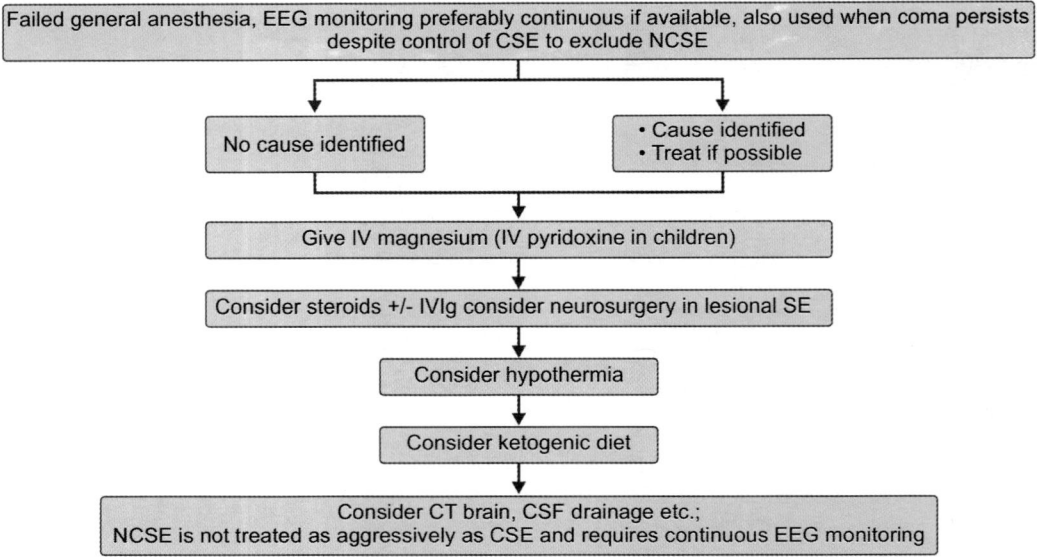

EEG, electroencephalogram; CSE, convulsive status epilepticus; NCSE, nonconvulsive status epilepticus; SE, status epilepticus; CT, computed tomography; CSF, cerebrospinal fluid; IVIg, intravenous immunoglobulin; IV, intravenous.

Flowchart 3: Therapeutic approach to super-refractory status epilepticus

TABLE 1: Medications used in status epilepticus and their dosages

Drugs and route	Dose	Maximum	Rate	Frequency	Complications	Special mentions
Lorazepam (IV, SL, IO)	0.1 mg/kg	4 mg	<2 mg/min	Q 10 min twice can be given	Respiratory depression, hypotension	Must be refrigerated and diluted before administration
Midazolam (IV, buccal, nasal)	0.1–0.2 mg/kg	5 mg	<2 mg/min	Q 5–10 min	Respiratory depression, hypotension	IV preparation can be given buccal
Diazepam (IV, IO)	0.3 mg/kg	10 mg	<2 mg/min	Q 5 min thrice can be given	Respiratory depression, hypotension	Administer as close to vein as possible without dilution
Diazepam (PR)	0.5 mg	10 mg	–	Q 5–10 min	Respiratory depression, hypotension	Use undiluted IV preparation
Phenytoin (IV, IO)	20 mg/kg	1,000 mg (30 mg/kg)	1 mg/kg/min	May give another 5 mg if required	Hypotension, arrhythmia	Given in nonglucose containing solution

Continued

Continued

Drugs and route	Dose	Maximum	Rate	Frequency	Complications	Special mentions
Fosphenytoin (Prodrug)	20 mg phenytoin equivalents 1 phenytoin equivalents = 1.5 fosphenytoin equivalents	–	3 mg/kg/min	May give another 5 mg if required	Advantage of administering the drug at a faster rate, to control seizures, without causing cardiac complications and thrombophlebitis as found with phenytoin	Less toxic when extravasated
Phenobarbital (IV, IO)	20 mg/kg	600 mg (30 mg/kg)	1 mg/kg/min	–	Respiratory depression	Choice in neonates
Valproate	20–40 mg/kg	60 mg/kg	20 mg/kg/min infusion over 20 min	BD dose	Hepatotoxicity	Diluted in normal saline/ringer lactate
Levetiracetam	10–30 mg/kg	30–40 mg/kg	Infusion over 15 min	BD dose	Relatively safe drug	Dilute in normal saline/ringer lactate/5% dextrose

IV, intravenous; IO, intraosseous; SL, sublingual; PR, per rectum; BD, twice a day.

ventilator support and other hemodynamic supports, as tolerated. Monitor patient closely for anticipated problems and unanticipated deteriorations in the transition period. Once patient tolerates the weaning of life support measures, antiepileptic infusions and general condition improves, gradually initiate oral feeds, consider changing medications to oral preparations, and consider rehabilitating as needed, and plan for shifting out of pediatric intensive care unit for further management.

CONCLUSION

Convulsive status epilepticus is more common in children and especially in the infantile period. Febrile SE carries the best prognosis and the causative role of CSE itself on mesial temporal sclerosis and subsequent epilepsy or the influence of age, duration, or treatment on outcome of CSE remains largely unknown.

Nonconvulsive status epilepticus is commoner than previously thought and requires continuous electroencephalographic monitoring.

KEY LEARNING POINTS

- Status epilepticus requires a skilled approach to management, to ensure survival of the patient and to minimize the sequelae associated with it due to respiratory and hemodynamic compromise
- Diagnosis and correction of the cause of convulsions is equally important as is the control of seizures

SUGGESTED READINGS

1. Berg AT, Berkovic SF, Brodie MJ, Buchhalter J, Cross JH, van Emde Boas W, et al. Revised terminology and concepts for organization of seizures and epilepsies: report of the ILAE Commission on Classification and Terminology, 2005-2009. *Epilepsia.* 2010;51:676-685.
2. Meldrum B, Brierley JB. Prolonged epileptic seizures in primates: ischemic cell change and its relation to ictal physiological events. *Arch Neurol.* 1973;28:10-17.
3. Maytal J, Shinnar S, Moshe SL, Alvarez LA. Low morbidity and mortality of status epilepticus in childhood. *Pediatrics.* 1989;83:323-331.

CHAPTER 16

Super-refractory Status Epilepticus

Ramesh Konanki, Lokesh Lingappa

INTRODUCTION

Super-refractory status epilepticus (SRSE) is defined as "status epilepticus (SE) that continues or recurs 24 hours or more after the onset of anesthetic therapy, including those cases where SE recurs on the reduction or withdrawal of anesthesia". It is an uncommon but important clinical problem with high mortality and morbidity rates. More severe the precipitating insult (for instance, in SE after trauma infection or stroke), the more likely is the SE to become super-refractory. Nevertheless, SRSE also occurs frequently in previously healthy patients without obvious cause.

Management of super-refractory epilepsy is a medical challenge.

CASE 1

A 9-year-old girl presented with history of fever which subsided with symptomatic treatment in 2 days. The child was well for next 5 days and then had focal seizures with secondary generalization, with initial seizure lasting for 4–5 minutes followed by unresponsiveness and another seizure after 1 hour.

She was treated by a primary care pediatrician with intravenous lorazepam, 10 mg (child's body weight 20 kg), followed by intravenous phenytoin, 200 mg, over 1 hour. In view of persistence of seizures, valproate (20 mg/kg) was also given; maintenance was continued. For the next 5 days, child was having persistent seizures with unresponsiveness.

In view of persistent seizures, she was referred to our tertiary care center for further management. The child was found to be in a state of unconsciousness, febrile, dyspneic (but maintaining airway and saturations of 98% with 10 L oxygen), and hemodynamically stable.

As seizures were not controlled, she sequentially received intravenous phenytoin, 400 mg (20 mg/kg), intravenous sodium valproate 600 mg (30 mg/kg), and intravenous levetiracetam, 800 mg (40 mg/kg) over next 60 minutes. As seizures were persisting, she was loaded with intravenous phenobarbitone 400 mg (20 mg/kg). Her respirations were shallow and there was an impending respiratory failure, she was intubated and mechanically ventilated. Yet, she continued to have seizures. At this stage, intravenous midazolam infusion was started at a rate of 4 µg/kg/min. The infusion was titrated upwards by 2 µg/kg/min every 3–4 min till a maximum of 30 µg/kg/min over next 45 minutes. The seizures became less frequent at intervals of 10–15 minutes. After about 2 hours of seizure-free period, she started having seizures again; either left or right focal seizures, each lasting for 2–3 minutes.

On examination, the vital parameters were normal on mechanical ventilation. General examination was unremarkable for any neurocutaneous markers, skin rash, lymphadenopathy, etc. Child was stuporous, no cranial nerve palsies, no meningeal signs, and unremarkable systemic examination.

With a provisional diagnosis of meningoencephalitis, the child was started on intravenous ceftriaxone; acyclovir; azithromycin (for suspected atypical organisms); and antiepileptic drugs (AEDs) including sodium valproate, levetiracetam, phenobarbitone were continued.

The evaluation revealed normal complete blood counts, liver and renal function tests, serum electrolytes, blood sugar, lactate, calcium, and magnesium. The computed tomography (CT) of brain (day 1 of admission) was normal.

Cerebrospinal fluid (CSF) analysis on day 3 had shown 40 cells (all lymphocytes), normal sugar, and protein. The CSF culture was sterile, polymerase chain reaction (PCR) for herpes simplex virus (HSV) was negative, anti-N-methyl D-aspartate (NMDA) receptor antibodies were negative. The magnetic resonance imaging (MRI) of brain (on day 5 of admission) had shown symmetric hyperintense signal changes and edema involving both medial hippocampi suggesting possibilities of postictal edema or viral encephalitis (Fig. 1).

The midazolam infusion was continued for 24 hours seizure-free period. The child was also monitored for electrographic seizures and nonconvulsive status epilepticus (NCSE) after starting the midazolam infusion. On tapering of midazolam infusion, child had seizure recurrence for which enteral topiramate was loaded at a dose of 10 mg/kg and maintenance dose (7.5 mg/kg/day) was continued. In view of persisting seizures, intravenous lacosamide was added, in spite of which there was no control of seizures. The child was also started on intravenous methylprednisolone (30 mg/kg/day for five doses) in view of suspected autoimmune phenomenon responsible for refractory status epilepticus (RSE).

Despite being on five AEDs (valproate, levetiracetam, phenobarbital, lacosamide, and topiramate), and methylprednisolone, child was still having 20–30 brief clinical seizures daily, each lasting for 10–30 seconds. The electroencephalogram (EEG) showed frequent electrographic seizures, some of which were not accompanied by clinical seizures (Fig. 2). Throughout this, the child has been encephalopathic (drowsy, not responding to verbal commands, not indicating needs, etc.). Hence, treatment options of intravenous immunoglobulin (IVIG 2 g/kg), cyclophosphamide (monthly), rituximab (4 weekly doses), and ketogenic diet were considered. After discussing with family, one dose of cyclophosphamide was given, along with initiation of ketogenic diet. The daily clinical seizure frequency reduced gradually to 4–5 seizures by day 5 after starting cyclophosphamide, and seizure-free from day 7 onwards. The AEDs and ketogenic diet were continued.

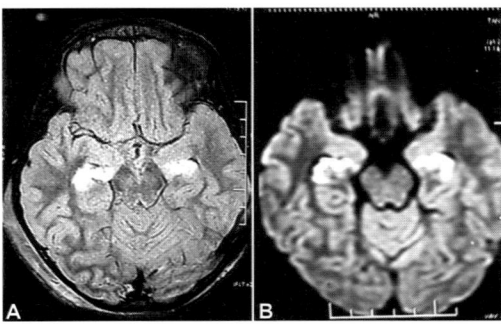

Figure 1: T2-fluid attenuated inversion recovery axial sequence showing hyperintense signal changes involving bilateral medial temporal regions. Diffusion weighted imaging showing areas of restricted diffusion involving bilateral medial temporal regions

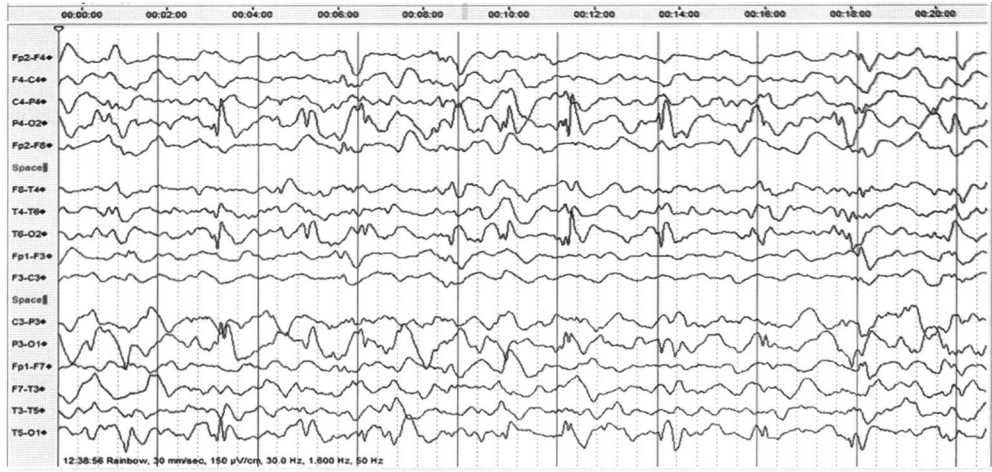

Figure 2: Electroencephalogram showing continuous, generalized sharp-slow wave complexes of 1–2 Hz suggestive of nonconvulsive status epilepticus *(For color version, see Plate 1)*

CASE REVIEW IN A NUTSHELL

This girl, aged 9 years, previously by and large healthy (except for underweight), presented with fever for 2 days, and recurrent seizures 5 days later. Seizures progressed to RSE not controlled even with four AEDs. Her neurological and systemic examination was unremarkable except encephalopathy. With a provisional diagnosis of meningoencephalitis, the child was started on intravenous ceftriaxone, acyclovir, and azithromycin. She was subsequently mechanically ventilated and treated with intravenous midazolam infusion (up to 30 µg/kg/min) without success, necessitating thiopentone infusion. The evaluation revealed normal complete blood counts, liver and renal function tests, serum electrolytes, blood sugar, lactate, calcium, magnesium, and CT of brain. The CSF analysis revealed 40 cells (lymphocytes), normal sugar, and protein; culture was sterile, PCR for HSV was negative, anti-NMDA receptor antibodies were negative. The MRI of brain (on day 5 of admission): symmetric hyperintense signal changes and edema involving both medial hippocampi suggesting possibilities of postictal edema or viral encephalitis. The child was also started on intravenous methylprednisolone (30 mg/kg/day for 5 doses) in view of suspected autoimmune phenomenon. Along with convulsive, child also had NCSE on continuous EEG monitoring. She was then treated with one dose of cyclophosphamide and ketogenic diet was initiated. The daily seizure frequency reduced gradually to 4–5 seizures by day 5 after starting cyclophosphamide, and seizure-free from day 7 onwards.

INTERACTIVE TOPIC REVIEW

Q. What are status epilepticus, refractory status epilepticus and super-refractory status epilepticus?

Status epilepticus

It refers to "a seizure lasting more than 30 minutes or recurrent seizures lasting more than 30 minutes without regaining consciousness in between the seizures".

However, the more practical definition has shortened the time cutoff to 5 minutes, i.e., generalized convulsive SE in children aged more than 5 years refers to seizures lasting more than 5 minutes, or two or more discrete seizures between which there is incomplete recovery of consciousness.[2]

For all practical purposes, all children arriving in the emergency room convulsing are considered to be in.

Refractory status epilepticus

When seizures persist despite the administration of two appropriate anticonvulsants at acceptable doses, with a minimum duration of SE of 60 minutes, it is called "RSE". The RSE may be seen in up to 25% patients and cause significant morbidity and mortality.

Super-refractory status epilepticus

It is defined as SE that continues or recurs 24 hours or more after the onset of anesthetic therapy, including those cases where SE recurs on the reduction or withdrawal of anesthesia.[7]

Q. What is the optimal evaluation in a child presenting with refractory status epilepticus for the first time?

Evaluation: The purpose of investigations include identifying etiology, identifying complications of SE and its treatment, and monitoring the seizure control. Identifying an etiology helps in treating the underlying cause as well as predicting the outcome. The extent of evaluation depends on the age, history, (premorbid development, past history of seizures, febrile seizures, likely cause of seizures, etc.), and physical examination (Table 1). The investigations and treatment should proceed simultaneously. The likelihood of finding a cause is higher in younger children (infections, acute metabolic disturbances, etc.).

Blood investigations like complete blood count, blood sugar, electrolytes, calcium, and magnesium are mandatory in all children with SE. A lumbar puncture should always be considered in a child presenting with fever and SE. Neuroimaging is also mandatory in all cases

TABLE 1: Evaluation of a child presenting with status epilepticus (new-onset cases)

Likely etiology	Investigations	Comments
Acute metabolic disturbances	Blood sugar, electrolytes, serum calcium, magnesium	• Commonest and treatable causes, especially in infants
Infection related causes (febrile seizures and brain infections)	Complete blood counts, blood culture, cerebrospinal fluid analysis and culture	• In infants <1 year, meningitis needs to be ruled out before diagnosing as febrile seizure
Suspected encephalitis or focal lesions (Inflammatory granuloma, focal cortical dysplasia, heterotopias, etc.), and traumatic brain injury	Neuroimaging (CT/MRI)	• CT has limited role for example, in traumatic brain injury, calcified granulomas, and when child is unstable for shifting to MRI • MRI is the preferred modality in majority of the cases
–	Electroencephalogram	• Indicated in all cases of SE; timing depends on the indication (detailed in the text)

CT, computed tomography; MRI, magnetic resonance imaging.

where the etiology of SE is not clear from earlier blood investigations and clinical evaluation. Except in hemodynamically unstable children and following head trauma, MRI is the preferred modality in all cases. Serum AED levels may be considered in known case of epilepsy presenting with breakthrough SE.

Q. What are the causes of refractory status epilepticus?

The common causes for new-onset refractory status epilepticus in children are prolonged febrile seizures (febrile SE) and infections and inflammatory conditions of the central nervous system. Among known cases of epilepsy, the etiologies are slightly different and include previous structural injury, mesial temporal sclerosis, and inborn errors of metabolism (Box 1).

Q. What are the initial drugs for seizures for convulsive status epilepticus in children?

Early identification and rapid treatment is associated with better efficacy of AEDs and better outcome, and longer duration of SE is associated with worse outcomes. The first and second line drugs used in pediatric SE are described below (Table 2).

BOX 1: Causes of new-onset status epilepticus in children

Febrile status epilepticus
- Acute symptomatic causes
  - Bacterial/viral meningitis and encephalitis
  - Autoimmune encephalitis
  - Fever induced refractory epileptic encephalopathy in school-aged children
  - Acute metabolic disturbances of sugar, electrolytes, and calcium
  - Trauma
  - Cerebrovascular accidents
- Remote symptomatic causes
  - Sequelae of perinatal hypoglycemia/hypoxic-ischemic encephalopathy
  - Sequelae of prior traumatic brain injury/central nervous system infection/stroke
  - Structural malformations of brain
  - Mesial temporal sclerosis
  - Inborn errors of metabolism

First line drugs

Benzodiazepines are the first line drugs for seizure control in SE. The preferred medications based on efficacy and side effect profile are: intravenous lorazepam, intravenous midazolam, intravenous diazepam. Other routes of administration in emergency include intramuscular (all benzodiazepines), intranasal (midazolam, lorazepam), and rectal

SECTION 4: Neurology

TABLE 2: Drugs used in pediatric status epilepticus

Drug	Dosage and route of administration	Comments
Midazolam	0.2 mg/kg/dose IV/IM/nasal (maximum 5 mg)	Nasal sprays available (one puff = 500 µg)
Diazepam	0.2–0.3 mg/kg/dose IV/IM/rectal (maximum 10 mg)	IV should be given either as slow injection over 4–5 min or as infusion (cardiorespiratory monitoring is desirable) Separate rectal preparations available (2.5 and 5 mg)
Lorazepam	0.1 mg/kg/dose IV (maximum 4 mg)	Give slowly; respiratory depressant effect; long-acting among the three benzodiazepines used in status epilepticus treatment
Phenytoin	20 mg/kg (maximum 1,000 mg) diluted in normal saline; IV infusion @ 1 mg/kg/min; given at least over 20 min	Cardiac monitoring is mandatory during the infusion; can cause arrhythmias and hypotension
Fosphenytoin	20 mg/kg phenytoin equivalents; IV; can be given at faster rate up to 3 mg/kg/min	Fewer hemodynamic side effects; can be given IM when IV access is not available
Pheno-barbitone	20 mg/kg diluted in normal saline; IV infusion @ 1–1.5 mg/kg/min; given at least over 20 min	Higher risk of respiratory depression and sedation; may be avoided in encephalopathic children if ventilation facilities are not available
Sodium valproate	20–30 mg/kg @ 2–3 mg/kg/minu as IV infusion	Contraindicated in liver disease, thrombocytopenia, and suspected metabolic etiology
Levetiracetam	20–40 mg/kg @ 3–5 mg/kg/min IV infusion	Antiepileptic drug with minimal side effects; higher rates of infusion up to 5 mg/kg/min also well-tolerated
Topiramate	10 mg/kg enteral loading Maintenance 5 mg/kg/day enteral	Hyperpyrexia due to decreased sweating, metabolic acidosis are notable side effects in acute period
Lacosamide	Loading 3–5 mg/kg over 20 min Maintenance 2–10 mg/kg/day IV or enteral	Approved for older children for use in refractory partial epilepsies as add-on therapy Excellent safety profile and bioavailability

IV, intravenous; IM, intramuscular.

(diazepam, midazolam). The risk of respiratory depression increases with higher doses of benzodiazepines.

Second line drugs

Following the benzodiazepines, phenytoin, fosphenytoin (prodrug of phenytoin) and pheno-barbitone are the most commonly used drugs with proven efficacy. More recently, sodium valproate and levetiracetam are being used following phenytoin and/or phenobarbitone, or even earlier in some situations.

The choice of drugs among these depends on the availability and setting. For example, in a setting with no pediatric intensive care unit (PICU) facilities, levetiracetam may be preferred over phenobarbitone as levetiracetam has least respiratory depressant effect. For a presumed febrile SE in an infant, phenobarbitone and levetiracetam may be preferred over phenytoin or valproate.

Levetiracetam

Among the newer drugs, levetiracetam has the best side effect profile. The other advantages with levetiracetam are availability of intravenous preparation that can be used infused at much faster rate compared with other AEDs, and least drug interaction when used as part of polytherapy.

Sodium valproate
It has been used in children failing to respond to benzodiazepine and phenytoin and found to be equal or more effective.

Lacosamide
A broad spectrum antiepileptic drug, it has been primarily approved for use in older children and adults with refractory partial epilepsies. However, the recent studies including case reports and small case series have demonstrated safety and similar efficacy in infants and children. The advantage with lacosamide is the availability of intravenous formulation, thus adding another drug for SE management. The unique mechanism of action (inactivation of slow inactivating voltage-gated sodium channels) is another advantage in management of SE.

Topiramate
It has been found to be useful in refractory epilepsies in infants and children. Oral loading (10 mg/kg) has been used in SE management with reasonable success. Topiramate also has neuroprotective properties, hence being used widely even in neonates with seizures and encephalopathy.

Q. What is "nonconvulsive status epilepticus"?
It is a term used to denote a range of conditions in which electrographic seizure activity is prolonged and results in nonconvulsive clinical symptoms. Patients are considered to have NCSE if they have repetitive or prolonged patterns of continuous spike and wave discharges lasting more than 30 minutes on EEG that have shown a clear change from their baseline (interictal) or an evolution of the EEG pattern. The NCSE may be seen in 20–35% of children who had convulsive SE and is an important predictor of short-term outcomes. More children with RSE have been found to have associated NCSE than children with shorter duration status.

Q. What are the treatment strategies for super-refractory status epilepticus?
The definition of RSE highlights the treatment implications of this emergency. The commonly used definitions are failure of two or three appropriately chosen AEDs to control seizures, or failure to control seizures by 60 minutes from onset. The underlying assumption of both definitions is the fact that the neuronal injury and pharmacoresistance increase with time, and the number of drugs used is a surrogate for time lapsed. A more operational definition of RSE is "persistent electroclinical or electrographic seizures after administration of two appropriate AEDs at acceptable doses". The treatment is said to be successful if all seizure activity is eliminated without recurrence for at least 24 hours. Hence, the goals of managing a case of RSE include cessation of all seizures (electroclinical and electrographic), prevent seizure recurrence, and identify and treat the complications due to RSE or its treatment. The two prerequisites for optimal management of these children are availability of PICU and availability of EEG monitoring facilities. The algorithm for management of SE including RSE is given in (Fig. 3).

Electroencephalography: Utility and indications
The EEG monitoring of a child with SE is the standards of care today. Both the "routine" EEG, i.e., short-duration EEG of 30–60 minutes as well as continuous EEG monitoring are recommended based on the duration of SE and degree of encephalopathy of the child.
- Electroencephalography helps in identifying the focal/generalized nature of SE
- Interictal patterns like periodic lateralizing epileptiform discharges have localizing value and give etiological clues
- Continuous EEG monitoring is the only way to identify NCSE, i.e., electrographic seizures without clinical seizures. Control of both clinical and electrographic seizures is the goal of therapy in such cases
- Electroencephalography monitoring is also needed to monitor the achievement of burst-

Step 1
< 5 min
- IV access: IV midazolam 0.2 mg/kg or IV lorazepam 0.1 mg/kg (maximum 5 mg)
- No IV access: Nasal/buccal midazolam 0.2 mg/kg or rectal diazepam 0.3 mg/kg

Step 2
5–20 min
- Repeat benzodiazepine @ same dose as above and
- IV phenytoin 20 mg/kg over at least 20 min or IV fosphenytoin 30 mg/kg phenytoin equivalents over at least 15 min

Step 3
>20 min
- IV phenobarbitone 20 mg/kg over 20 min or
- IV sodium valproate 30 mg/kg over 15–20 min or
- IV levetiracetam 30–40 mg/kg over 5–15 min
- If seizures persist/recur after this, repeat the same antiepileptic drug at half dose

Step 4
- If pediatric intensive care unit and mechanical ventilation available: Start IV midazolam infusion @ 3–5 µg/kg/min; titrate every 2–3 min by 2 µg/kg/min till seizure control (maximum 30 µg/kg/min) or
- IV thiopentone 3–5 mg/kg bolus; infusion @ 1 mg/kg/h; titrate till seizure control (maximum 10 mg/kg/h)
- Mechanical ventilation not available: Load with one of phenobarbitone/valproate/levetiracetam that was not used in step 3 above or topiramate 10 mg/kg enteral

- After 24 h of electroclinical seizure-free period with/without burst suppression on EEG: Taper midazolam/thiopentone over next 24–36 h
- EEG monitoring throughout step 3 and 4 to identify nonconvulsive status epilepticus

IV, intravenous; EEG, electroencephalography.

Figure 3: Management of status epilepticus in children

suppression pattern, the electrographic target of therapy in children with SRSE
- Electroencephalography also helps to rule out nonepileptic movements including psychogenic nonepileptic events (pseudoseizures).

Hence, continuous EEG monitoring is indicated in all children who have prolonged unconsciousness following clinical seizure cessation (suspected NCSE), and to monitor success of anesthetizing agents in SRSE.

Anesthetizing drugs

The two commonly used drugs are midazolam, thiopentone, high-dose phenobarbitone, and propofol in that order. The drug dosages are given in table 3.
- Anesthetizing drugs should only be used in setting with facilities of PICU, continuous hemodynamic monitoring, ventilation, and EEG monitoring
- Titration of dose should be rapid; not more than 3–5 minutes should lapse before escalating the dose upwards in case of persistence of seizures
- The aim is to suppress both clinical and electrographic seizures. Achievement of burst-suppression pattern on EEG indicated electrographic seizure remission
- After achieving clinical and electrographic seizure remission, maintain the same doses for at least 24 hours seizure-free period, before tapering anesthetizing drugs
- The tapering of anesthetizing drugs should be done over at least 24–48 hours.

The commonly used anesthetizing drugs are midazolam and thiopentone. The major drawback of midazolam is the high rate of recurrence during the tapering. Whereas with thiopentone, major problems are related to drug related side effects like immunosuppression and susceptibility to infections and respiratory depression. There is some evidence that ketamine is safe and effective in up to two-thirds of children.

TABLE 3: Anesthetizing drugs used in refractory status epilepticus and super-refractory status epilepticus

Drug	Dose and administration	Comments
Midazolam	• Loading dose: 0.3–0.4 µg/kg • Start infusion @4–5 µg/kg/min. Escalate the dose by 2 µg/kg/min every 3–5 min till seizure control is achieved. Maximum up to 30 µg/kg/min	• The onset of action is quicker. Maximum dose should be reached within 45–60 min • Major disadvantage is high rate of relapse during tapering or after stopping the infusion
Thiopentone	• Loading dose: 5 mg/kg • Maintenance: Start @1 mg/kg/h; escalate every 5 min by 0.5 mg/kg/h; maximum up to 10 mg/kg/h	• Pediatric intensive care unit and ventilation facilities are mandatory • Higher rates of respiratory depression and hypotension • Increased risk of nosocomial infections due to immunosuppressant effects
Phenobarbitone	• 20–30 mg/kg/day (high dose)	• Similar side effects as thiopentone
Propofol	• Loading dose: 1–2 mg/kg • Maintenance: Start @1 mg/kg/h • Escalate up to 10–15 mg/kg/h	• Quicker onset of action • Higher risk of propofol infusion syndrome, especially when used with corticosteroids, ketogenic diet • Higher relapse rates on withdrawal
Ketamine	• Loading dose: 1 mg/kg intravenous; infusion @5–10 µg/kg/min; titrate up to 60 µg/kg/min	• Should be given with midazolam to prevent emergent reactions

Immunomodulatory therapies

Status epilepticus attributed to inflammatory conditions and immune mediated mechanisms may respond to immunomodulatory therapies like high dose corticosteroids, IVIG, and drugs like cyclophosphamide and rituximab. For example, autoimmune conditions associated with SE [anti-NMDA receptor antibody encephalitis, anti-voltage gated potassium channel encephalitis, Hashimoto's encephalopathy] respond well to these therapies either singly or in combination.

Of these, intravenous methylprednisolone and IVIG are the commonly used drugs and well tolerated by children. Among the second line drugs, rituximab has proven efficacy in conditions like anti-NMDA receptor encephalitis,[44] the encephalitis associated with antibodies against the NMDA receptor. However, the limitation is the longer time taken for onset of its effect, i.e., about 6-8 weeks. In contrast, cyclophosphamide has onset of action within a week, but has more side effects on hematological parameters. Hence, depending on the severity of SE and time frame available for seizure control, one should choose the appropriate regimen of immunomodulatory treatments.

Ketogenic diet

The common, proven indications for ketogenic diet are infantile and early-onset epileptic encephalopathies like West syndrome and Lennox-Gastaut syndrome. Among acute conditions, SE associated with inflammatory pathologies like fever induced refractory epileptic encephalopathy in school-aged children, presumed viral encephalitis, and NCSE may be responsive to ketogenic diet.

Surgery

Depending on the nature of pathology (focal or diffuse), the epilepsy surgery may be curative (focal or lobar resection, hemispherectomy) or palliative (corpus callosotomy, functional hemispherectomy). In all children with new-onset SE, efforts should be made to rule out surgically remediable causes like focal cortical dysplasias and heterotopias.

Hypothermia

Therapeutic hypothermia (25–30°C) along with diazepam and general anesthesia has been shown to suppress cerebral electrical activity and of benefit in SE and neuroprotection in patients undergoing cardiac surgery.

CONCLUSION

Status epilepticus must receive early and aggressive treatment for successful outcome. Else, there is a grave risk of its changing over to SRSE with poor outcome. Continuous EEG monitoring is the standard of care when managing children with refractory and SRSE. Combination of therapies (AEDs, anesthetizing drugs, immunomodulatory therapies, and ketogenic diet) may be needed for the best possible outcome in super-refractory epilepsy.

KEY LEARNING POINTS

- Early and aggressive treatment of status epilepticus (SE) is crucial for successful outcome. The longer it takes to control SE, more difficult will it become to control further, and poor will be the outcomes
- Continuous electroencephalography monitoring is the standard of care when managing children with refractory and super-refractory status epilepticus (SRSE)
- Combination of therapies (antiepileptic drugs, anesthetizing drugs, immunomodulatory therapies, and ketogenic diet) may need to be tried for the best outcome in children with SRSE.

SUGGESTED READINGS

1. Novy J, Logroscino G, Rossetti AO. Refractory status epilepticus: a prospective observational study. *Epilepsia.* 2010;51:251-256.
2. Owens J. Medical management of refractory status epilepticus. *Semin Pediatr Neurol.* 2010;17:176-181.
3. Shorvon S, Ferlisi M. The treatment of super-refractory status epilepticus: a critical review of available therapies and a clinical treatment protocol. *Brain J Neurol.* 2011;134: 2802-2818.
4. Yasiry Z, Shorvon SD. The relative effectiveness of five antiepileptic drugs in treatment of benzodiazepine-resistant convulsive status epilepticus: a meta-analysis of published studies. *Seizure.* 2014;23:167-174.

Raised Intracranial Pressure

CHAPTER 17

Rakshay Shetty, Dinesh Chirla

INTRODUCTION

An acutely sick child with altered level of consciousness can present a significant management challenge. Unconsciousness or coma can result from a wide variety of clinical disease processes, both traumatic and nontraumatic, and each has their unique requirements in terms of treatment and management. These children often require invasive ventilation for airway protection, as well as ongoing ventilatory support for the underlying disease process. Majority of these conditions are prone to intracranial hypertension and its presence generally spells poor prognosis. Intractable elevated intracranial pressure (ICP) can lead to death or devastating neurological damage either by reducing cerebral perfusion pressure (CPP) and causing cerebral ischemia or by compressing and causing herniation of the brainstem or other vital structures. Prompt recognition and aggressive management is crucial in order to intervene appropriately.

CASE 1

A 6-year-old previously healthy boy fell through the screen of a third-floor window of an apartment on to concrete below. He was unconscious and was rushed to nearby children's hospital by an auto. On arrival in the emergency room, he was unresponsive to voice and posturing to painful stimulus. Cervical spine immobilization was undertaken with an appropriately sized semi-rigid collar. His initial vital signs were respiratory rate of 23/min, oxygen saturations of 97% in air, a heart rate of 82/min, a blood pressure of 118/64 mmHg, and a Glasgow Coma Scale (GCS) score of 5 (E1/V1/M3). Pupils were reacting sluggishly and breathing pattern was normal.

Oxygen was administered, intravenous (IV) access obtained and blood sent for routine trauma panel (complete blood count, blood group and screen, urea and electrolytes, creatinine, glucose, liver function tests, and also serum amylase). He was intubated with a size 5-cuffed oral endotracheal tube (ETT) using a rapid sequence technique and hyperventilation was initiated. End-tidal carbon dioxide ($ETCO_2$) confirmed correct ETT position. An orogastric tube was also inserted.

The initial chest X-ray and cervical spine plain films were normal. The secondary survey failed to identify other significant injuries. He was placed on a transport ventilator [respiratory rate (RR) 25, tidal volume 8 mL/kg, 5 cm H_2O positive end expiratory pressure] and taken immediately to the radiology department for an urgent head computed tomography (CT). Hyperventilation was continued as a rescue maneuver until a diagnosis was made. He was given 1 g/kg mannitol during the transfer to the CT scanner. The CT scan of the head showed a skull fracture near the vault, effaced basal cisterns, evidence of diffuse axonal injury, and blood in the subarachnoid, subdural, and epidural spaces.

An abdominal and pelvic CT scans was normal. Neurosurgeon was contacted who advised that there was no acute surgical lesion and the child was transferred to pediatric intensive care unit (PICU).

Upon arrival at the PICU, he was connected to volume control mode of ventilation with tidal volume of 8 mL/kg, RR of 30/min and fraction of inspired oxygen of 40%. Child was continued on $ETCO_2$ monitoring with the goal to maintain it between 30 and 40 mmHg and SpO_2 of more than 96%. Right radial arterial line was inserted. Intensivist placed an intraparenchymal ICP pressure transducer in the right frontal region 2 cm lateral to the midline. His initial ICP was 25 mmHg. His CPP was 62 mmHg. Transcranial Doppler was performed to have a gross idea on perfusion and cerebral autoregulation. Since autoregulation was preserved, it was decided to manage the child as per CPP based protocol with the goal to keep CPP above 60 mmHg. A femoral central venous catheter was placed. He remained on infusions of morphine at 20 µg/kg/min, sedated and paralyzed intermittently with lorazepam and rocuronium as required to manage ICP spikes or for fighting the ventilator or coughing and suctioning. Continuous electroencephalogram (EEG) was also arranged on the day of admission to exclude subclinical seizure activity. Continuous rectal temperature monitoring was also initiated and goal was to maintain core body temperature below 37.5°C. Full enteral feeds were established by day 2. He was started on normal saline (NS) maintenance fluid.

His ICU course was complicated by episodes of raised ICP greater than 20 mmHg with drop in CPP below target and seizure-like activity, despite the midazolam infusion and phenytoin. Despite adequate volume resuscitation using NS targeting a central venous pressure of 8–10 mmHg, an infusion of nor epinephrine at 0.1 µg/kg/min was required to maintain a CPP more than 60 mmHg. Normothermia was maintained and mannitol and 3% hypertonic saline (HTS) were given intermittently for spikes in ICP affecting CPP. Serum osmolarity and serum sodium was regularly monitored.

A repeat CT scan was performed on day 2 and day 4. Day 4 CT scan demonstrated hypodense regions in the left frontal and thalamic regions. Eventually, the ICP normalized by day, sedation was weaned and the child was allowed awakening. He was extubated on day 6 and was transferred to the ward next day. He had right-sided weakness and an improving right facial palsy at the time of the transfer.

CASE REVIEW IN A NUTSHELL

This case highlights the importance of neuromonitoring in identifying and managing raised ICP in a child with severe traumatic brain injury (TBI). Advances in neuromonitoring have facilitated in better understanding of neurophysiology and appropriate application of interventions. Role of neuromonitoring has been more clearly defined for TBI. Though raised ICP is also seen in other types of brain injuries like encephalitis, hypoxic–ischemic injury, metabolic encephalopathies, stroke and intracerebral bleed, role of neuromonitoring have not been clearly established. However, recent reports suggest that neuromonitoring particularly ICP monitoring might be beneficial in central nervous system (CNS) infections and also in certain metabolic encephalopathies. Understanding of the interplay between cerebral blood flow (CBF), cerebral metabolism, cerebral autoregulation and ICP is crucial for effective implementation of neurointerventions.

INTERACTIVE TOPIC REVIEW

Q. What are the initial management steps for a child with neurological emergencies?

- Establish airway and give high flow oxygen by mask
- Measure blood pressure and resuscitate with NS/inotropes if low; do not reduce immediately if high
- Perform blood sugar testing and give dextrose if low
- Assess level of consciousness using the modified GCS (Table 1)
- Assess brainstem function and decide whether the patient has evidence of central or uncal herniation
- Lift the eyelids and look for tonic deviation of the eyes or nystagmus
- Examine the fundi for papilledema (rarely seen in acute encephalopathy; absence does not exclude intracranial hypertension),

CHAPTER 17: Raised Intracranial Pressure

TABLE 1: Modified Glasgow Coma Scale

Score	Infants	Children <4 years	Age 4–14 years
Eye opening			
4	Spontaneous	Spontaneous	Spontaneous
3	To speech	To speech	To verbal command
2	To pain	To pain	To pain
1	No response	None	None
Verbal response			
5	Coos, babbles	Oriented-social smile, follows objects, converses	Oriented
4	Irritable cry	Confused, disoriented, aware of environment, consolable cries	Disoriented
3	Cries to pain	Inappropriate words, inconsolable persistent cries	Inappropriate words
2	Moans to pain	Inappropriate sounds, agitated, restless, inconsolable	Incomprehensible
1	No response	No response	No response
Motor response			
6	Normal spontaneous movement	Normal spontaneous movement	Obeys verbal command
5	Withdraws to touch	Localizes pain	Localizes to painful stimuli
4	Withdraws to pain	Withdraws to pain	Withdrawal
3	Abnormal flexion	Abnormal flexion	Abnormal flexion (decorticate)
2	Abnormal extension	Abnormal extension	Extension (decerebrate)
1	No response	No response	No response.

retinal hemorrhages, and macular star suggestive of hypertension
- If modified GCS is less than 8 or there is evidence of herniation, intubate and ventilate
- If modified GCS is between 12 and 14, or intubation is not possible immediately and there is evidence of progressive uncal or central herniation give mannitol 0.25 g/kg
- If there is tonic deviation of the eyes or nystagmus, assume subtle status epilepticus and give a benzodiazepine and/or fosphenytoin.

Q. How do you identify a child with impending herniation?

In conditions with diffuse cerebral edema, herniation of cerebral contents follows a progressive systematic pattern. Due to differences in pressure between the forebrain compartment and the posterior fossa, one (uncal herniation) or both (diencephalic and midbrain or upper pontine herniation syndromes) temporal lobes may herniate through the tentorium. Similarly, if there is a pressure difference between the posterior fossa and the spinal canal, the brain may herniate through the foramen magnum [lower pontine and medullary herniation syndromes (Fig. 1)]. Central or uncal herniation through the tentorium is compatible with intact survival; herniation through the foramen magnum is not. These syndromes, and the changes from one to the next which signify progressive herniation, are recognizable clinically. Serial examination of the posture, response to pain, tone, peripheral reflexes, and plantar response, pupil size and

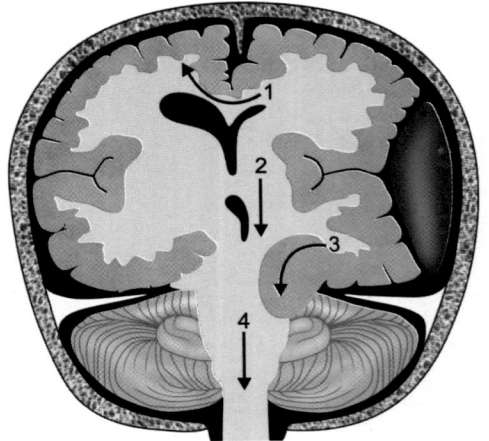

Figure 1: Sites of brain herniation: 1.Subfalcine; 2. Transtentorial; 3. Uncal (transtentorial); 4. Tonsillar

TABLE 2: Details of clinical examination findings of herniation syndromes

Uncal	• Unilateral fixed dilated pupil • Unilateral ptosis • Minimal deviation of eyes on oculocephalic/oculovestibular testing • Hemiparesis
Diencephalic	• Small or midpoint pupils reactive to light • Full deviation of eyes on oculocephalic/oculovestibular testing • Flexor response to pain and/or decorticate posturing • Hypertonia and/or hyperreflexia with extensor plantars • Cheyne-Stokes respiration
Midbrain/upper pontine	• Midpoint pupils, fixed to light • Minimal deviation of eyes on oculocephalic/oculovestibular testing • Extensor response to pain and/or decerebrate posturing • Hyperventilation
Lower pontine	• Midpoint pupils, fixed to light • No response on oculocephalic/oculovestibular testing • No response to pain or flexion of legs only • Flaccidity with extensor plantars • Hyperventilation
Medullary	• Pupils dilated and fixed to light • Slow, irregular, or gasping respiration • Respiratory arrest with adequate cardiac output

response to light and respiratory pattern allows us to identify herniation syndromes (Table 2). It is, however, important to remember that the signs of the diencephalic stage of central herniation may be mimicked by drugs, toxins, encephalitis and metabolic abnormalities, as well as during seizures and in postictal phase. In the acute situation, however, it is always better to assume that central herniation is imminent and take appropriate action, rather than waiting for clear evidence of progression through the stages, which may occur very rapidly. Recovery is extremely unlikely if the patient has reached the lower pontine or medullary stage, so that if children are seen with some or all of the signs, either of uncal herniation or of the diencephalic or mid-brain or upper pontine phases of central herniation, emergency management of presumed raised ICP is mandatory.

Q. What are the indications of intubation?

- GCS more than 8
- Acute increased in ICP needing hyperventilation
- Hypoxia
- Hypercarbia
- Inability to protect airway
- Severe thoracic or airway trauma
- Prior to transport of patient
- Combative patients prior to CT scan.

Q. How to intubate a child with raised ICP?

Rapid sequence intubation should be done in these patients. It is very important to realize that intubating a child with raised ICP is a dangerous procedure. Child can herniate to death if appropriate steps are not followed to decrease noxious stimulus.

Medications chosen should not decrease blood pressure, should lower cerebral metabolic rate, should not increase ICP and provide good analgesia. Medications like lidocaine, thiopentone, etomidate and propofol decrease cerebral metabolic rate and can be used during rapid sequence induction. However, propofol should be avoided in presence of hypotension. Recent studies suggest use of Ketamine in the presence of hypotension, as it has not shown to increase ICP if patient already has raised ICP. Similarly, it is better to avoid usage of depolarizing muscle relaxant drugs like succinyl choline as it can cause acute surge in ICP.

Q. How to manage impending herniation?

Impending herniation is an emergency. If not attended immediately, it can lead to death. Child should be immediately hyperventilated and an osmotic agent like mannitol or HTS should be administered. All correctable aggravating factors like agitation, seizures, fever, hypotension, etc. should address meanwhile and if needed decompression needs to be planned.

Q. What is the pathophysiological basis for the management of a child with raised ICP?

The skull is a rigid container with three key component constituents: (1) brain tissue, (2) cerebral blood and (3) cerebrospinal fluid (CSF). The Monro-Kellie doctrine states that the sum of intracranial volumes is constant and therefore an increase in any one of these compartments must be offset by an equivalent decrease in the other two. Under normal conditions the pressure within the cranial space is in equilibrium. Should pressure from one constituent increase, compensation occurs (up to a point) by reduction in volume of another constituent and a subsequent rise in ICP. This generally involves shifts of CSF and venous blood out of the cranium to compensate for the added volume. Once this compensatory reserve is exhausted, pressure increases and brain shifts may occur and result in herniation. The compliance curve is expressed by plotting

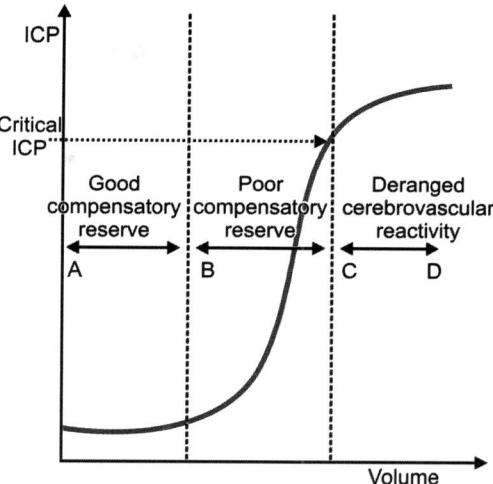

ICP, intracranial pressure.

Figure 2: Intracranial pressure-volume curve: The curve has three parts: (1) A flat part representing good compensatory reserve (A-B), (2) an exponential part representing reduced compensatory reserve (B-C), and (3) a final flat part representing terminal derangement of cerebrovascular responses at high ICP (C-D)

the ICP against an expanding volume. Once the compensatory reserve is exceeded the increase in pressure for a given increase in volume will rise dramatically (Fig. 2). The CPP is the main determinant of CBF. Normally, CBF is coupled to metabolic demand of tissue, with normal flow greater than 50 mL/100 g/min. Less than 20 mL/100 g/min is considered the ischemic threshold. The process of cerebral autoregulation maintains CBF between CPP ranges of approximately 50–150 mmHg in adults. Outside these ranges CBF becomes pressure-dependent. As shown in figure 3, when CPP is less than the lower threshold for autoregulatory compensation, CBF progressively decreases with CPP, resulting in ischemia.

Q. What are neuroprotective measures?

Neuroprotective measures focuses on decreasing cerebral metabolic rate and maintaining appropriate CBF.

Neuroprotective measures followed in our unit for a child with raised ICP is listed here:

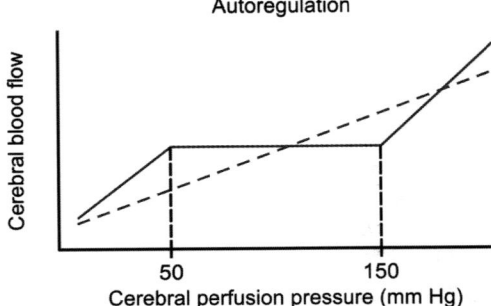

Figure 3: Cerebral autoregulation curve: In the normal relationship (solid line), with cerebral blood flow (CBF) held constant across a wide range of cerebral perfusion pressure (50 ± 150 mmHg). In disease states (e.g., vasospasm, ischemia, intracranial mass lesion), CBF may become pressure passive (dotted line)

- Head in neutral position, with head of bed elevated 30°
- Normovolemia: Isotonic solutions for intravascular volume support (0.9% NS)
- Normotension (age-related norms) for ICP targeted treatment
- Normothermia: 36–36.5°C. Do not cool to less than 36°C
- Analgesia with morphine and sedation with intermittent lorazepam boluses or midazolam infusion
- Arterial line for blood pressure monitoring
- ICP Monitor: Preferably external ventricular drain (EVD), if not intraparenchymal pressure transducer
- EVD transducer positioned 20 cm above the tragus
- Set both transducers for ICP and arterial line at level of the tragus and calculate CPP
- Target CPP more than 40 mmHg for children less than 10 years of age for ICP targeted therapy. For CPP targeted therapy, CPP more than 40 mmHg in infants and more than 60 mmHg in older children
- Use vasopressor infusion to maintain BP: Noradrenaline (norepinephrine)
- Fluids at normal maintenance (maintain normovolemia)
- Normal serum electrolytes: Serum sodium 140–150 mmol/L with HTS
- Avoid free water infusions and rapid changes in serum sodium levels
- Routine blood work: Electrolytes and blood gases every 6 hours for initial 48 hours
- Commence enteral feeding within the first 24 hours
- Repeat head CT routinely after 24–48 hours.

Q. How do I monitor a neurologically injured child?

Monitoring of a neurologically injured child is categorized as below:
- Neurological examination: Pupils, reflexes, muscle tone, new focal deficits
- General systemic monitoring: Arterial blood pressure, heart rate, respiratory rate, body temperature, arterial blood gases, laboratory tests
- Imaging monitoring modalities: CT-scan, magnetic resonance imaging, positron emission tomography scan, cerebral angiography
- Multimodal cerebral monitoring: ICP/CPP, brain tissue oxygen pressure, jugular venous oxygen saturation ($SjvO_2$), oxygen extraction, EEG, evoked potentials, transcranial Doppler flow, microdialysis (lactate/pyruvate/glutamate levels) near-infrared spectroscopy.

Q. What are the indications of ICP monitoring?

Intracranial pressure monitoring is appropriate in infants and children with severe TBI [Glasgow Coma (GCS) score ≤8].

The presence of open fontanels and/or sutures in an infant with severe TBI does not preclude the development of intracranial hypertension or negate the utility of ICP monitoring.

Intracranial pressure monitoring is not routinely indicated in infants and children with mild or moderate head injury. However, a physician may choose to monitor ICP in certain conscious patients with traumatic mass lesions or in patients for whom serial neurologic examination is precluded by sedation, neuromuscular blockade, or anesthesia.

Q. What are the types of ICP monitoring systems available?

Though various hods for ICP monitoring are available, in clinical practice, only the following two are employed:
1. Intraventricular catheter
2. Intraparenchymal catheter tip microtransducer system.

The gold-standard method involves a catheter inserted into the lateral ventricle via a burr hole (right frontal) (Fig. 4).

Q. Is ICP monitoring safe?

The main concerns are the risks of infection, bleeding, device accuracy and drift of measurement over time.

Infection rates have been consistently shown to be low (0.3-1.5%) in pediatric studies investigating both intraparenchymal and intraventricular devices, where devices were left in situ for a median of 3 days. A large adult study found that the infection risk increased after 5 days of insertion to a rate of 5-7% in case of intraventricular drains.

The risk of bleeding has been reported to be up to 4 times higher with intraventricular drains than intraparenchymal devices (17.6% versus 6.5%). In patients at risk of bleeding, e.g., those with fulminant hepatic failure and severe coagulopathy, monitoring could be undertaken from subdural region. Overall, studies have proven ICP monitoring to be safe and accurate.

Q. What is the basis of CPP targeted therapy?

Cerebral perfusion pressure is the difference between mean arterial pressure (MAP) and ICP. It represents the pressure under which the brain is perfused. In the management of patients with cerebral pathology, CPP is generally used as a correlate of global CBF.

Traditionally, management of severe head injury has depended on rigorous control of raised ICP. Early studies in TBI documented improved outcome with aggressive ICP control. However, pathological studies have shown evidence of ischemia in about 90% of patients who died of TBI implicating ischemia as a major cause of unfavorable outcome. Ultra early evaluation of CBF following head injury has documented lowest CBF values during the first 6 hours following injury, with about a third of them having CBF values less than 18 mL/100 g/min, a threshold that represents cerebral ischemia.

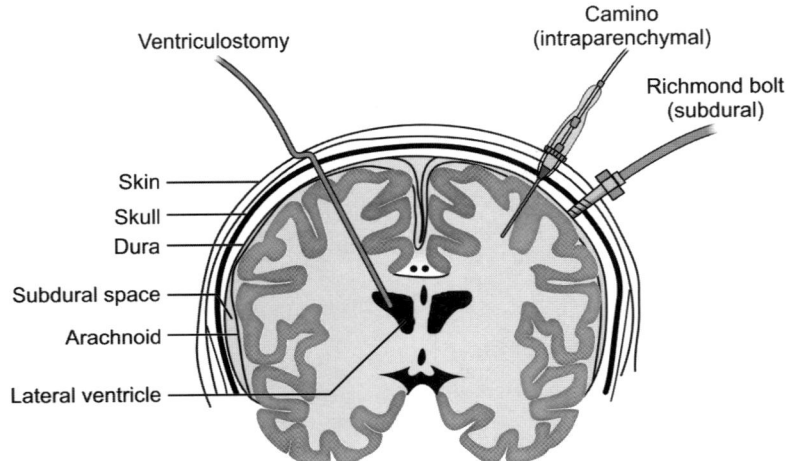

Figure 4: Sites for intracranial pressure monitors: Ventriculostomy allows both intracranial pressure monitoring and therapeutic drainage of cerebrospinal fluid (CSF), subdural and intraparenchymal monitors cannot be used to drain CSF

Cerebral perfusion early after injury has been correlated with the long-term neurological outcome. In studies where episodes of cerebral oxygen desaturation have been monitored by jugular venous oxygen saturation, a good correlation has been found between the number of episodes of cerebral oxygen desaturation and the long-term neurological outcome. In a serial evaluation of CBF in 125 patients monitored by transcranial Doppler, and Xe133, a triphasic CBF response has been noticed with hypoperfusion occurring on the day of injury and a prolonged delayed hypoperfusion from day 4 through day 14. Based on the evidence of the critical role played by cerebral ischemia in causing poor neurological outcome, it has been postulated that maintenance of optimal CBF is necessary to protect the brain from secondary insults.

In normal brain, autoregulation maintains CBF within normal limits over a wide range of CPP. Impairment of autoregulation in a patient with brain injury results in passive increase in CBF when CPP is increased. While this may be one argument in support of CPP-based therapy, the major advantage of CPP therapy seems to lie in its ability to decrease the ICP. According to the hypothesis of vasodilatory cascade, a reduction in CPP–either as a result of an increase in ICP or a decrease in MAP–causes cerebral vasodilation in an attempt to maintain CBF. This normal autoregulatory response increases cerebral blood volume (CBV) and ICP resulting in further reduction of CPP. Thus, a vicious cycle of progressive CPP reduction is set up. An increase in arterial pressure, under these circumstances, increases CPP, causes cerebral vasoconstriction and reduces CBV. The associated decrease of ICP enhances the CPP further, thus setting up a favorable cycle of events that progressively improve the CPP and CBF.

Q. What are the CPP targets in children?

The CPP targets have been well studied in adults. For CPP targeted therapy, CPP between 60 and 70 mmHg seems to provide the best outcomes. CPP higher than 70 mmHg can increase the incidence of acute lung injury and mortality. For ICP targeted therapy, CPP is generally maintained at physiological threshold.

Chambers et al. have suggested age-related CPP targets (0–2 years >40 mmHg, 2–6 years >53 mmHg, 7–10 years >63 mmHg, 11–15 years >66 mmHg, 16 years >70 mmHg) for ICP targeted protocols. For CPP targeted therapy, targets in children have not been clearly defined. We use 50 mmHg for infants and 60 mmHg for other age groups.

Q. Is CPP targeted therapy better than ICP targeted therapy?

In CPP based therapy, higher CPP is targeted as autoregulation is shifted towards right side in the injured brain. This decreased CBV and, hence, reduces ICP. However, in ICP targeted therapy, ICP is the primary target and CPP is maintained above physiological threshold.

Both therapies are useful. Key question is if cerebral autoregulation is preserved or not. As explained above, CPP targeted therapy works only when cerebral autoregulation is preserved. If cerebral autoregulation is absent, high CPP can lead to higher ICP due to pressure passive circulation. However, it makes lots of physiological sense to use CPP based protocol when cerebral autoregulation is preserved and it has shown to improve outcomes as mentioned previously.

Q. How to manage a child with raised ICP if I don't have ICP monitoring facilities?

If ICP monitoring facilities are not available, it might be safer to follow ICP targeted protocol, which aims at maintaining normotension and use of osmotherapy. Child should be observed clinically for early detection of herniation syndromes listed earlier. They would need more frequent neuroimaging like CT head. Using high normal BP like in CPP targeted therapy might be hazardous as it can potentially increase ICP if autoregulation is absent. CPP targeted protocol should not be implemented if ICP monitoring facilities are not available.

Q. Can ICP be measured noninvasively?

Yes. However, they are not as accurate as invasive measurement. Optic nerve sheath diameter measurement (ONSD) holds the most promise. Studies indicate that ONSD more than 5.9 mm was predictive of elevated ICP. Transcranial Doppler has also been used to detect raised ICP; however, there is lack of clarity regarding which parameters to use. Tympanic membrane displacement is another technique that has been studied.

Q. How to manage acute rises in ICP?

Acute surges in ICP need to be approached in systematic manner. It is very important to find out the reason for ICP surge to effectively implement treatment. Acute surge in ICP can occur because of increase in CBV as in agitation, seizures, fever, hypercarbia and hypoxemia. It can also occur due to increase in CSF volume if there is hydrocephalus or due to increase in cerebral edema.

Out of these reasons, osmotherapy will work only for cerebral edema. Increase in blood volume is effectively tackled by hyperventilation and hydrocephalus by CSF drainage (Table 3).

Q. How important is continuous body temperature management?

Continuous core body temperature monitoring is very important in children with brain injury. Hyperthermia increases the cerebral metabolic rate for oxygen and glucose that results in increased CBF and in turn increased CBV and raised ICP. It also potentiates secondary cellular cascade injury. It is associated with a longer length of stay and a poorer neurological state at discharge. Children suffering from an acute neurologic insult need to be maintained at normothermia. A cooling blanket may be employed if warranted.

On the contrary, hypothermia in animal models has turned out to be protective, following a variety of acute neurologic insults. However, no human clinical studies in patients with TBI have demonstrated benefit on long-term outcome, including ac recent international HYP-

TABLE 3: An approach to manage acute surges in intracranial pressure

Step 1	Ensure: The airway is secured, ventilation is appropriate, CO_2 is in normal range The blood pressure is in the normal range The patient is not hyperthermic, agitated and having a seizure.
Step 2	CSF drainage: If ventricular drain is in place if can be opened and allowed to drain for 5 minutes. In some patients if may be necessary to leave the drain open continuously. If this occurs it is important to turn the 3-way stopcock every 10–15 minutes to record the actual ICP. The role of CSF drainage is to reduce the intracranial fluid volume, thereby lowering ICP
Step 3	Mannitol: If opening the extraventricular drain fails to lower the ICP because the CSF is not draining, administer mannitol 0.25–1 g/kg. Maintain normovolemia at all times, and follow electrolytes closely. Discontinue mannitol if hyperthermia develops
Step 4	Hypertonic Saline: If the patient is hyponatremic (Na <135 mmol/L), hypertonic saline should be considered as an alternative to mannitol (1–5 mL/kg 3% saline infused over 10–20 minutes). Avoid large changes in serum sodium and maintain serum osmolality <320 mmol/L
Step 5	Hyperventilation to $PaCO_2$ 30–35 mmHg only during acute resuscitation for raised intracranial pressure or guided by Jugular venous saturation and cerebral flow studies

HIT study. Furthermore, such complications as dyselectrolytemia, arrhythmias, coagulopathy, enhanced infections, etc., may accompany rapid rewarming can further exacerbate the axonal insult that results from TBI. Understandably, as of now, induced hypothermia is best avoided for the management of TBI.

Q. Is HTS better than mannitol as osmotic agent?

Mannitol and HTS are both effective for the control of increased ICP after severe head injury, but have not been shown to improve outcome. HTS is increasingly used rather than mannitol because it remains within the vascular compartment longer than mannitol and so is useful in treating hypovolemic patient. It also has a better reflection co-efficient across the blood-brain barrier (BBB), i.e., it tends to cross the BBB less. HTS can also be used to treat hyponatremia, which untreated can worsen brain edema. Mannitol lowers the ICP 1–5 minutes after IV administration, and its peak effect is at 40 minutes. Mannitol reduces ICP by reducing blood viscosity. CBF is maintained through reflex vasoconstriction and CBV and ICP decrease. Mannitol also reduces ICP by an osmotic effect due to the gradual movement of water from the parenchyma into the circulation. This effect develops more slowly (over 15–30 minutes), persists for up to 6 hours and requires an intact BBB, if not can worsen vasogenic edema.

Q. What are the treatment strategies available for refractory raised ICP?

- Hypothermia
- Lumbar drainage may be considered as an option only in the case of refractory intracranial hypertension with a functioning ventriculostomy, open basal cisterns, and no evidence of a major mass lesion or shift on imaging studies
- Surgical treatment with decompressive craniectomy.

CONCLUSION

Raised ICP is an important contributor to poor outcomes in certain neurological emergencies. Understanding of pathophysiology of raised ICP is very important to apply appropriate neurointervention. ICP monitoring is of great value in children with raised ICP with certain diagnoses and it helps in implementing CPP targeted therapy when autoregulation is intact. Essence of treating a child with raised ICP is to optimize CPP, oxygenation, and metabolic substrate delivery and to avoid cerebral herniation events.

KEY LEARNING POINTS

- Initial resuscitative efforts in the emergency department and ongoing critical care support are aimed at the maintenance of normoxia, normocarbia, normovolemia, and normothermia
- Hypoventilation and hypotension should be identified and corrected early. It is important to avoid free water administration and closely monitor serum sodium
- Routine mild or prophylactic hyperventilation ($PaCO_2$ <35 mmHg) should be avoided. Hyperventilation should be restricted only to children showing signs of cerebral herniation or acute neurologic deterioration
- Mannitol therapy should be reserved for euvolemic children with acute neurological deterioration to allow time for diagnostic investigations or in children with an ICP monitor demonstrating acute elevations in an elevated baseline ICP
- CPP targeted therapy can improve outcomes and should be implemented only if ICP monitoring facilities are available and if child has intact cerebral autoregulation.

SUGGESTED READINGS

1. Adelson PD, Bratton SL, Carney NA, Chesnut RM, du Coudray HE, Goldstein B, et al. Guidelines for the acute medical management of severe traumatic brain injury in infants, children, and adolescents. Chapter 17. Critical pathway for the treatment of established intracranial hypertension in pediatric traumatic brain injury. *Pediatr Crit Care Med.* 2003;4:S65-67.
2. Biros MH, Heegaard W. Prehospital and resuscitative care of the head-injured patient. *Curr Opin Crit Care.* 2001;7:444-449.
3. Bratton SL, Chestnut RM. Brain Trauma Foundation, American Association of Neurological Surgeons, Congress of Neurological Surgeons, Joint Section on Neurotrauma and Critical Care, AANS/CNS, Guidelines for the management of severe traumatic brain injury. VIII. Intracranial pressure thresholds. *J Neurotrauma.* 2007;24:S55-58.
4. Cecil S, Chen PM, Callaway SE, Rowland SM, Adler DE, Chen JW. Traumatic brain injury: advanced multimodal neuromonitoring from theory to clinical practice. *Crit Care Nurse.* 2011;31:25-36.
5. Kirkham FJ. Non-traumatic coma in children. *Arch Dis Child.* 2001;85:303-312.
6. Kochanek PM, Carney N, Adelson PD, Ashwal S, Bell MJ, Bratton S, et al. Guidelines for the acute medical management of severe traumatic brain injury in infants, children, and

adolescents–Second edition. *Pediatr Crit Care Med.* 2012;13:S1-82.
7. Morris KP, Forsyth RJ, Parslow RC, Tasker RC, Hawley CA, UK Pediatric Traumatic Brain Injury Study Group, et al. Intracranial pressure complicating severe traumatic brain injury in children: monitoring and management. *Intensive Care Med.* 2006;32:1606-1612.
8. Smith M. Monitoring intracranial pressure in traumatic brain injury. *Anesth Analg.* 2008;106:240-248.
9. Tameem AB, Krovvidi HR. Cerebral physiology. *Contin Educ Anaesth Crit Care Pain.* 2013;13:113-118.
10. Weintraub D, Williams BJ, Jane J Jr. Decompressive craniectomy in pediatric traumatic brain injury: A review of the literature. *Neuro Rehabilitation.* 2012;30:219-223.

CHAPTER 18

Acute Febrile Encephalopathy

Sheffali Gulati, Harsh Patel

INTRODUCTION

Acute febrile encephalopathy is defined as fever, seizures, and/or altered consciousness. It is a common presentation in children in tropical developing countries. Outcomes range from complete recovery through varying degrees of neurological disability, which slowly resolve or remain permanent to death from either the acute illness or complications. Whilst bacterial meningitis accounts for a proportion of children affected, the etiology in many remains unclear but includes malaria, and probably, viral encephalitis is a neurological emergency. Etiological workup and initial resuscitation and stabilization of a child with acute febrile encephalopathy are simultaneous process. A thorough workup is warranted for determining the etiological condition. Early and prompt management of complications, underlying etiology, and rehabilitative care, impacts the overall prognosis.

CASE 1

A previously well 6-year-old boy presented with fever for 3 days and 4–5 episodes of vomiting on 2nd day of illness for which he visited local doctor and advised symptomatic management. He developed lethargy and increased somnolence since day 3 of illness and had prolonged generalized seizure which lasted for about 30 minutes on morning of 4th day of illness. He was brought to emergency department after 45 minutes of status epilepticus and had decorticated posturing at presentation suggestive of raised intracranial pressure (ICP). His airway was stabilized with rapid sequence intubation and was put on mechanical ventilation and transferred to pediatric intensive care unit.

He was diagnosed as acute encephalitis syndrome (AES) with raised ICP and started on intravenous acyclovir, ceftriaxone, and artesunate. His raised ICP was managed with intravenous sedation (midazolam infusion), head-end elevation, mannitol, and 3% hypertonic saline infusion and maintenance of normotension, normothermia, and electrolytes levels. Artesunate was stopped after negative malaria card test and normal peripheral smear examination.

His cerebrospinal fluid (CSF) showed pleocytosis of 50 cells predominantly lymphocytes with CSF sugar 56 mg/dL (blood sugar 87 mg/dL) and CSF protein was 65 mg/dL. His magnetic resonance imaging (MRI) done on 10th day of illness showed hyperintense signals in fluid attenuated inversion recovery (FLAIR) and T2-weighted images in bilateral thalamus (left is more than right) and bilateral substantia nigra with patchy cortical involvement of left parieto-occipital area. His intravenous acyclovir was stopped after negative herpes simplex virus-polymerase chain reaction (HSV-PCR) and his serum serology for Japanese encephalitis virus was positive. He was ventilated for total 7 days and gradually recovered and remained seizure-free throughout stay.

He was discharged after 22 days of hospital stay in minimal conscious state after parental training of proper nursing care, physiotherapy, tracheotomy care, and feeding.

CHAPTER 18: Acute Febrile Encephalopathy

CASE REVIEW IN A NUTSHELL

This 6-year-old boy presented with acute onset of encephalopathy and status epilepticus following viral prodromal illness of fever and vomiting. This clinical profile is consistent with AES. Resuscitative care in emergency department and subsequent care at intensive care unit of this child underscore the prompt need for recognition and treatment of raised intracranial tension. Child underwent electroencephalography (EEG) on the day of admission to look for nonconvulsive status epilepticus (NCSE) as he was presented soon after convulsive status epilepticus. After stabilization, his CSF study was done which pointed to infective etiology, probably viral causes. Later, his peculiar MRI brain findings had narrowed down differentials to a few and positive serology result had confirmed the diagnosis as Japanese encephalitis (JE).

In the absence of any specific therapy for JE, supportive management was continued which improved survival of patient. Hence, rationale use of available investigations leads us to confirmatory diagnosis in majority cases of acute febrile encephalopathy.

CASE 2

A previously well 18-month-old girl presented with fever and cough for 2 days. On day 3 of illness, she had right focal seizure for 10 minutes. Followed by she developed altered sensorium and abnormal behavior in the form of agitation and episodes of inconsolable cry. The same day she was hospitalized with diagnosis of acute febrile encephalopathy and was given intravenous ceftriaxone, acyclovir, and artesunate. With negative rapid malaria card test and normal peripheral thick and thin smear, artesunate was stopped.

Her CSF study done, 1st day of admission showed 30 cells lymphocytes with 100 red blood cells (a nontraumatic tap). Cerebrospinal fluid sugar was 47 mg/dL (blood sugar 78 mg/dL) and CSF protein was 71 mg/dL.

Her contrast-enhanced computed tomography brain on day 3 of illness was normal. Subsequent an MRI brain scan on next day showed features consistent with focal encephalitis with left fronto-temporal lobe involvement. One week later, the PCR results confirmed herpes simplex type 1 infection. She completed 3 weeks of acyclovir. Her sensorium was improved after day 3 of hospitalization and remained seizure-free throughout stay. After 24 days of hospital stay at discharge, she was in her premorbid state.

During her second admission after a relative asymptomatic period of 4 weeks, she admitted with fever, encephalopathy, and movement disorder. Possibility of parainfectious autoimmune encephalitis would be high in such presentation as repeat MRI brain showed no new lesions and her CSF HSV-PCR was negative ruling out relapse. Hence, her CSF and serum N-methyl D-aspartate (NMDA) antibodies sent and were turned out to be positive. She was given prompt and aggressive immunotherapy and responded well.

Developmental state. She was remained in regular follow-up after discharge and was doing well.

Two months after discharge, she suddenly became encephalitic and readmitted with behavioral change, mutism, and choreoathetoid movements. She had facial dyskinesia and numerous nonpurposeful movements, but no fever or rash. Her MRI brain was repeated, showed no new lesion or demyelination but had gliotic changes in the same left frontotemporal region suggestive of sequelae of previous insult. With acute encephalopathy with marked movement disorder and absence of high grade fever, a possibility of autoimmune encephalitis was kept in backdrop of previous HSV encephalitis. Her CSF and serum NMDA receptor antibody turned out to be positive. She was started on aggressive immunotherapy and received simultaneous intravenous immunoglobulin and intravenous methylprednisolone pulse in standard dosages followed by oral steroids and gradually her encephalopathy improved over 12 weeks after starting immunotherapy, and her dyskinesia subsided with return of normal speech.

CASE REVIEW IN A NUTSHELL

This 18-month-old girl, having fever, focal seizure, and altered sensorium, satisfied criteria for febrile encephalopathy. She was managed on same principles as are highlighted in case 1. Prompt recognition and management of raised ICP and seizures are essential for successful management of a child with acute febrile encephalopathy.

During her second admission after a relative asymptomatic period of 4 weeks, she admitted with fever, encephalopathy, and movement disorder. Possibility of parainfectious autoimmune encephalitis would be high in such presentation as repeat MRI brain showed no new lesions and her CSF HSV-PCR was negative ruling out relapse. Thus, her CSF and serum NMDA antibodies were sent and turned out to be positive. She was given prompt and aggressive immunotherapy and responded well. Autoimmune encephalitis should be thought of inappropriate clinical situations as discussed below due to treatment implications. Tumor vigil is imperative in any child having autoimmune encephalitis.

INTERACTIVE TOPIC REVIEW

Q. What is acute encephalitis syndrome?

Acute encephalitis syndrome is a term used by World Health Organization for syndromic surveillance in the context of JE which is a broad term, which not only includes viral infective causes but other bacterial etiology, demyelination syndromes, metabolic, and toxic agents.

Encephalopathy

Encephalopathy is a clinical syndrome of altered mental status, manifesting as reduced consciousness or altered behavior mainly due to diffuse disease of brain either affecting its structure or function.

Encephalitis

Encephalitis means an inflammation of the brain parenchyma, presenting as diffuse and/or focal neuropsychological dysfunction. Although it is a pathological diagnosis, but surrogate clinical or imaging markers can be helpful as an evidence of inflammation.

Acute encephalitis syndrome

A case of AES is defined as a person of any age, at any time of year with the acute onset of fever and a change in mental status (including symptoms such as confusion, disorientation, coma, or inability to talk) (not explained by fever alone), and/or new onset of seizures (excluding simple febrile seizures).

Q. What are the salient points in history while assessing a child of suspected acute febrile encephalopathy?

Focused history and examination are vital and invaluable tools in the assessment of a child of suspected encephalitis presenting to the emergency.
Salient points in history are as follows:
- Presence of current or recent febrile illness with flu-like symptoms or gastrointestinal symptoms
- History of altered behavior or cognition, personality change, or altered consciousness; onset, progression and extent of involvement
- History of new-onset seizures and any focal neurological symptoms
- Any history of rash (e.g., varicella zoster, measles, roseola, *Enterovirus*)
- Any history of similar illness in others in the family or neighborhood (e.g., measles, mumps, influenza)
- Travel history to epidemic area (e.g., arboviral encephalitis, JE, rabies)
- Any history of recent vaccination [e.g., acute disseminated encephalomyelitis (ADEM)] or contact with animals (e.g., rabies)
- Contact with fresh water (e.g., leptospirosis) or exposure to mosquito or tick bites (e.g., cerebral malaria, arboviruses, Lyme disease, tick-borne encephalitis)
- History of factors predisposing for immune suppression (recent intake of steroids, chemotherapy, severe acute malnutrition, measles infection)
- Human immunodeficiency virus risk factors
- History of trauma, any drug ingestion, or toxin exposure
- History of similar episodes in past with or without febrile illness (metabolic causes e.g., organic acidemias, urea cycle disorders, mitochondrial cytopathies, channelopathies, etc.)

Q. What are the salient features on clinical examination while assessing a child with acute febrile encephalopathy?

Careful and detailed clinical examination is an essential part in management of child with acute febrile encephalopathy. A tactful general

CHAPTER 18: Acute Febrile Encephalopathy

physical examination can provide valuable etiological clues. Pallor may indicate cerebral malaria or intracranial bleed. Icterus can be seen in leptospirosis, hepatic encephalopathy, or cerebral malaria. Parotitis and orchitis point toward mumps as etiology. Skin rashes usually indicate meningococcemia, dengue, measles, rickettsial diseases, varicella, arboviral diseases, and enteroviral encephalitis (hand-foot-mouth disease). Petechiae and ecchymosis could be seen in meningococcemia, dengue, and viral hemorrhagic fevers. Injection marks are seen in drug abuse and animal bite marks are seen in rabies or snake bite while insect bites can be seen in arboviruses (eschar mark is characteristic of scrub typhus).

Neurological examination should be focused on following points:
- Assessment of encephalopathy and its severity [Full Outline of UnResponsiveness (FOUR) score or/and modified Glasgow Coma Scale (GCS) (Appendices A and B) are preferable for objectivity and usefulness in decision-making]
- To look for signs of raised ICP and herniation syndromes like altered papillary size and responses, raised blood pressure, bradycardia, altered respiratory pattern, abnormal posture (decorticate or decerebrate), papilledema
- Focal neurological deficits (cranial nerve involvement, hemiparesis, abnormal posturing) and movement disorders including parkinsonism
- Signs for subtle motor seizures—tonic eye deviation, nystagmus, subtle clonic movements of face or fingers, and evidence of prior seizures (tongue bite, injury).

Q. What are the critical steps in management of a child with acute febrile encephalopathy?

Acute encephalitis syndrome is a medical and neurological emergency, requiring immediate life support, control of seizures (if any), proper investigation for identification of cause, and when available, institution of specific therapy. While initial resuscitation and stabilization of a child is the utmost priority, identification of cause (clinical evaluation and investigations) and treatment plans should be carried out simultaneously (Flowchart 1).

The critical steps are as follows:
- Step 1: Rapid assessment and stabilization (securing airway, breathing, circulation, control of seizures, and raised ICP)
- Step 2: Detailed history and focused clinical examination
- Step 3: Investigations (serum, blood, and other body fluids, CSF, MRI (preferable) or CT scan of brain, nasopharyngeal or throat swab)
- Step 4: Empirical treatment (intravenous acyclovir, ceftriaxone, and artesunate injections).

Q. When should we consider lumbar puncture in a patient presented with acute febrile encephalopathy?

All the patients presented with acute febrile encephalopathy should undergo lumbar puncture for CSF examination as soon as they stabilize after ruling out any clinical contraindication (listed below). In a clinical situation, when lumbar puncture is not possible in a given patient at first, the condition should be reviewed every 24 hours and lumbar puncture should be performed at earliest whenever it is safe to do so. If an initial lumbar puncture is nondiagnostic, a second lumbar puncture should be performed 24–48 hours later. Whenever lumbar puncture is contraindicated, a neuroimaging study should be performed. Being invasive procedure, minimum 3–5 mL CSF should be taken during lumbar puncture. Cerebrospinal fluid should be examined for cytology, biochemistry, Gram-stain, Ziehl-Neelsen stain for acid fast bacilli, bacterial culture, latex agglutination, PCR for HSV-1 and -2, immunoglobulin M antibodies for JE and for dengue serology or PCR. Concurrent blood sugar must be measured to look for the CSF to blood sugar ratio. If required later, 1–2 mL CSF should be stored for other additional studies.

Table 1 presents typical CSF fndngs in different infective pathologes.

Clinical contraindications to lumbar puncture are listed below:

SECTION 4: Neurology

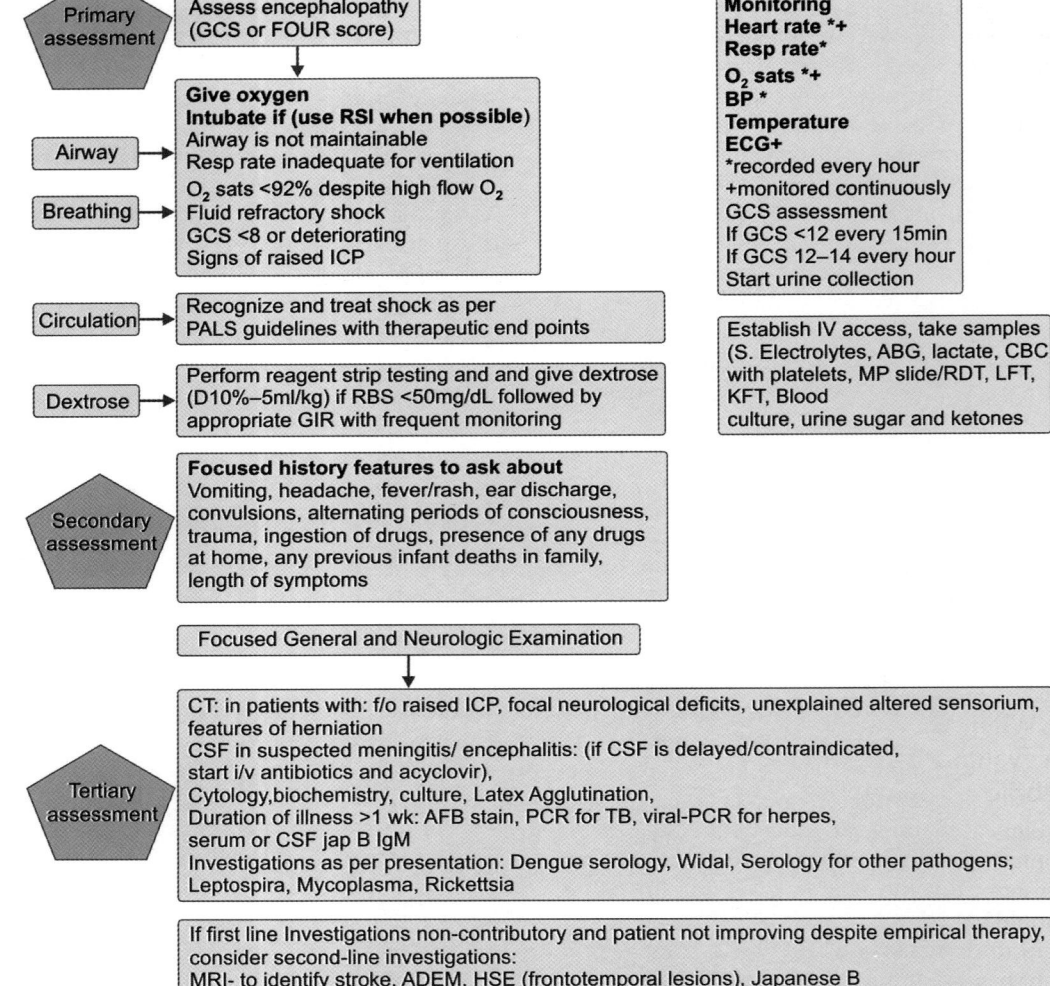

Flowchart 1: Algorithm for the management of a child with acute febrile encephalopathy using pediatric advanced life support format

TABLE 1: Typical cerebrospinal fluid findings in various infective pathologies

Investigation	Normal	Bacterial	Viral	Tubercular	Fungal
Opening pressure	10–20 cm	High	Normal/high	High	High/very high
Color	Clear	Turbid	Clear/cloudy	Cloudy/cob web formation	Clear/cloudy
Cells	<5	50–50,000	5–1,000	Usually <500	0–1,000
Differential count	Lymphocytes	Polymorphs	Lymphocytes	Lymphocytes	Lymphocytes
Cerebrospinal fluid/plasma glucose	50–66%	Low (<40%)	Normal	Low–very low (<30%)	Normal–low
Protein(g/L)	<0.45	High (>1)	Normal–high (0.5–1)	High–very high (1–5)	Normal–high (0.2–5)

- Moderate-to-severe impairment of consciousness (GCS <13) or fall in GCS of >2
- Focal neurological signs (including unequal, dilated, or poorly responsive pupils)
- Abnormal posture or posturing
- Papilledema
- After seizures until stabilized
- Relative bradycardia with hypertension and/or abnormal "doll's eye" movements
- Presence of shock
- Coagulopathy
- Local infection to the site of lumbar puncture.

Q. Where does the neuroimaging stand in evaluation of a child with acute febrile encephalopathy?

If clinical features of raised ICP or any other clinical contraindication to lumbar puncture present, computed tomography (CT) brain should be performed as soon as possible. It may help to detect shift of brain compartments or tight basal cisterns, due to mass lesions and/or focal or diffuse cerebral edema or infarct. A CT brain may help to clinch alternative diagnosis altogether (e.g., tumor, neurocysticercosis, or tuberculoma, etc.). Whenever coagulopathy or thrombocytopenia or intracranial bleed suspected, noncontrast CT brain should be done; barring these conditions, CT scan with contrast is preferable. Neuroimaging provides additional information but it can never be a replacement for CSF study. If CT scan does not show any radiological contraindication to lumbar puncture, it should be done in a given child as soon as possible. If facility available and patient condition permits, MRI brain (with contrast and diffusion weighted images) should be performed as early as possible in all the children with acute febrile encephalopathy, especially when the diagnosis is uncertain. An MRI is more sensitive in detecting the early changes and helpful to identify etiology or alternative diagnosis (e.g., ADEM) in certain circumstances (Table 2).

Q. When should we order an electroencephalogram in a child with acute febrile encephalopathy?

There is no need for EEG in all patients with suspected encephalitis; however, in patients with mildly altered behavior, if it is uncertain whether there is a psychiatric or organic cause, an EEG can be performed to look for encephalopathic changes. An EEG may be very helpful in all the children with acute febrile encephalopathy having subtle motor seizures or after prolonged convulsive status epilepticus to rule out NCSE.

Periodic lateralized epileptiform discharges, once considered pathognomonic EEG changes of HSV encephalitis, they are now recognized in other viral encephalitis and noninfectious conditions, and it is accepted that there are no EEG changes diagnostic of HSV encephalitis.

Q. What is the role of empirical therapy in management of a child with acute febrile encephalopathy?

Empirical therapy should be started without waiting for results. Third-generation cephalosporin ceftriaxone (100 mg/kg/day in two divided

TABLE 2: Typical magnetic resonance imaging findings in various etiology of acute febrile encephalopathy in children

Etiology	Magnetic resonance imaging findings
Herpes simplex virus encephalitis	• Early MRI changes occur in the cingulate gyrus and medial temporal lobe, and include gyral edema on T1-weighted images, and hyperintensity on T2-weighted and T2 fluid attenuated inversion recovery images • Diffusion-weighted MRI may be especially sensitive to early changes • Later there may be hemorrhage better detected by susceptibility weighted images
Japanese B encephalitis	• Abnormal T2 hyperintensity in thalamus and basal ganglia including substantia nigra
Varicella zoster encephalitis	• Immunocompetent children: The most common pathogenesis is a large vessel vasculitis having ischemic or hemorrhagic infarct seen on MRI and angiography. Cerebellitis is also common. • Immunocompromised children: Multifocal leukoencephalopathy is more common
Mycoplasma pneumoniae	• Nonspecific. Focal cortical and deep white matter lesions with areas of demyelination
Enterovirus	• Abnormal signal intensity in the brainstem, especially dorsal pons, medulla, midbrain, and dentate nuclei of the cerebellum and may involve thalami and basal ganglia
Acute disseminated encephalomyelitis	• Diffuse poorly demarcated cerebral white matter lesions (usually large >1–2 cm), deep-gray matter lesions also can be present.

MRI, magnetic resonance imaging.

dosages) or cefotaxime (150–200 mg/kg/day in 2–3 divided dosages) should be adequate. In situations where cephalosporins resistance high or pneumococcal infections suspected, vancomycin should be used as adjuvant therapy. Antibiotic therapy can be later changed to sensitivity pattern or can be stopped if no evidence of bacterial meningitis is forthcoming.

All the children with acute febrile encephalopathy should be given IV acyclovir if viral encephalitis is suspected. It can be stopped if alternative diagnosis is made or HSV PCR negative and MRI normal. In scenarios where possibility of HSV is very high, IV acyclovir can be continued for till repeat CSF results or MRI available or can be given full course.

Empirical antimalarial (artemisinin-based combination therapy) must be started if clinical suspicion of cerebral malaria. It can be stopped if the peripheral smear and rapid diagnostic tests are negative.

TABLE 3: Specific treatment of herpes simplex encephalitis

Birth to 3 months of age	Children >3 months
Intravenous acyclovir • 20 mg/kg TDS for at least 21 days	Intravenous acyclovir • 3 months–12 years: 500 mg/m^2 TDS for 21 days • Over 12 years: 10 mg/kg TDS for 21 days

TDS, three times daily.

Specific treatment of herpes simplex encephalitis is mentioned in table 3. A child having varicella zoster virus (VZV) encephalitis should be given intravenous acyclovir 15 mg/kg three times daily for 15 days. Varicella zoster virus cerebellitis is a self-limiting condition, so usually does not require any specific treatment and child having stroke due to VZV vasculopathy can be given oral steroids (prednisolone) 2 mg/

kg (up to 80 mg) for 3–5 days in acute period. Pleconaril and intravenous immunoglobulin (IVIg) are having some evidence of beneficial effect in enterovirus encephalitis. Some anecdotal reports suggest the use of IVIg in treatment of Japanese B encephalitis.

Q. What is autoimmune encephalitis? When should we think of it in a child with acute febrile encephalopathy?

In very recent years, autoimmune encephalitis has emerged as potentially treatable neurological disorder with discovery of new neuronal surface and antineuronal antibodies. Moreover, the clinical phenotypes of these recently described disorders are still expanding; at times, it is difficult to differentiate them from other causes of acute febrile encephalopathy.

Acute encephalitis should be strongly suspected in a given child if he or she presents with
- Acute or subacute (<12 weeks) onset of symptoms (subacute is more common)
- Evidence of central nervous system (CNS) inflammation (at least one of following):
  ○ Cerebrospinal fluid (lymphocytic pleocytosis, CSF-specific oligoclonal bands or elevated immunoglobulin G index)
  ○ Magnetic resonance imaging features suggestive of autoimmune encephalitis (e.g., mediotemporal lobes FLAIR/T2 hyperintensities in case of a limbic encephalitis-like syndrome; or enhancement of cerebellar sulci, basal ganglia, or subcortical white matter) or
  ○ Functional imaging (hypermetabolism on fluorodeoxyglucose-positron emission tomography or hyperperfusion on single-photon emission computed tomography in the acute-subacute phase)
  ○ Inflammatory neuropathology (lymphocytic infiltrates or other signs of immune activation) on brain biopsy.

History of other antibody mediated disorders (e.g., myasthenia gravis), organ-specific autoimmunity, connective tissue disorders, preceding infections, febrile illness, or viral disease-like prodromes provide supportive evidence for autoimmune pathophysiology in a given child. Other potential causes of encephalopathy (e.g., relevant infective etiology, trauma, toxic, metabolic, tumors, demyelinating, or histories of previous CNS disease) should be ruled out before embarking upon diagnosis of acute autoimmune encephalitis.

Apart from supportive therapy, immunotherapy is backbone of treatment of autoimmune encephalitis. There is no clear guideline for immunotherapy due to lack of good quality evidence. Majority centers worldwide are using intravenous methylprednisolone pulse (30 mg/kg/day for 5 doses) along with either IVIg 2 g/kg/day (over 3–5 days) or plasmapheresis (3–5 cycles daily or alternate days) as a first line immunotherapy. After completion of first line immunotherapy, if there is no improvement or clinical deterioration, second line immunotherapy agents like intravenous rituximab or intravenous cyclophosphamide can be used. Usually, these patients may take few weeks to months for significant recovery. Most of them require long-term immunosuppressive therapy as oral steroids or steroid-sparing agents like azathioprine, mycophenolate mofetil, methotrexate. In view of strong association of autoimmune encephalitis with neoplasm, a comprehensive tumor screening should be done at first attack and should be continued annually or at specific intervals during follow-up of these patients.

Salient clinical features of established antibody associated autoimmune encephalitis more commonly seen in pediatric age group are discussed in table 4. Paraneoplastic syndromes are also having autoimmune pathophysiology and are commonly associated with antineuronal antibodies (e.g., anti-Hu, anti-Ri, anti-Ma2, amphiphysin, etc.) which are not so common in pediatric population.

TABLE 4: Established antibody associated autoimmune encephalitis syndrome

Antigen	Age	Clinical features	Cerebrospinal fluid findings	Magnetic resonance imaging findings	Tumor association	Disease course
NMDA receptor	Infancy–elderly, frequently 2–40 years	Multistage corticosubcortical encephalopathy having behavioral disturbance, psychosis, catatonia, seizures, aphasia, movement disorders including orolingual dyskinesias, central hypoventilation, dysautonomia	Up to 90% abnormal—CSF lymphocytosis, CSF oligoclonal bands, and elevated protein	Up to 50% abnormal; medial temporal lobe hyperintensity, focal cortical T2-weighted/FLAIR hyperintensity	Ovarian (or other) teratomas in ≤50%	Responds well to early immunotherapies and early tumor removal but nonparaneoplastic cases can be chronic and tend to relapse
Voltage gated potassium channel (leucine-rich glioma inactivated 1 and contactin associated protein-like 2)	Median 60 years but known in pediatric age group also	Faciobrachial dystonic seizures, limbic encephalitis, epilepsy (often tonic seizures), myoclonus, sleep disorders, neuromyotonia	Up to 40% abnormal findings same as NMDA receptor	40–85% medial temporal lobe FLAIR high signal	20–40% (lung, thymus)	Often monophasic without need for continuing immunosuppression but prognosis confounded by tumor when present
Glutamic acid decarboxylase	5–69 years	Temporal lobe epilepsy with mild cognitive involvement, progressive encephalomyelitis with rigidity, stiff person syndrome	Abnormal in up to 60% cases	Same as NMD receptor	Typically nonparaneoplastic	In case reports, immunotherapy led to substantial improvement

FLAIR, fluid-attenuated inversion recovery; NMDA, N-methyl-D-aspartate.

APPENDIX

Appendix A: Modified Glasgow Coma Scale

Category	Score	Response <1 year		Response >1 year
Eye opening	4	Spontaneous		Spontaneous
	3	To shout		To speech
	2	To pain		To pain
	1	None		None
Best motor response	6	Normal movement		Obeys command
	5	Localizes pain		Localizes pain
	4	Flexion withdrawal		Flexion withdrawal
	3	Flexion abnormal (decorticate)		Flexion abnormal (decorticate)
	2	Extension (decerebrate)		Extension (decerebrate)
	1	None		None
Best verbal response		0–23 months	2–5 years	>5 years
	5	Smiles/coos/cries, appropriate	Appropriate words/phrases	Orientated
	4	Cries/screams, consolable	Inappropriate words	Confused response
	3	Irritable/inconsolable	Cries/screams	Inappropriate words
	2	Grunts/agitated	Grunts	Incomprehensible
	1	None	None	None

Note:
- Apply knuckles to sternum and observe arms
- Arouse patient with painful stimulus if necessary

Appendix B: Full Outline of UnResponsiveness score

Category	Response	Score
Eye response	Eyelids open or opened, tracking, or blinking to command	4
	Eyelids open but not tracking	3
	Eyelids closed, opens to loud voice, not tracking	2
	Eyelids closed, opens to pain, not tracking	1
	Eyelids remain closed with pain	0
Motor response	Thumbs up, fist, or peace sign to command	4
	Localizing to pain	3
	Flexion response to pain	2
	Extensor posturing	1
	No response to pain or generalized myoclonus	0
	Status epilepticus	–
Brainstem reflexes	Pupil and corneal reflexes present	4
	One pupil wide and fixed	3
	Pupil or corneal reflexes absent	2
	Pupil and corneal reflexes absent	1
	Absent pupil, corneal and cough reflex	0
Respirations	Not intubated, regular breathing pattern	4
	Not intubated, Cheyne-Stokes breathing pattern	3
	Not intubated, irregular breathing pattern	2
	Breathes above ventilator rate	1
	Breathes at ventilator rate or apnea	0

KEY LEARNING POINTS

- History and physical examination are important tools in the evaluation of a child with acute febrile encephalopathy
- Cerebrospinal fluid study should be considered in all the patients after initial resuscitation and in absence of procedural contraindications
- Computed tomography (CT) scan brain can be where facility available in presence of clinical features of raised intracranial pressure (ICP) or other contraindications to lumbar puncture are present. Magnetic resonance imaging brain is preferred over CT scan and should be considered when patient is stabilized
- Empirical therapy should be given while results are awaited with addition of antimalarial or antiviral agents in appropriate clinical situations
- Early recognition and prompt management of raised ICP and seizures are necessary
- High index of autoimmune encephalitis should be kept in mind while dealing with a child of acute febrile encephalopathy as it has important treatment implications.

CONCLUSION

Acute febrile encephalopathy is a neurological emergency. Etiological workup and initial resuscitation and stabilization of a child with acute febrile encephalopathy are simultaneous process. Cerebrospinal fluid study, brain imaging, and other tests guided by history and physical examination should be offered for exact determination of etiology in a child with acute febrile encephalopathy. Early and prompt management of complications, underlying etiology, and rehabilitative care are important parameters to decide overall prognosis. It is imperative to have high index of suspicion of autoimmune encephalitis while evaluating a child with acute febrile encephalopathy due to important treatment implications.

SUGGESTED READINGS

1. Bowker RP, Stephenson TJ, Baumer HJ. Evidence-based guideline for the management of decreased conscious level. *Arch Dis Child Pract Ed.* 2006;91:Ep115-Ep122.
2. Kirkham FJ. Guidelines for the management of encephalitis in children. *Dev Med Child Neurol.* 2013;55:107-110.
3. Kneen R, Michael BD, Menson E, Mehta B, Easton A, Hemingway C, et al. Management of suspected viral encephalitis in children—Association of British Neurologists and British Paediatric Allergy, Immunology and Infection Group national guidelines. *J Infect.* 2012;64:449-477.
4. Raj D, Gulati S, Lodha R, Status epilepticus. *Indian J Pediatr.* 2011;78:219-226.
5. Sharma S, Mishra D, Aneja S, Kumar R, Jain A, Vashishtha VM, et al. Consensus guidelines on evaluation and management of suspected acute viral encephalitis in children in India. *Indian Pediatr.* 2012;49:897-910.
6. Sharma S, Kochar GS, Sankhyan N, Gulati S. Approach to the child with coma. *Indian J Pediatr.* 2010;77:1279-1287.
7. Vincent A, Bien CG, Irani SR, Waters P. Autoantibodies associated with diseases of the CNS: new developments and future challenges. *Lancet Neurol.* 2011;10:759-72.
8. Wijdicks EF, Balmet WR, Maramattom BV, Manno EM, McClelland RL. Validation of a new coma scale: The FOUR Score. *Ann Neurol.* 2005;58:584-593.

Acute Flaccid Paralysis

CHAPTER 19

Sheffali Gulati, Biswaroop Chakrabarty

INTRODUCTION

Acute flaccid paralysis (AFP) is defined clinically by hypotonic weakness of limbs with variable involvement of sensorium, cranial nerves, respiratory muscles, and sensory and autonomic nervous system.

Although there is no defined time period for evolution of symptoms and signs and their progression to nadir, it is usually mentioned in days to weeks. The reason for this is that by keeping it flexible, chances of missing out epidemiologically relevant cases from the point of view of polio surveillance will be negligible. In addition, it is imperative to correctly diagnose these cases early as a significant proportion responds to immunotherapy, thereby reducing associated morbidity and mortality.

CASE 1

A premorbidly normal, 9-year-old boy presented with progressive weakness of all four limbs for last 1 week and deviation of angle of mouth to right side for 4 days. He had a febrile illness with cough and coryza, lasting for 5 days, 4 weeks back. There was no history of associated fever, pain in the limbs, altered sensorium, other cranial nerve deficit, abnormal sensation, jerky eye movements, or bladder or bowel complaints. His birth and family history were uneventful and he was immunized for age. There was no history of recent immunization, animal bite, exposure to heavy metals or toxins-like organic solvents, acute diarrhea, abdominal pain, discoloration of urine, or tick bite.

On examination, he had tachycardia, normal respiratory rate and rhythm, and normal blood pressures. His anthropometric parameters were within age appropriate limits and there was no evidence of nutritional deficiency on general physical examination. Salient positive findings on nervous system examination were right lower motor neuron facial nerve palsy, flaccid are flexic quadriparesis [lower limb involvement (0–1/5) more than upper limb (3–4/5)] with no diaphragmatic or intercostal muscle weakness and terminal neck rigidity. Rest of the neurological and systemic examinations were within normal limits.

Investigations: AFP reporting was done immediately. Cerebrospinal fluid examination revealed albumin-cytological dissociation in the form of elevated protein (120 mg%) with normal sugar and no pleocytosis. Nerve conduction study (NCS) showed delayed distal motor and sensory latencies and reduced conduction velocities with normal amplitude of sensory and motor nerve action potentials consistent with the diagnosis of acute inflammatory demyelinating polyneuropathy (AIDP). Urine for porphobilinogen was not done as the neuropathy was demyelinating and not axonal.

Treatment: He was given intravenous immunoglobulin (IVIg) 2 g/kg divided over 5 days. Over this 1 week, his illness reached a plateau. His cardiac, respiratory, and autonomic status were regularly monitored with no noted complications. On day 7, at discharge, his tachycardia resolved.

> Outcome: Within next 2 weeks, his power in the limbs improved significantly. By 4 weeks, he became ambulatory with normal upper limb power with some minor residual gait impairment. However, he continued to be hyporeflexic. He was on regular physiotherapy.

CASE REVIEW IN A NUTSHELL

Any AFP case presenting to the hospital is an emergency. It is imperative to know all the common clinical differentials to reach a correct diagnosis as it has treatment complications. As this child was premorbidly normal, the following entities were considered:
- Guillain-Barré syndrome (GBS)
- Acute infectious or parainfectious myelitis
- Botulism
- Diphtheria
- Myositis.

As there was no bladder and bowel involvement, and sensory deficit or a level myelitis was not considered and magnetic resonance imaging (MRI) spine with contrast not done. Nerve conduction study was done and AIDP variant of GBS was diagnosed. In view of no acute diphtheria like illness, absence of palatal palsy and the child being fully immunized, possibility of postdiphtheritic polyneuropathy was unlikely. Although there was facial neuropathy, absence of other cranial nerve involvement and ascending nature of the paralysis, ruled out botulism. Absence of significant pain went against myositis.

It is very important to rule out other causes in history and examination like animal or insect bite, exposure to heavy metals and other toxins, disease states precipitating hypokalemia like acute diarrhea, and metabolic causes like porphyria. This was done appropriately in the current case.

Tachycardia seen in the current case denotes autonomic neuropathy. It is mandatory to monitor these children for development of arrhythmias. The neck rigidity encountered was secondary to meningeal inflammation because of radiculitis seen in AIDP.

Treatment with IVIg was the correct decision as the child was nonambulatory with cranial neuropathy and the disease was in a progressive state. The disease process reached a plateau within 2 weeks of illness.

INTERACTIVE TOPIC REVIEW

Q. What are the anatomical and etiological correlates of a patient with acute flaccid paralysis?

Anatomical and etiological correlates of a patient with AFP have been described in table 1.

TABLE 1: Anatomical and etiological correlates of a patient with acute flaccid paralysis

Anatomical site	Etiology
Anterior horn cell	*Enterovirus* including polio
Dorsal root ganglia	Herpes, rabies
Spinal cord	Acute transverse myelitis, space occupying lesions, vascular events, trauma
Radicles and peripheral nerves	Guillain-Barré syndrome, chronic inflammatory demyelinating polyneuropathy, human immunodeficiency virus infection, diphtheria, rabies, tick bite, borreliosis, heavy metals (lead, arsenic, thallium, gold), chemotherapeutic agents (vinca alkaloids, cisplatin), organic solvents including glue sniffing, critical illness, hypokalemic (acute symptomatic and familial), vitamin B12 deficiency
Neuromuscular junction	Myasthenic crisis, organophosphorus poisoning, drugs (aminoglycoside), botulism, snake envenomation, critical illness
Muscle	Connective tissue disorder, acute infectious myositis

Q. What are the salient steps in the initial management of a child with acute flaccid paralysis?

All cases of AFP should be treated like medical emergency. Initiation of these steps should be ensured even before making a correct etiological diagnosis.
- Cardiovascular monitoring: In view of underlying autonomic dysfunction, these patients are prone to develop arrhythmias. Ideally, electrocardiographic monitoring should be done in all AFP patients
- Respiratory care: Monitoring of respiration to look for rapid breathing, use of accessory muscles, and shallow or paradoxical respiratory efforts should be done regularly. Initiation of assisted respiratory support at the correct time is crucial for positive outcome in these patients
- Hypokalemia and snakebite, should be ruled because of treatment implications
- Ruling out underlying spinal cord lesion: Early ruling out of spinal cord disease is mandatory to facilitate immobilization, administration of corticosteroids, and neurosurgical intervention in the patient whenever indicated
- Monitoring for bulbar weakness: Bulbar dysfunction in the form of pooling of secretions, weak cough, nasal regurgitation, and intonation should be regularly checked. Nasogastric feeding considered wherever appropriate.

Q. What is the epidemiological relevance of a case of acute flaccid paralysis?

Acute flaccid paralysis surveillance is the cornerstone of the global polio eradication initiative, resolved by the World Health Organization (WHO) in 1988. In that regard, AFP is defined as a paralytic illness in children less than 15 years of age or any age when polio is suspected. It is mandatory to report all AFP cases to the WHO in patients less than 15 years of age and all these cases should be investigated within 48 hours of reporting. Two stool samples at 24–48 hours apart intervals should be collected, transported, and tested for poliovirus at WHO accredited laboratories. Then they are followed till 60 days to look for any residual paralysis. The sensitivity of AFP reporting is objectively defined by the proportion of:
- Cases with both the stool samples collected within 2 weeks after onset of paralysis (ideally >80%)
- Nonpolio AFP cases in children less than 15 years of age (at least 1/100,000 children in 1 year).

In India, the National Polio Surveillance Project was started in 1997 and it has been declared polio-free in January 2014. The last confirmed case of wild type poliomyelitis was reported on 13th January 2011.

Q. What are the clinical pointers toward correct diagnosis in a case of acute flaccid paralysis?

The clinical pointers toward, correct diagnosis in a case of AFP have been described in table 2.

Q. What is the role of laboratory investigations in a patient with acute flaccid paralysis?

Keeping in mind the various etiological possibilities in a patient with AFP, the following investigations should be done on a case-to-case basis:
- Acute flaccid paralysis reporting and surveillance (already discussed)
- Magnetic resonance imaging spine with contrast (to rule out any spinal cord lesion)
- Electrophysiology: NCS in suspected GBS case and repetitive nerve stimulation test in suspected cases of myasthenia (rarely they may present in crisis as AFP)
- Cerebrospinal fluid examination (in GBS, albuminocytological dissociation is documented beyond the 1st week)
- Serum potassium (to rule out hypokalemic states)
- Serum creatinine phosphokinase (if viral myositis is suspected)
- Serum vitamin B12 and peripheral smear (if clinical picture suggestive)

TABLE 2: Clinical pointers toward correct diagnosis

Disease	Progression to nadir	Distribution	Deep tendon reflexes	Sensory involvement	Bladder and bowel involvement	Fever	Systemic features	Etiological clues
Guillain-Barré syndrome	2–4 weeks	Symmetric, ascending, generalized, cranial nerve involvement (commonly 7th), occasionally early respiratory weakness	Absent	May be present	May be seen	Occasional	Meningeal signs may be seen	Preceding prodromal illness or immunization
Acute transverse myelitis	Hours to few days	Symmetric, generalized, respiratory involvement in cervical cord involvement	Absent (in spinal shock phase), brisk below the level of lesion later	Sensory level present	Early	May be seen	Meningeal signs may be seen	Preceding prodromal illness or immunization
Enteroviral illness including polio	Hours to few days	Asymmetric, pure motor involvement with proximal predominance	Absent	Absent	Absent	Present	Meningeal signs, prodromal features	May be precipitated by intramuscular injection
Rabies	2–4 weeks	Symmetric, ascending, generalized	Absent	Present	May be seen	Present	Presence of bite mark	History of animal bite
Postdiphtheritic polyneuropathy	2–4 weeks	Symmetric, descending, generalized, cranial neuropathy (commonly 9th and 10th), occasionally early respiratory weakness	Absent	Present	May be seen	Absent	Cardio-myopathy	Preceding history of fever with bull neck and membranous pharyngitis

Continued

Continued

Disease	Progression to nadir	Distribution	Deep tendon reflexes	Sensory involvement	Bladder and bowel involvement	Fever	Systemic features	Etiological clues
Botulism	Hours to few days	Symmetric, descending, generalized, cranial neuropathy (ocular and bulbar), occasionally early respiratory weakness	Absent	May be seen	Absent	Absent		
Tick bite paralysis	2–4 weeks	Symmetric, generalized, cranial neuropathy (ocular)	Absent	Absent	Absent	Absent	Bite mark	Travel to tick endemic areas
Viral myositis	Hours to few days	Symmetric, generalized, tender muscles	Normal or reduced	Absent	Absent	Present		Features of nonspecific viral illness
Hypokalemic periodic paralysis	Hours to few days	Symmetric, proximal predominance with early neck flexor and respiratory weakness	Absent	Absent	Absent	Absent		Temporal relation to postprandial state or physical exertion

- Urine for porphobilinogen (in suspected porphyria cases)
- Urine and serum toxicology screen (if there are clues to heavy metal toxicity)
- Lyme's serology (for treatment related implications).

Q. What are the essential steps in the management of a child with acute flaccid paralysis?

The key components in management are:
- Initial emergency management and stabilization (already discussed)
- Definitive therapy:
  - Intravenous immunoglobulin (2 g/kg/day, divided over 4–5 days) is indicated in GBS and myasthenic crises
  - Pulse IV methylprednisolone (30 mg/kg/day, maximum 1 g) is given in cases of myelitis
  - Antimicrobials: It is indicated in infectious causes like human immunodeficiency virus and Lyme's disease
  - Anti-snake venom in cases of suspected envenomation
  - Intravenous potassium in cases of hypokalemia
  - Definite treatment for vitamin B12 deficiency, porphyria, and heavy metal toxicity (lead, arsenic), if clinical picture and investigations suggestive
- Supportive care:
  - Physical and occupational therapy: In the acute phase, to prevent development of contractures stretching is advised. If the patient recovers with sequelae, physical and occupational therapy is advised
  - Bladder and bowel care: In cases of persistent urinary retention, clean intermittent catheterization is advised. If constipation sets in, nutritional modifications and laxatives are given. Enema is indicated in nonresponders and those with palpable fecaliths
  - Prevention of pressure sores: Regular change of position in nonambulatory patients should be practised and bed with air-filled mattresses should be used
  - Nutrition: Adequate intake of calorie and protein with appropriate mineral and vitamin supplementation should be ensured
  - Pain management: Pain secondary to neural or meningeal inflammation is treated by drugs such as gabapentin and carbamazepine.

Q. Define Guillain-Barré syndrome.

Guillain-Barré syndrome is a postinfectious disorder of autoimmune origin characterized by peripheral neuropathy (sensory, motor, or both) with or without involvement of autonomic nervous system, respiratory muscles, and cranial nerves.

Q. What proportion of patients have history of antecedent infection and which are the common infections associated with Guillain-Barré syndrome?

Up to two-thirds of patients have history of antecedent infection in the last 3 weeks. The common pathogens are *C. jejuni*, *Cytomegalovirus*, Epstein-Barr virus, *Mycoplasma pneumoniae*, and *Haemophilus influenzae*. Among the vaccines, influenza and hepatitis B are most commonly implicated.

Q. Enumerate the various subtypes of Guillain-Barré syndrome.

On the basis of clinical and electrophysiological findings, GBS has been divided into subtypes:
- Acute inflammatory demyelinating polyneuropathy: This is characterized by demyelinating pattern on NCS (reduced conduction velocity, prolonged distal latencies, and preserved amplitudes of sensory and motor nerves)
- Acute motor axonal neuropathy (AMAN)/acute motor sensory axonal neuropathy (AMSAN) This variant has reduced motor (AMAN) and sensorimotor (AMSAN) action potential amplitudes with preserved conduction velocity and distal latencies

- Miller Fisher variant: This is characterized by the triad of ataxia, ophthalmoplegia, and areflexia
- Miller Fisher variant overlap syndromes: There may be an overlap of cranial neuropathies and limb weakness
- Bickerstaff encephalitis: In this entity, along with cranial neuropathy and limb weakness, altered sensorium is also seen.

Q. Describe the salient steps in the pathogenesis of Guillain-Barré syndrome.

In the serum of GBS patients, antibodies to gangliosides are found, which play significant role in maintaining structural integrity of peripheral nerve cell membranes. Molecular mimicry also contributes exemplified by homology of lipo-oligosaccharides in *C. jejuni* cell membranes and gangliosides. Host factors, like human leukocyte antigen and single nucleotide polymorphisms, may also be associated in this pathway. The final common pathway is through complement activation and formation of membrane attack complex.

Q. Enumerate the serum antiganglioside antibodies described in Guillain-Barré syndrome.

Serum antiganglioside antibodies described in GBS have been listed in table 3.

Q. Describe the salient points in the natural history of Guillain-Barré syndrome.

Most patients reach the nadir of disease progression by 2-4 weeks. The plateau phase may continue for weeks to months. Up to 25% may need artificial ventilation.

Q. Describe the role of immunotherapy in the management of Guillain-Barré syndrome.

Use of IVIg or plasma exchange (5 sessions of complete exchange over 2 weeks) leads to improvement in long-term disability, reduces the need for mechanical ventilation and overall mortality. However, they are useful early in the disease course within the first 4 weeks, particularly first 2 weeks. There is no benefit of one over the other or in combination when compared to either alone. Steroids alone or in combination have not been found to be effective.

Q. What are the indications for immunotherapy in Guillain-Barré syndrome?

Immunotherapy is indicated in all non-ambulatory patients. Patients who deteriorate after initial improvement or stabilization may benefit with a repeat course of immunotherapy. However, in those who continue to deteriorate after first course of immunotherapy with no interim stabilization or improvement, a repeat course has not been proven to be beneficial.

Q. What are the indications for admission to an intensive care unit?

- Rapidly progressive weakness with impending respiratory failure
- Bulbar dysfunction with high chances of aspiration
- Severe autonomic dysfunction.

CONCLUSION

Acute flaccid paralysis is an emergency clinical situation. From the perspective of polio surveillance, it is a notifiable condition as advocated by WHO. It is of utmost importance to stabilize these patients and to provide emergency care at presentation. This should be followed by correct clinical diagnosis, judicious use of investigations, and appropriate management.

TABLE 3: **Serum antiganglioside antibodies described in Guillain-Barré syndrome**

Subtype	Antibodies
Acute motor axonal neuropathy/acute motor sensory axonal neuropathy	GM1, GM1b, GD1a, GalNac-GD1a
Miller Fisher variant	GQ1b, GD3, GT1a

KEY LEARNING POINTS

- Acute flaccid paralysis (AFP) is clinically characterized by variable weakness of limbs with occasional involvement of respiratory muscles, cranial, sensory, and autonomic nerves.
- Acute flaccid paralysis surveillance and reporting is advocated by World Health Organization because of its significance in poliomyelitis
- The etiology of AFP varies according to the anatomical site of the lesion
- Acute flaccid paralysis is a clinical emergency. Initial stabilization in the emergency room is of utmost importance
- Correct diagnosis with the aid of necessary clinical examination and laboratory investigations is of utmost importance for appropriate management
- Management is three-pronged in the form of initial emergency stabilization, definitive treatment, and supportive care.

SUGGESTED READINGS

1. Chakrabarty B, Gulati S. Approach to acute flaccid paralysis. In: Gupta P, Menon PSN, Lodha R (Eds). *PG Textbook of Pediatrics*. New Delhi: CBS; 2015.
2. Marx A, Glass JD, Sutter RW. Differential diagnosis of acute flaccid paralysis and its role in poliomyelitis surveillance. *Epidemiol Rev*. 2000;22:298-316.
3. Singhi SC, Sankhyan N, Shah R, Singhi P. Approach to a child with acute flaccid paralysis. *Indian J Pediatr*. 2012;79: 1351-1357.
4. Vandoorn PA, Ruts L, Jacobs BC. Clinical features, pathogenesis, and treatment of Guillain-Barré syndrome. *Lancet Neurol*. 2008;7:939-950.

CHAPTER 20

Metabolic Crisis

Sheffali Gulati, Ranjith K Manokaran

INTRODUCTION

Incidence of neurometabolic disorders is about 3–4 per 1,000 live births. Unlike in India, where sepsis and asphyxia account for a majority of newborn emergencies, inborn errors of metabolism (IEM) account for about 20% of cases of acute illnesses in newborns.

CASE 1

An 80-hour-old female newborn presented to the emergency room with the complaints of lethargy for 1 day, poor feeding, and seizures. Baby was born full term by normal vaginal delivery. Apgar scores were 9, 9, and 9 at 1, 5, and 10 minutes, respectively. Birth weight was 2.8 kg. Baby was feeding well till 2 days of life.

There was family history of two early neonatal deaths. First baby was normal till day 3 of life then the baby developed lethargy, breathing difficulty, and poor feeding. It was labeled as late onset sepsis (? meningitis). He died on day 4 of life.

The second sibling was also a female baby. It was also a full-term normal vaginal delivery; her birth weight was 2.7 kg. On day 3 of life, baby developed refusal to feed and also had seizures. She was also suspected to be having sepsis. Baby died on day 5 of life. On examination, the baby was sick looking, hypothermic, and had cold and clammy extremities. She also had tachypnea and respiratory distress. Anterior fontanel was at level. There was no evidence of any dysmorphism. There was no organomegaly.

Baby was stuporous, hypertonic, deep tendon reflexes were brisk. Spontaneous movements were reduced. Blood sugar and ionized calcium were normal. Sepsis screen was negative (twice). Cerebrospinal fluid examination was acellular with sugar and protein being normal. On blood gas analysis, there was no acidosis, electrolytes were normal. Arterial lactate was normal. Ultrasonography of head was showing normal study. Blood ammonia was elevated 480 µmol/L (Ref: 50–80 µmol/L). A diagnosis of urea cycle disorder was made.

CASE 1 REVIEW IN A NUTSHELL

This newborn presented with neonatal encephalopathy and seizures. There was a period of apparent normalcy. Family history of early neonatal deaths is highly suggestive of some inherited metabolic disorder. Negative sepsis screen and normal cerebrospinal fluid studies are suggestive of a non-infectious etiology. Absence of metabolic acidosis with severe hyperammonemia was a strong pointer towards a diagnosis of urea cycle disorder. Elevated ammonia levels are toxic to brain. Management of hyperammonemia essentially comprises of steps to prevent protein catabolism, to remove the excessively accumulated ammonia, to reduce the formation of toxic metabolites by decreasing substrate availability, and limit the protein intake by stopping feeds in the acute phase. Provide adequate calories by dextrose infusion and lipids. Immediate measures to clear ammonia in severe case can be carried out by peritoneal dialysis. Lifelong management including dietary restrictions may be required in some disorders. Liver transplantation may be beneficial in some forms of urea cycle disorders.

CASE 2

A 2-week-old baby girl, who was born to a primigravida mother presented with the complaints of poor feeding and vomiting for 3 days. She also developed tonic seizures for 1 day. It was a full-term normal vaginal delivery at home. Baby cried immediately after birth. On examination, the baby was sick looking and lethargic. Tone was increased in all four limbs. Abnormal sucking and cycling movements were noticed. There was intermittent opisthotonic posturing.

Blood sugar was 37 mg/dL. Arterial blood gas analysis revealed pH 7.37, pCO_2 37, HCO_3 18. Arterial lactate was 2.2 mmol/L. Blood ammonia was 65 μg/dL.

Urine ketones were strongly positive. Dinitrophenylhydrazine testing was positive.

Computed tomography scan of head showed severe brain edema with prominent brainstem and cerebellar swelling.

Tandem mass spectrometry showed increased levels of leucine, isoleucine, valine, and alloleucine.

Urine gas chromatography showed increased excretion of lactate, 2-hydroxyisovalerate, 2-hydroxyisocapronate, 3-hydroxyisovalerate, valine, leucine, and isoleucine.

A diagnosis of classic neonatal maple syrup urine disorder was made. Baby was started on low protein diet, thiamine, and phenobarbitone.

CASE 2 REVIEW IN A NUTSHELL

This newborn presented with neonatal encephalopathy and seizures. On metabolic evaluation, except for hypoglycemia, there was neither metabolic acidosis nor hyperammonemia. Urine dinitrophenylhydrazine test was positive. This is suggestive of maple syrup urine disease (MSUD). Tandem mass spectrometry (TMS) is a diagnostic test for aminoacidopathies. Aminoacidopathies should be suspected in any child with IEM like presentation with normal blood gases and blood ammonia. In this case, TMS showed elevated branched chain aminoacids suggestive of classic neonatal MSUD. The management of classic neonatal MSUD is initial stabilization followed by life long therapy in the form of dietary modifications. Some forms of MSUD may respond to thiamine supplementation. Liver transplantation may be curative in some cases.

CASE 3

A 5-month-old male born out of a nonconsanguineous marriage without any history of adverse perinatal events presented with global developmental delay, refractory seizures, generalized and myoclonic seizures since 2 months of age.

There was no history of hearing or visual deficits. Child presented to emergency with complaints of lethargy, poor feeding, and fast breathing. There was no history of fever.

On examination, child was afebrile. Pulse rate was 148/min. Peripheral pulses were thready. Capillary refill time was 3–4 seconds. Respiratory rate was 44/min (acidotic). Blood pressure was 78/38 mmHg. Weight was 4 kg. Head circumference was 37 cm (~ −2 SD). Erythematous macular rash was appreciable in the extremities. Rest of the systemic examination was normal.

Central nervous system: GCS – E2M4Vcry. Fundus examination was normal. There were no meningeal signs or any cranial nerve deficit. There was generalized hypotonia and brisk deep tendon reflexes.

Child was resuscitated in emergency with intravenous fluids and inotropic support. He required intubation (in view of deteriorating sensorium and worsening shock). He was administered hydrocortisone, bicarbonate infusion, and broad spectrum antibiotics. Antiepileptic medications were continued.

Hemoglobin and blood counts were in normal range. Serum electrolytes and renal function testing were normal. Random blood sugar was 70 mg/dL. Arterial blood gas showed Ph -7.11/Po2-112/Pco2-17/Hco3-35/Base excess -23/Chloride - 98 suggestive of severe metabolic acidosis. Lactate was elevated to 7.3 (1.1–2.3 mmol/L). Serum ammonia was 124 μmol/L. Urine were positive for ketones. Cerebrospinal fluid was not suggestive of meningitis. Serum valproate level was normal. Organic acids profile revealed increased 3-methylcrotonylglycine and propionyl glycine pointing to multiple carboxylase deficiency.

Child was started on biotin and carnitine, child showed gradual improvement with supportive therapy and biotin. Serum biotinidase level was 1 nmol/mL/min (normal >5 nmol/mL/min). On follow up, seizure frequency gradually decreased; became seizure free after 2 weeks of discharge; antiepileptics were tapered and stopped after 2 years. Gradually child started gaining of milestones. Skin lesions resolved completely.

CASE 3 REVIEW IN A NUTSHELL

This infant presented with developmental delay and seizures. There was an episode of acute decompensation at 5 months of age. On metabolic evaluation, there was profound metabolic acidosis. There was hyperlactatemia and mild hyperammonemia. Organic acidurias generally present with hyperammonemia and high anion gap metabolic acidosis. Presence of erythematous macular rash is specific for multiple carboxylase deficiency. Urine organic acid profile is tested by urinary gas chromatography mass spectrometry. Organic acidurias are an important class of inherited metabolic disorders arising due to defect in intermediary metabolic pathways.

INTERACTIVE TOPIC REVIEW

Q. When to suspect a metabolic cause?

High index of suspicion is a must for arriving at a diagnosis of a metabolic crisis. If missed, it may prove fatal. In neonates and infants, one should suspect a neurometabolic etiology, in case of the following situations.
- Deterioration after a period of apparent normalcy in newborns
- Rapidly progressive encephalopathy and seizures (unexplained)
- Neonatal sepsis like presentation with negative sepsis screen
- Persistent or recurrent vomiting, peculiar body/urine odor
- Parental consanguinity, family history of similar illness/neonatal deaths
- Acute fatty liver or hemolysis, elevated liver enzyme levels, and low platelet count during pregnancy
- Severe metabolic acidosis, ketosis, and hypoglycemia.

Q. What is the list of investigations which need to be performed for a child with suspected neurometabolic etiology?

- Complete blood count: (Neutropenia and thrombocytopenia seen in propionic and methylmalonic acidemia)
- Arterial blood gases and electrolytes
- Blood glucose
- Plasma ammonia (normal values in newborn: 90–150 µg/dL or 64–107 µmol/L)
- Arterial blood lactate (normal values: 0.5–1.6 mmol/L)
- Liver function tests
- Urine ketones
- Urine reducing substances
- Serum uric acid (low in molybdenum cofactor deficiency).

Q. What are the precautions one should take before collecting samples?

Preferably, all samples necessary should be taken before any specific treatment is started. Lactate sample should be arterial, 2-hour fasting. It should be taken in a preheparinized syringe. Ammonia sample should be taken after at least 2-hour fasting. Ammonia should be taken in an Ethylenediaminetetraacetic acid (EDTA) container. Sample should be transported in ice and immediately tested. Avoid air mixing. Sample should be free flowing.

Q. What is biochemical autopsy?

- Blood: 5–10 mL; frozen at –20°C; heparinized (chromosomal studies) and EDTA (deoxyribonucleic acid studies)
- Urine: Frozen at –20°C
- Cerebrospinal fluid: Frozen at –20°C

- Skin biopsy: Including dermis in culture medium or saline with glucose (4–8°C)
- Liver/muscle biopsy: Histopathology, electron microscopy, and enzyme studies
- Kidney or heart biopsy (if indicated)
- Clinical photograph (especially in presence of dysmorphism)
- Infantogram (skeletal abnormalities).

Q. What are the components of supportive care in a child with suspected metabolic crisis?

Supportive care is sometimes as essential as the definitive therapy. It is important to stabilize the metabolic disturbances in the child so as to prevent mortality and minimize the morbidity; maintain normothermia; correct dehydration, acidosis, and dyselectrolytemias, and maintain euglycemia. Treatment of infection should be carried out with broad spectrum antibiotics. Mechanical ventilation may be commenced if required. Treatment of seizures is also of paramount importance to prevent additional neurological insult. It is preferable to avoid valproate as it may increase ammonia levels. Valproate has also been reported to cause fatal hepatotoxicity in some mitochondrial disorders.

Q. What is the management of hyperammonemia?

Management of hyperammonemia essentially comprises of steps to prevent protein catabolism and to remove the excessively accumulated ammonia. To reduce the formation of toxic metabolites by decreasing substrate availability, limit the protein intake by stopping feeds in the acute phase. Provide adequate calories by dextrose infusion at the glucose infusion rate of 8–10 mg/kg/min. Start lipids at 0.5 g/kg/day (up to 3 g/kg/day). Immediate measures to clear ammonia in severe case can be carried out by peritoneal dialysis. Hemodialysis is better than peritoneal dialysis, but hemodialysis is not feasible in younger children. Exchange transfusion is not useful in the management of hyperammonemia.

Exploit alternate pathways for nitrogen excretion. Sodium benzoate combines with glycine to form hippurate which can be easily excreted in the urine. Sodium benzoate can be given (intravenous/oral) loading dose 250 mg/kg followed by maintenance doses of 250–400 mg/kg/day in 4 divided doses. Similarly, phenylbutyrate combines with glutamine to form phenylacetylglutamine. Sodium phenylbutyrate (not available in India) can be given as a loading dose 250 mg/kg followed by 250–500 mg/kg/day in 4 divided doses. Arginine (oral or intravenous) 300 mg/kg/day can be given. Arginine is contraindicated in arginase deficiency. L-carnitine (oral/intravenous) 100–200 mg/kg/day can be added to treatment to facilitate ammonia removal. intravenous preparation of carnitine is not available in India.

Q. What is the cutoff value for hyperammonemia?

For the neonatal age, the cutoff levels are given below:
Normal level:
- Healthy neonate less than 110 μmol/L
- Sick neonate up to 180 μmol/L.
    In neonates, suspect inborn error of metabolism when the ammonia level is more than 200 μmol/L.

For infants and children:
- Normal 50–80 μmol/L.
    In neonates and children, suspect inborn error of metabolism when the ammonia is more than 100 μmol/L.
    Conversion: μmol/L = μg/dL × 0.59.

Q. How to approach a case of hyperammonemia?

The case of hyperammonemia has been studied as given in flowchart 1.

Q. How to classify metabolic disorders based on the available investigations?

The metabolic disorders based on the available investigation have been given in table 1.

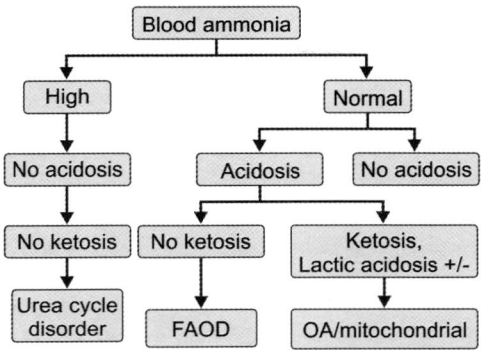

OA, organic acidemia; FAOD, fatty acid oxidation disorder.
Flowchart 1: Case of hyperammonemia

TABLE 1: Metabolic disorders based on the available investigation

Acidosis	Ketosis	Arterial lactate	Ammonia (>80 µg/dL)	Diagnosis
−	+	−	−	MSUD
+	+	±	±	Organic acidurias
+	+	+	±	Lactic acidosis
−	−	−	+	Urea cycle disorder
−	−	−	−	NKH, PD

MSUD, maple syrup urine disease; NKH, nonketotic hyperglycinemia; PD, pyruvate dehydrogenase deficiency.

Q. How to further workup a case of urea cycle defect?

The workup of a case of urea cycle defect has been explained through flowchart 2.

Q. What are clinical pointers for organic acidemia?

Age at onset and clinical features of organic acidemias may be variable. They may be acute/intermittent/chronic in presentation. Common symptoms are lethargy, poor feeding, coma, vomiting, seizures, developmental delay, ataxia, and dystonia. Specific odors in urine and cerumen may have specific clues to certain disorders. Classical metabolic abnormalities seen in metabolic acidosis, lactic acidosis, ketosis, hyperammonemia, and hypoglycemia. Blood counts may reveal neutropenia especially in cases of methylmalonic acidemia, isovaleric acidemia, propionic acidemia, and 3-methylcrotylglutaric acidemia.

Neuroimaging may reveal cerebral edema, atrophy, or hypomyelination. Basal ganglia changes signal changes may be seen in isovaleric acidemia, methylmalonic acidemia, and propionic acidemia (metabolic stroke). White matter changes are seen in multiple carboxylase deficiency/biotinidase deficiency. Cerebellar hemorrhages may be seen in isovaleric acidemia, methyl malonic acidemia, and propionic acidemia.

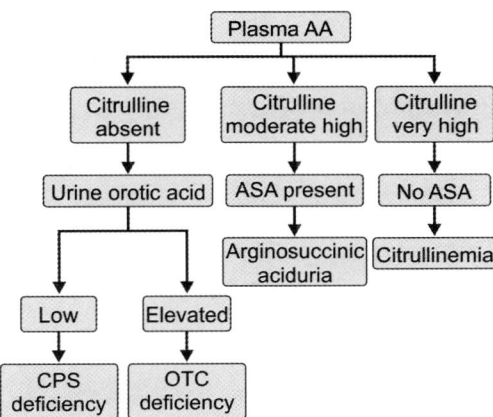

AA, aminoacidogram; ASA, arginosuccinic acid; CPS, carnitine palmitoyl synthase; OTC, ornithine transcarbamylase deficiency.
Flowchart 2: Urea cycle defect

Q. How to confirm diagnosis of organic acidemia?

Definitive diagnosis of organic acidemias can be established by enzyme analysis in cultured skin fibroblasts.

Q. What is the treatment of suspected organic acidemias?

Acute phase:
- Hydration
- Adequate calories
- Correction of metabolic acidosis, hypoglycemia, and hyperammonemia

- Carnitine
- Dialysis.

Following recovery:
- Low protein diet (1–1.5 g/kg/day)
- Special diets
- Avoiding fasting
- Chronic alkali therapy
- Carnitine (50–100 mg/kg/day).

Specific:
- Multiple carboxylase deficiency: Biotin (5–20 mg/day)
- Methylmalonic acidemia: Vitamin B12 (1 mg/day)
- Maple syrup urine disease: Thiamine (10–200 mg/day)
- Isovaleric acidemia: Glycine (250 mg/kg/day).

Q. What is the role of genetic counseling in such disorders?

The inheritance pattern is important to determine the risk of recurrence. Most of them are autosomal recessive inheritance and they carry a recurrence risk of 25% in subsequent pregnancies. In this era, advanced techniques are available for prenatal diagnosis. Prenatal diagnosis can be established based on enzymatic, metabolic, or molecular diagnosis. Even preimplantation embryonic diagnosis is being researched.

CONCLUSION

Inborn errors of metabolism are usually underdiagnosed but are important causes of neonatal and childhood mortality and morbidity. They can mimic common neonatal and childhood illnesses. High index of suspicion should be kept in such clinical scenario. Simple investigations are required for classification and management. Baseline metabolic workup includes blood ammonia, arterial blood gas, arterial lactate, and urinary ketones. Accurate diagnosis is necessary for proper treatment and genetic counseling. Early diagnosis is important to prevent irreversible neurological damage in neurometabolic crisis. Some conditions like multiple carboxylase deficiency can be managed by simple measures like the supplementation of the required cofactor. Newborn screening for IEM should be a part of newborn care and it helps in the earliest possible recognition of disorders to prevent the most serious consequences by timely intervention.

KEY LEARNING POINTS

- ☞ High index of suspicion is the key for approach to inborn errors of metabolism (IEMs)
- ☞ Period of apparent normalcy, encephalopathy/seizures, sepsis like presentation, family history and consanguinity are strong clinical pointers
- ☞ Sample should be taken in an appropriate manner and biochemical autopsy should be performed postmortem in any case of suspected IEM
- ☞ Supportive care, specific dietary modifications and cofactor supplementation are the cornerstones of management
- ☞ Prenatal diagnosis can be established by enzymatic, metabolic or molecular diagnosis and appropriate genetic counseling should be offered to the affected families.

SUGGESTED READINGS

1. All India Institute of Medical Sciences. (2014). Inborn errors of metabolism presenting in newborn period. [online] WHO website. Available from: http://www.newbornwhocc.org/clinical_proto.html [Accessed June 2016].
2. Blaser S, Feigenbaum A. A neuroimaging approach to inborn errors of metabolism. *Neuroimag Clin N Am*. 2004;14:307-329.
3. Cataltepe SU, Levy HL. Inborn errors of metabolism. In: Cloherty JP, Eichenwald EC, Stark AR, (Eds). *Manual of Neonatal Care*. 6th edn. Philadelphia: Lippincott Williams & Wilkins; 2008:558-573.
4. Leonard JV, Morris AAM. Diagnosis and early management of inborn errors of metabolism presenting around the time of birth. *Acta Pediatr*. 2006;95:6-14.
5. Nordli DR, De Vivo DC. Classification of infantile seizures: implications for identification and treatment of inborn errors of metabolism. *J Child Neurol*. 2002;17:3S3-7; discussion 3S8.
6. Summar M. Current strategies for the management of neonatal urea cycle disorders. *J Pediatr*. 2001;38:S30-S39.
8. Leonard JV, Morris AAM. Urea cycle disorders. *Semin Neonatol*. 2002;7:27-35.
9. de Baulny HO, Saudubray JM. Branched-chain organic acidurias. *Semin Neonatol*. 2002;7:65-74.
10. Wolf NI, Bast T, Surtees S. Epilepsy in inborn errors of metabolism. *Epileptic Disord*. 2005;7:67-81.
11. Kabra M. Dietary management of inborn errors of metabolism. *Indian J Pediatr*. 2002;69:421-426.

CHAPTER 21

Bacterial Meningitis

Suraj Gupte, Gautami Anand, Robert Brakeman

INTRODUCTION

Meningitis refers to the inflammation of the meninges overlying the brain and the spinal cord. It is one of the most dreadful emergencies met with in pediatric practice. The fatality rate is high. Two types are generally recognized:
1. Pyogenic or bacterial: *Haemophilus influenzae*, pneumococcal, meningococcal, staphylococcal, streptococcal, and *Escherichia coli* infection
2. Aseptic: Tuberculous, viral, fungal, and protozoal (toxoplasmosis, amebic).

Bacterial meningitis accounts for around 5% of the pediatric admissions in our country. It results from either primary infection of the meninges or spread from a nearby pyogenic focus. At times, metastatic spread from a distant focus also causes this disease. In our country, *H. influenzae* and pneumococcus are the leading causative agents. Meningococcus and Staphylococcus are less common. *Escherichia coli* is infrequent indeed, except in neonatal meningitis. *Haemophilus influenzae*, in particular, affects mostly the infants and young children who have not received *H. influenzae* type b (Hib) vaccine.

CASE 1

An 8-month-old girl on treatment for acute otitis media with oral co-amoxiclav, presented with generalized seizures (just stopped a while before reporting, to the hospital) preceded by vomiting, lethargy and irritability. She had received vaccines as per national immunization schedule, including Hib vaccine.

Examination: Well built and well nourished infant (weight 8.2 kg, length 68 cm), quite drowsy, arousable on painful stimuli.
- Temperature: 40°C
- Respiration: 54/min (irregular)
- Pulse: 110/min
- Blood pressure: 110/80 mmHg
- Anterior fontanel: Bulging and tense
- Neck rigidity: Present
- Cranial nerves: No abnormality detected
- Tendon reflexes: Exaggerated
- Plantars: Extensor
- Petechiae: No
- Fundus: Normal.

Investigations:
- Hemoglobin: 11.5 g/dL, normocytic normochromic picture
- Total leukocyte count: 5,400/mm^3
- Differential leukocyte: Polymorphonuclear neutrophils—78%, lymphocytes—19%, eosinophil—1%, monocytes—2%
- Computed tomography scan: No abnormality detected
- Cerebrospinal fluid: Hazy and under pressure; protein—600 mg/dL; sugar—45 mg/dL, cells—400/mm^3, predominantly polymorphonuclear neutrophils.

Treatment: In addition to symptomatic measures and supportive measures, she was started on intravenous (IV) ceftriaxone. Since she had received requisite doses of Hib vaccine, steroids were not given. Response was satisfactory.

CASE REVIEW IN A NUTSHELL

This 8-month-old's problem started with acute otitis media, which is a known cause of central nervous system (CNS) infection. The onset of nausea, vomiting, and generalized seizures certainly pointed to involvement of CNS. Physical examination provided evidence-favoring meningitis. Cerebrospinal fluid examination virtually established the diagnosis of bacterial meningitis. Hence, it was a good decision to start him on intravenous ceftriaxone. The decision to withhold steroid was well-founded in view of the fact that the child had received Hib vaccine. Pneumococcal conjugate vaccine had not been given.

INTERACTIVE TOPIC REVIEW

Q. Is the term meningitis rationally correct in clinical practice?

Strictly speaking, the term meningitis is a misnomer. It is virtually impossible that inflammation is limited to the meninges only. Meningoencephalitis is a better nomenclature.

Q. What is age-wise microbial pattern in meningitis?

The age-wise microbial pattern in meningitis is given in box 1.

Q. What are the clinical features?

As a rule, the onset is sudden with high fever, vomiting, restlessness, irritability, headache,

> **BOX 1: Agewise etiology of pyogenic meningitis**
> **Under 2 months**
> - Gram-negative orgainisms, especially *Escherichia coli*
> - Group B β-*Streptococcus hemolyticus*
> - *Listeria monocytogenes*
>
> **2 months to 6 years**
> - *Haemophilus influenzae*
> - Pneumococcus
> - *Neisseria meningitides*
>
> **Beyond 6 years**
> - Pneumococcus
> - *Neisseria meningitides*

and often convulsions. In newborns and small infants, pyogenic meningitis may have insidious onset with meagre symptoms like refusal to take feed, fever, and irritability. Some may have convulsions. These, especially in the presence of bulging anterior fontanel, should arouse suspicion of meningitis.

Physical examination may reveal neck stiffness, and positive Kernig and Brudzinski signs. Cranial nerve palsies and papilledema are present in some cases. Hemiplegia may be noticed in a few cases who report late to the doctor.

Q. What are special features of meningococcal meningitis?

Meningococcal meningitis is characterized by the presence of a generalized purpuric rash which is only infrequently seen in dark-skinned children. Meningococcemia may, in certain cases, dominate the clinical picture of meningitis. Such cases become rapidly comatose and have toxemia, cyanosis and purple mottling of the skin.

Q. Do you mean the Waterhouse-Friderichsen syndrome?

Yes, that is right.

Q. Is a skin rash exclusively a feature of meningococcal meningitis?

No. Such a rash may also be seen in pneumococcal meningitis, influenza (type B), and some other viral infections.

Q. What should be the diagnostic approach?

Lumbar puncture is a "must" in any child in whom meningitis is suspected.

Cerebrospinal fluid is generally under increased pressure and frankly turbid or little opalescent.

Cell count is greatly increased, a large proportion of these being polymorphs. Cerebrospinal fluid proteins are greatly increased. However, sugar is considerably reduced, invariably below 30 and often as low as 10–20 mg/dL.

Cerebrospinal fluid culture should be done for identifying the causative organisms and their antibiotic sensitivity, provided such facilities are available.

Nitroblue tetrazolium test is a useful adjunct to differentiate it from tuberculous meningitis; so is countercurrent immunoelectrophoresis.

Q. Suppose the child with suspected bacterial meningitis is very unstable and needs resuscitation. Should cerebrospinal fluid culture be obtained in his case before initiating antibiotic(s)?

No, not really. Appropriate antibiotics should be started immediately. Lumbar puncture can wait until the child is resuscitated.

Outline the therapeutic approach

Antibiotic therapy

Empirical: Initial treatment of choice is empirical employing a third-generation cephalosporin, ceftriaxone or cefotaxime (intravenously).

Alternative choice is ampicillin, given intravenously in a dose of 100–400 mg/kg/day as such or in combination with chloramphenicol. The low dose of ampicillin is only for newborns under 7 days of age. In them, it should be combined with an aminoglycoside (say, gentamicin or amikacin).

If the patient is hypersensitive to penicillin, ampicillin should not be given. Chloramphenicol 50–100 mg/kg/day is the next best agent. In a newborn, either it should be avoided or given in a low dose, i.e., 25 mg/kg/day, because of the risk of serious toxicity (Gray-baby syndrome).

Combination of chloramphenicol and penicillin continues to find favor with some clinicians.

Specific: After availability of culture and sensitivity report, suitable change in antibiotic therapy may be made as per box 2 provided that response to empirical therapy is unsatisfactory.

In case clinical response to therapy is satisfactory, antibiotic therapy may be stopped without a second lumbar puncture.

> **BOX 2: Recommended intravenous antibiotics in acute bacterial meningitis based on culture and sensitivity report**
> - Pneumococcal meningitis
>   - First choice: Penicillin G
>   - Alternative: Cefotaxime or ceftriaxone
> - Meningococcal meningitis
>   - First choice: Penicillin G
>   - Alternative: Cefotaxime or ceftriaxone
> - *Haemophilus influenzae* meningitis
>   - First choice: Ceftriaxone or cefotaxime
>   - Alternative: Ampicillin + chloramphenicol
> - Staphylococcal meningitis
>   - Penicillin G in case of penicillin-sensitive pathogens
>   - Vancomycin in case of penicillin-resistant pathogens
> - Listeria meningitis
>   - Ampicillin + amikacin/netilmicin/gentamicin
> - Pseudomonas meningitis
>   - First choice: Ceftazidime + amikacin, netilmicin or gentamicin
>   - Second choice: Piperacillin or ticarcillin
>   - Meropenem
>   - Cefepime

In most cases, duration of therapy is 10–14 days. Pseudomonoas and other Gram-negative meningitis may need a longer course.

Intrathecal administration of antibiotics, particularly initially, may be considered in neonates and patients with advanced disease.

Rising intracranial pressure may be controlled by intravenous mannitol.

Corticosteroids

A short course of steroids (dexamethasone, 0.15 mg/kg /dose intravenously every 6 hourly for 3 days; the first dose more than 15 minutes before starting antibiotics) in *H. influenzae* meningitis and pneumococcal meningitis is recommended in postneonatal cases. Its benefits include reduction in frequency of neurological complications such as deafness (sensorineural), interenal hydrocephalus, and behavioral problems. Overall mortality is not affected by this therapy.

Controlling seizures
Anticonvulsant agents such as intravenous diazepam and/or phenytoin are usually needed to control seizures.

Controlling raised intracranial pressure
Mannitol 0.5 g/kg of 20% solution is given intravenously stat and then every 4–6 hour. Total administration must not exceed 6 doses.

Controlling blood pressure
Dopamine or dobutamine as vasopressors is useful in controlling associated hypotension.

Supportive measures
- Maintenance of hydration, nutrition (intravenous drip is almost indispensable for first few days), vitamin supplements and good nursing care
- Syndrome of inappropriate secretion of antidiuretic hormone warrants cutting down of maintenance fluids by one-third
- Good nursing care.

Q. What is the prognosis?
The outlook has now considerably improved with the availability of modern antibiotics. Most of the mortality is confined to neonatal meningitis.

Q. What are the complications?
The complications include:
- Subdural effusion/empyema
- Brain-abscess
- Hydrocephalus
- Deafness, blindness, ocular paralysis.

Q. Any sequelae?
The sequelae include mental retardation, epilepsy, speech problems, hearing loss (due to labyrinthitis, or direct inflammation of auditory nerve), visual impairment, varying pareses, hydrocephalus, diabetes insipidus, obesity, and precocious puberty.

Q. Finally, what should be the algorithmic approach to child with suspected bacterial meningitis?
Flowchart 1 presents an algorithmic approach in suspected bacterial meningitis.

CONCLUSION
Meningitis, a dreadful emergency in pediatric practice, caries a high fatality rate with considerable sequelae in the survivors. Bacterial meningitis results from either primary infection of the meninges or spread from a nearby pyogenic focus and, occasionally from metastatic spread from a distant focus also causes this disease. In India, *H. Influenzae* and *S. pneumonia* (pneumococcus) are the leading causative agents.

KEY LEARNING POINTS
- Meningitis is inflammation of the membranes (meninges) overlying the brain and the spinal cord
- Two types are generally recognized, Pyogenic or bacterial and aseptic (viral, tuberculous. parasitic, fungal)
- *Haemophilus influenzae* and *S. pneumonia* (pneumococcus) are the leading causative agents in India in grownup children
- Meningococcus and Staphylococcus are causative pathogens in certain circumstances
- *E. coli* is infrequent indeed, except in neonatal meningitis
- *Haemophilus influenzae*, in particular, affects mostly the infants and young children who have not received Hib vaccine
- CSF analysis is mandatory for the diagnosis
- Therapy depends on the etiology.

CHAPTER 21: Bacterial Meningitis

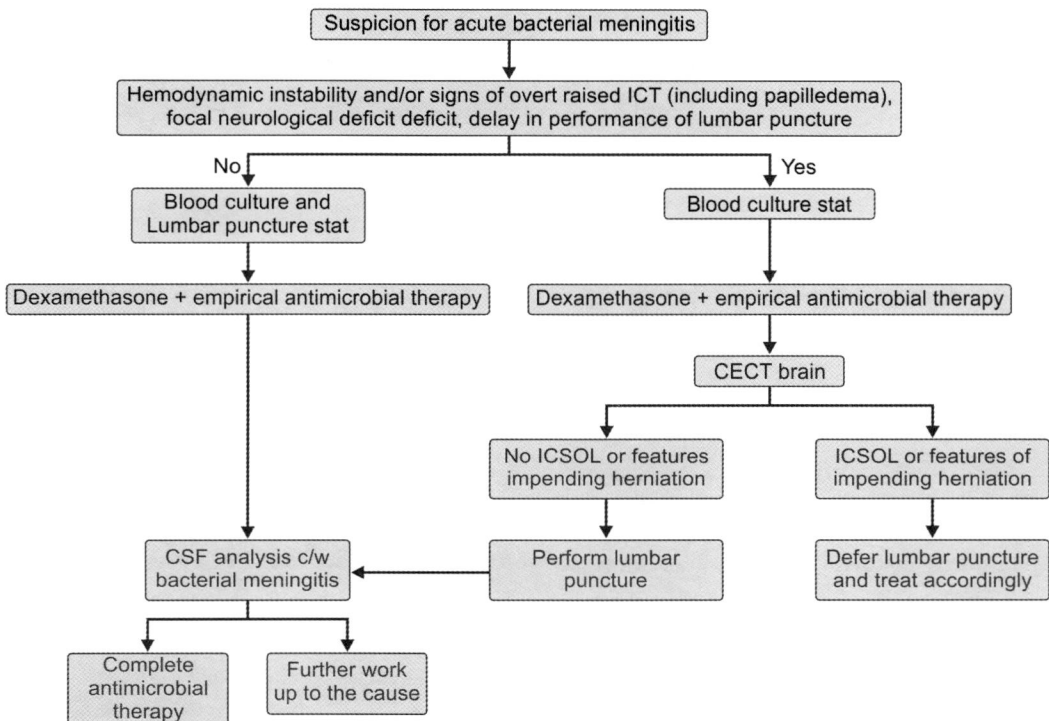

*ICT, intracranial temperature; †CECT, contrast-enhanced computed tomography; ‡ICSOL, intracranial space occupying lession; §CSF, Cerebrospinal fluid.

Flowchart 1: Algorithmic approach to suspected bacterial meningitis

Source: Gulati S. Central nervous system infections. In: Gupte S, Gupte SB, Guptre M (Eds). *Recent Advances in Pediatrics: (Immunology, Infections and Immunization)*. New Delhi: Jaypee Brothers Medical Publishers; 2013:143-188.

SUGGESTED READINGS

1. Brouwer Mc, Mcintyre P, Prasad K, van de Beek D. Corticosteroids for acute bacterial meningitis. *Cochrane Database Syst Rev.* 2013:CD004405.
2. Gulati S, Singh LB, Gupte S, Chowdhary BB. Pediatric neurology. In: Gupte S (Ed). *The Short Textbook of Pediatrics*, 12th edn. New Delhi: Jaypee Brothers Medical Publishers; 2016:506-548.
3. Gulati S. Central nervous system infections. In: Gupte S, Gupte SB, Guptre M (Eds). *Recent Advances in Pediatrics (Immunology, Infections and Immunization)*. New Delhi: Jaypee Brothers Medical Publishers; 2013:143-188.
4. Newman R, Newland J. In: Cobana MD, Brakeman P, Curran ML (Eds). *The 5-minute Pediatric Consult*, 7th edn. New Delhi: Wolters Kluwer; 2012:576-577.

SECTION 5
Pulmonology

CHAPTER 22

Respiratory Distress

BP Karunakara, Sumitha Nayak

INTRODUCTION

Respiratory distress is defined as increased respiratory rate with increased work of breathing. The increased work of breathing is characterized by chest retraction (defined as paradoxical indrawing of lower one-third of the chest wall during inspiration), with or without flaring of the alae nasi, stridor, grunting, and wheezing.

It is difficult to detect respiratory distress in infants and young children. Close monitoring of the respiratory rate usually gives a clue to the development of distress. Even in a crowded outpatient room or in the emergency room (ER), the respiratory rate (RR) can be counted for 1 full minute. Infants and children with a RR more than or equal to 60/min should be considered as those requiring urgent and immediate care. Respiratory rate more than 60/min is a good predictor of hypoxia in infants less than 2 months of age.

The normal respiratory rate varies in different ages during childhood. Knowledge of this information is important in the assessment and interpretation in children. Table 1 shows the age-related rates of respiration in children.

TABLE 1: Normal age-related respiratory rates

Age	Respiratory rate (breaths/min)
Premature	40–70
0–3 months	35–55
3–6 months	30–45
6–12 months	25–40
1–3 years	20–30
3–6 years	20–25
6–12 years	14–22
12 years+	12–18

CASE 1

A 6-month-old girl was brought to the ER with history of fever, cold, and cough of 2–3 days, followed by hurried breathing since 1 day. History of reduced activity and feeding were present. On examination in the ER, the child was febrile; temperature 101°F, RR 68/min; nasal flaring and chest retractions were present. There was no cyanosis and bilateral scattered rhonchi were found on chest examination. Other systems examination was noncontributory.

Following standard interventions, the infant responded with gradual improvement in breathing and normalization in 48 hours. The infant was weaned off oxygen as the condition improved and was started on feeds. She was discharged after 3 days in the hospital.

CHAPTER 22: Respiratory Distress

CASE REVIEW IN A NUTSHELL

The patient is a young infant who developed acute upper respiratory symptoms followed by lower respiratory symptoms and signs suggesting that the child is suffering from acute lower tract disease, possibly acute bronchiolitis. The common etiological agents include respiratory syncytial virus (RSV), influenza, parainfluenza, Epstein-Barr virus, and others. The presence of rhonchi in an infant with or without crepitations points toward the probability of acute viral bronchiolitis.

Intervention required in ER are administration of humidified O_2 (10 L/min via oxygen hood), and intravenous maintenance fluids, and paracetamol drops were given to maintain the temperature below 100°F. The infant responded with gradual improvement in breathing and normalization in 48 hours. The infant was weaned off oxygen as the condition improved and was started on feeds. The infant was discharged after 3 days in the hospital.

Q. What are the clinical features that point toward respiratory distress in a child?

There are several symptoms and signs that may point toward the appearance of distress in a child. Tachypnea and chest retractions are the two most important clinical features. Others are as mentioned in table 2.

TABLE 2: Signs and symptoms of respiratory distress

	Symptoms	Signs
Early	Restlessness, agitation	Lethargic, supracostal, subcostal, and intercostals retractions
	Change in breathing pattern	Flaring of alae nasi
	Fast breathing	–
	Disinterest in surroundings	Stridor, cyanosis-initially peripheral, later central also
Late	Weak cry	Drowsy, poorly responsive to stimuli
	Shallow respiratory effort	Grunting, jaw breathing

Q. What are the significance of these signs?

Each of the signs of respiratory distress indicates a pathological change in some areas of the respiratory tract. By picking up the signs accurately, it may be possible to estimate the location and severity of the disease.

Tachypnea or increased respiratory rate is a reliable predictor of significant hypoxia in the patient. Respiratory rate more than 60/min can be considered as an indicator for immediate administration of supplemental oxygen as they would be significantly hypoxic. Count the respiratory rate for 1 full minute, possibly by observation alone, without placing the stethoscope on the anterior chest wall, as this can stimulate some changes in the breathing pattern.

Bradypnea or decreased rate of breathing is usually associated with abnormal breathing patterns. This is an ominous sign that should draw immediate attention as it would be indicative of impending respiratory failure and apnea.

Chest retractions indicate increased respiratory effort, weak chest wall, or both. A significant chest retraction is the retraction of the lower one-third of the chest, and it significantly correlates with underlying parenchymal lung disease. Retractions may be suprasternal, which most often suggests an upper airway obstruction. It could also be present with upper airway anomalies, especially in younger infants.

Stridor indicates respiratory effort that is made against the closed glottis in an attempt to keep the airways open. Stridor indicates an upper airway obstruction above the thoracic inlet.

Grunting indicates an effort made by the patient to maintain the functional residual capacity (FRC). The patient exhales against a partially closed glottis, in an attempt to keep the alveoli open. Conditions with reduced FRC like pneumonia, pulmonary edema, etc. and conditions with small airway diseases like bronchiolitis, etc. manifest with grunting.

Cyanosis indicates significant levels of right to left shunting that occurs when there is widespread atelectasis. This is a sign of severe hypoxia or respiratory failure and is an emergency situation.

Decreased tidal volume produces rapid and shallow respirations and indicates decreased lung compliance. Conditions with increased tidal volume like obstructive airway diseases produce deep respirations, which are less rapid.

Q. What are the causes of respiratory distress?

The common respiratory causes of distress include bronchopneumonia, bronchiolitis, asthma, croup, and foreign body aspiration. Nonrespiratory causes for distress include congestive cardiac failure secondary to congenital or rheumatic heart diseases, meningitis, encephalitis, and metabolic causes. Box 1 enlists the causes of respiratory distress in children.

> **BOX 1: Causes of respiratory distress**
> - Respiratory causes
>   - Central airway obstruction—choanal atresia, laryngomalacia, retropharyngeal abscess, foreign body aspiration, epiglottitis, mediastinal mass
>   - Peripheral airway obstruction—asthma, bronchiolitis, pneumonia, foreign body aspiration, cystic fibrosis, α-1 antitrypsin deficiency
>   - Alveolar diseases—lobar pneumonia, interstitial pneumonia, hyaline membrane disease, ARDS, pulmonary hemorrhage
>   - Thoracic chest wall defects—flail chest, kyphoscoliosis, asphyxiating thoracic dystrophy
> - Nonrespiratory causes
>   - Cardiovascular
>   - L→R shunts like VSD, ASD, PDA, AV canal defect, truncus arteriosus
>   - CCF secondary to coarctation of the aorta, aortic stenosis, mitral stenosis, hypoplastic left heart syndrome
>   - Cardiogenic shock due to myocarditis, myocardial infarction or left heart obstructions
>   - Central nervous system
>   - Increased intracranial pressure due to meningitis, encephalitis, space occupying lesions
>   - Toxic encephalopathy—drug induced, chemical induced, Reye's syndrome
>   - Neurogenic pulmonary edema—secondary to intracranial lesions, which stimulate the brain stem respiratory centers
>
> *Continued*

Continued

> - Metabolic
>   - Diabetic ketoacidosis
>   - Hyperammonemia—due to ammonia cycle disorders, Reye's syndrome
>   - Organic academia—metabolic disorders
> - Renal—renal tubular acidosis, renal hypertension
> - Miscellaneous
>   - CNS infections
>   - Brain stem and spinal cord trauma
>   - Transverse myelitis
>   - Poliomyelitis
>   - Guillain-Barré syndrome
>   - Muscular dystrophy
>   - Birth trauma
>   - Diaphragmatic hernia
>   - Phrenic nerve injury
>   - Eventration of diaphragm
>   - Myasthenia gravis
>   - Organophosphorus poisoning
>
> ARDS, acute respiratory distress syndrome; VSD, ventricular septal defect; ASD, atrial septal defect; PDA, patent ductus arteriosus; AV, atrioventricular; CCF, congestive cardiac failure; CNS, central nervous system.

Q. How to diagnose respiratory distress?

Clinical observation is the cornerstone for diagnosing respiratory distress. The tachypnea with increased work of breathing in the form of chest retractions indicates respiratory distress. Presence of other signs and symptoms add up to the clinical features.

Q. What investigations must be done in cases of respiratory distress?

The following investigations are required for diagnostic and therapeutic purposes:
- Routine blood counts, peripheral smear, acute phase reactants like erythrocyte sedimentation rate, C-reactive protein will reveal the presence of infections. In bacterial infections, total leukocyte counts are increased, but may be normal in cases of viral infections with normal levels of acute phase reactants
- Chest X-ray is an important investigation in the diagnosis of respiratory distress. Patchy consolidation in acute pneumonia,

diffuse nonhomogenous opacities in bronchopneumonia. In case of foreign body aspiration, there may be evidence of atelectasis. In bronchiolitis, the chest X-ray may be unremarkable. Chest wall deformities can be noted that may obstruct the respiratory functions. In congenital cardiac diseases, congestive cardiac failure, cardiac shunts, etc., the cardiac shape, size, and outline will be altered and point toward the diagnosis. X-ray of the neck in an extended position will assist in the diagnosis of croup. The steeple sign may be visible in this condition. Blood glucose estimation will point toward metabolic abnormalities like ketoacidosis that is causing respiratory distress. Serum electrolytes sodium, potassium, bicarbonate, chloride will reveal dyselectrolytemia that may occur due to the underlying disease process. Electrolyte levels must be monitored closely during acute illness and as long as the patient is on intravenous fluids
- Electrocardiogram in all leads and echocardiogram in case suspected cardiac causes.

Q. How to monitor respiratory status in a child with respiratory distress?

The important aspect of monitoring is clinical observation. A cost-effective and reliable method of monitoring is by using pulse oximetry, which helps in monitoring oxygen saturation and heart rate. Pulse oximetry is a noninvasive and safe method for monitoring patients who may develop respiratory distress. Pulse oximetry is an easy to use bedside monitoring device that measures the arterial hemoglobin O_2 saturation levels.

Q. What is the principle of working of the pulse oximeter?

The light absorption of oxyhemoglobin varies from that of deoxyhemoglobin at wavelengths of 660 nm which is of red light and 940 nm which is the wavelength of infrared light. The oximeter sensor is attached to the finger or toe, or in case of very young infants, it is attached to the foot. The differential absorption by the arterial blood of the two wavelengths emitted by the sensor is used to determine the oxygen saturation. The ratio of detected red and infrared intensities is calibrated empirically against the direct measurements of arterial blood oxygen saturation (SaO_2) to arrive at the pulse oximeter's estimate of arterial oxygen saturation (SpO_2). A plethysmographic waveform is also displayed that helps to distinguish artefacts from true signals.

Q. Are there any limitations for using pulse oximetry?

Pulse oximetry has limited use in case of associated pathological conditions like anemia, carboxyhemoglobinemia, methemoglobinemia, hypotension, and physiological conditions like vasoconstriction and motion artefacts. It is unreliable in those with poor pulsatile flow and poor perfusion to the extremities. Estimate of arterial oxygen saturation values greater than 95% are indicative of normal saturation.

Q. What is the role of blood gas analysis in cases of respiratory distress?

Blood gas analysis is a useful necessity in sick children and not in all children with respiratory distress. Hypoxia and/or respiratory acidosis are useful indicators of the condition of the disease and decide on need for oxygen, ventilator support, and others. With the administration of oxygen, these changes get reversed especially when there are no severe parenchymal lesions and no intrapulmonary shunting of blood. Central nervous system defects that impede the neuromuscular function and those that depress the respiratory center also have similar blood gas picture and they respond very well to oxygen supplementation.

Q. How to manage a patient with respiratory distress?

The primary goal of managing patients with respiratory distress is to maintain a patent airway and to provide supplemental oxygen. Tissue hypoxia is a life-threatening condition and must be treated aggressively.

- Ensure that the airway is patent and that the patient is comfortable
- Provide humidified oxygen to the patient.

Assess the need for supportive measures like oral or nasal airways to maintain the patency of the airway, need for bag and mask ventilation, and invasive and noninvasive ventilator support. Provide the support as needed. The minimum requirement for a child with respiratory distress is the administration of humidified oxygen.

Q. How is oxygen administered to the patient?

There are several ways of administering oxygen to the patient.

Oxygen prongs are easy to use but provide low levels of oxygen supplementation. As these are inserted into the anterior nares, the flow levels must be maintained at less than or equal to 5 L/min, as higher levels would result in irritation to the nares.

Higher oxygen flow rates between 5 and 10 L/min can be achieved by using a simple oxygen mask. This has open side ports and a valve less oxygen source. The amount of oxygen delivered varies with the size and fit of the mask, while the minute volume of the child determines how much oxygen is inhaled. In case where better and more precise oxygen delivery is desired, it is essential to use other varieties of masks. The venturi mask and partial or nonbreather masks are other oxygen delivery methods. The venturi mask and reservoir system has an adapter at the end. This mask entrains the room air and delivers flow rates between 5 and 10 L/minute of preset fractions of oxygen. Using the partial rebreather mask allows higher oxygen delivery as it allows for some mixing with the reservoir gas during exhalation.

Q. Is there a need for intravenous fluids?

The patients with respiratory distress are at risk of aspiration during fast breathing on administration of oral feeds. Hence, intravenous fluids reneeded till the breathing returns to normal. Provide maintenance fluids. Consider relaxing or restricting fluids depending upon dehydration or syndrome of inappropriate antidiuretic hormone secretion.

Q. Is there any other treatment that must be administered?

Based on the presence of the underlying pathology, the treatment must be modified accordingly.

In hospitalized patients, gentle suctioning of the secretions is required to decrease the obstruction caused by the tenacious secretions and sputum.

Antimicrobials

Patients with respiratory distress should be started on antibiotics, pending other laboratory reports. In case of suspected or proven viral etiology, there is no need to continue antibiotics. Choices of antibiotics include amoxicillin, amoxicillin-clavulanic acid, cefuroxime, and others. Parenteral antibiotics are indicated during the acute phase in order to obtain prompt and better results. In suspected cases of staphylococcal disease, start on cloxacillin or vancomycin (methicillin-resistant *Staphylococcus*). In atypical pneumonias, consider administration of erythromycin, azithromycin, or other macrolides.

Antivirals are required in few special situations. Respiratory syncytial virus infections can cause severe bronchiolitis, hence require specific antiviral medications. Ribavirin is an antiviral that is delivered through the oxygen hood, facemask, or endotracheal tube. It is given by a fine particle aerosol generator for 3–5 days. Some trials have shown the usefulness of ribavirin in the management of infections by RSV by reducing the duration of hospitalization and the need for mechanical ventilation. Palivizumab is another antiviral that has been licensed for usage as a prophylactic agent in high risk infants. This is a monoclonal antibody that helps in decreasing RSV infections.

Other treatments

Depending on the etiology, the specific management must be administered. Besides humidified oxygen and intravenous fluids, in moderate-to-severe respiratory distress due to bronchiolitis, saline nebulization may be useful in clearing the secretions. In cases of moderate-to-severe bronchospasm, nebulization with bronchodilators is useful. The frequency of nebulization must be titrated based on patient response. Consider steroid nebulization in cases of distress due to acute severe asthma. In case of acute severe asthma, the remaining management must be administered as per protocols.

Q. What is the eventual course and prognosis of the child?

The response to treatment of respiratory distress depends on the underlying pathology. In most cases of distress associated with pulmonary infections, the child responds to the treatment and there are no residual deficits. In nonpulmonary pathology, the underlying cause must be adequately treated, so that there is no recurrence of the distress. Central nervous system causes associated with weak muscle function as well as those cases with chest wall defects, metabolic disorders, and renal tubular acidosis may develop recurrent episodes of respiratory distress and need to be closely monitored.

Q. What if the patient does not improve with oxygen supplementation?

For those patients who do not improve with oxygen supplementation alone, consider non-invasive ventilator support or positive pressure ventilation.

CONCLUSION

Respiratory distress is a respiratory emergency. It is characterized by tachypnea and increased work of breathing—chest wall retractions, nasal flaring, tachypnea, stridor, grunting, and wheezing. Common causes include broncho-pneumonia, bronchiolitis, acute asthma, and others. Respiratory distress can be caused due to respiratory as well as nonrespiratory pathology. Pulse oximetry allows continuous monitoring of the respiratory rate, and blood gas analysis can provide the basis for corrections in the electrolyte deficits. Management includes administration of humidified oxygen, nebulized saline (bronchiolitis) and salbutamol nebulization/steroids for acute severe asthma, airway and ventilator support for severe cases and antibiotics for bacterial respiratory infections. The outcome depends on the underlying pathology, the rapidity of recognition and administration of supplemental oxygen and supportive care as well as the child's immune status.

KEY LEARNING POINTS

- Respiratory distress is defined as increased rate and work of breathing. Respiratory rate varies with the age, but rate more than 60 breaths/min can be considered tachypnea in any child
- Respiratory distress may occur due to respiratory as well as nonrespiratory causes
- Management includes administration of humidified oxygen, nebulized saline (bronchiolitis), and salbutamol nebulization/steroids for acute severe asthma, airway and ventilator support for severe cases and antibiotics for bacterial respiratory infections.

SUGGESTED READINGS

1. Jubran A. Pulse oximetry. *Intensive Care Med.* 2004;30: 2017-2020.
2. Rajesh VT, Singhi S, Kataria S. Tachypnea is a good predictor of hypoxia in infants under 2 months. *Arch Dis Child.* 2000; 82:46-49.
3. Sarnaik AP, Clark JA. Respiratory distress and failure. In: Kleigman RM, Stanton BF, St Geme III JW, Schor NF, (Eds). *Nelson Textbook of Pediatrics.* 20th edn. Philadelphia: Elsevier; 2016:314-321.
4. Sinex JE. Pulse oximetry: Principles and limitations. *Am J Emerg Med.* 1999;17:59-67.
5. Van de Louw A, Cracco C, Cerf C, Harf A, Duvaldestin P, Lemaire F, et al. Accuracy of pulse oximetry in the intensive care unit. *Intensive Care Med.* 2001;27:1606-1613.
6. Sekharan DV, Subramanyam L, Balachandran A. Arterial blood gas analysis in clinical practice. *Indian Pediatr.* 2001;38:1116-1128.

Acute Respiratory Distress Syndrome

CHAPTER 23

Anjul Dayal, Abhilasha Singh

INTRODUCTION

In infants and children, acute respiratory distress syndrome (ARDS) remains a significant cause of morbidity and mortality. Although any infant or child can develop ARDS, children who have experienced trauma, pneumonia, aspiration, or immune compromise are at increased risk. In-hospital settings, mortality related to these conditions is as high as 34–55%. Multiorgan failure is the terminal event causing death.

Acute respiratory distress syndrome often has to be differentiated from congestive heart failure, which usually has signs of fluid overload, and from severe pneumonia.

Treatment is by and large supportive. It includes mechanical ventilation, prophylaxis for stress ulcers, nutritional support, and pharmacotherapy of the underlying injury. Such factors as low tidal volume (V_T), high positive end-expiratory pressure, and conservative fluid therapy may improve outcomes.

Adoption of an open-lung ventilation strategy, characterized by sufficient positive end-expiratory pressure to avoid atelectasis, a V_T that is limited to less than 5–7 cc/kg/breath and a plateau pressure of 30 cm of water or less provide the greatest likelihood of survival and minimizes lung injury. The relative benefits of strategies such as high frequency oscillatory ventilation (HFOV), surfactant replacement therapy and inhaled nitric oxide (INO) are considered.

CASE 1

A 10-year-old girl, admitted for fever and cough with minimal respiratory distress. She was started on oxygen supplementation and antibiotics. Over next 2 days her respiratory distress worsened and she was intubated and was kept on ventilator. On ventilator, her saturations were not maintained on normal ventilator settings and her arterial oxygen pressure (PaO_2) decreased to 90 despite increasing the fraction of inspired oxygen (FiO_2) to 100%. Chest X-ray (CXR) showed left basal consolidation and diffuse bilateral infiltrates. She was sedated, paralyzed with atracurium and ventilated with low V_T and high positive end expiratory pressure with inspiratory-to-expiratory time ratio (I:E ratio) of 1:2. She was not maintaining saturation and she was ventilated in prone position. *Haemophilus influenzae* was grown from sputum and *Streptococcus* from blood cultures.

She was, therefore, commenced on injection cefotaxime. She remained unstable, requiring frequent proning to maintain her pH on hemoglobin saturation above 90%. Her X-ray worsened (Fig. 1) inspite of maximal ventilator pressures on conventional ventilation.

She was started on HFOV 4 days after admission to pediatric intensive care unit (PICU). Over the next 24 hours, her oxygenation improved with a PaO_2 of 180 and within next 3 days was possible to reduce the FiO₂ to 605. Her oxygen requirements continued to decrease as her oxygenation improved. She remained hemodynamically stable. After 5 days on HFOV, she was changed back to conventional ventilation. Her chest X-ray (CXR) improved and she was extubated and kept on noninvasive ventilation (NIV) through tight fitting face mask. She improved with radiographic clearing of the lungs and was shifted on to oxygen supplements via face mask. She was subsequently discharged after 12 days of hospital stay.

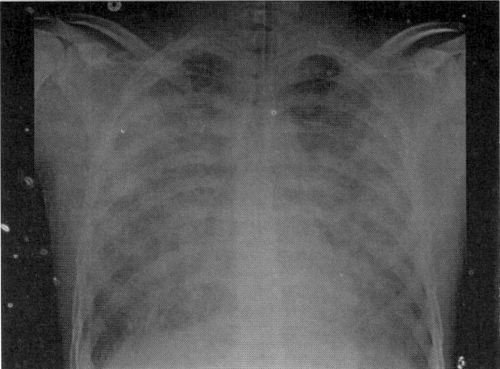

Figure 1: Chest X-ray showing bilateral homogeneous opacities suggestive of acute respiratory distress syndrome

CASE REVIEW IN A NUTSHELL

This 10-year-old girl with bad pneumonia developed ARDS with acute hypoxia and required to be ventilated. Due to the bad lungs, she was not able to maintain the saturations in spite of inspired oxygen of 100%. While on ventilator, she was sedated and paralyzed to maintain the ventilator–patient synchrony and was ventilated with lung protective strategy, i.e., keeping the positive end expiratory pressure high to prevent frequent collapse and distention of lung, thus preventing shearing force injury and also keeping a low V_T to prevent volutrauma of the lungs. She was also kept in prone position to improve the oxygenation, which improved oxygenation but not for prolonged sustained period.

In view of desaturation on this ventilatory mode, she was shifted on to HFOV. She improved on this ventilation. Her lung got adequately recruited. Her oxygen requirement was reduced.

Ventilation is the mainstay of treatment for ARDS. There are various strategies to improve the oxygenation by recruiting the lung without causing lung damage. In this case, lung protective strategy and high frequency ventilation was utilized.

INTERACTIVE TOPIC REVIEW

Q. What is the basic defect in ARDS?

The basic defect in ARDS is one of oxygenation rather than of ventilation, as a consequence of widespread alveolar collapse with resultant ventilation perfusion mismatch and hypoxemia.

The New Berlin 2012 definition of ARDS is:
- ARDS is now divided into three categories based on severity of hypoxemia:
  1. PaO_2/FiO_2 between 200 and 300 is defined as mild
  2. PaO_2/FiO_2 between 101 and 199 is defined as moderate
  3. PaO_2/FiO_2 of less than 100 is defined as severe
- The term "acute" now has a specified time frame of symptoms developing within one week of a known clinical insult. The CXR criterion is now more defined with the added phrase "bilateral opacities—not fully explained by effusions, lobar or lung collapse, or nodules"
- The CXR criteria is now more defined with the added phrase "bilateral opacities—not fully explained by effusions, lobar or lung collapse, or nodules"
- Pulmonary capillary wedge pressure reading is no longer required as part of the diagnosis as this is increasingly not used. Instead, this new definition requires that the respiratory failure cannot be explained fully by cardiac failure or volume overload.

Q. What is the pathophysiology of ARDS?

Acute respiratory distress syndrome is a noncadiogenic edema following lung injury.

To begin with, a direct pulmonary or indirect extrapulmonary insult causes a proliferation of inflammatory mediators that promote neutrophil accumulation in the microcirculation of the lung. Subsequently, the neutrophils activate and migrate in large numbers across the vascular endothelial and alveolar epithelial surfaces, releasing proteases, cytokines, and reactive oxygen species. The migration and mediator release causes pathologic vascular permeability, gaps in the alveolar epithelial barrier, and necrosis of Type I and II alveolar cells. In turn, there is pulmonary edema, hyaline membrane formation, and loss of surfactant that decrease pulmonary compliance and make air exchange difficult. Subsequently, collagen deposition, fibrosis, and worsening of the disease follow.

Q. Are there any histopathological stages of ARDS?

Acute respiratory distress syndrome can be divided into three histopathologic stages, as follows:
1. Exudative: Injury to lung endothelial cells and alveolar epithelial cells occurs during days 1–7 of the initial injury. Air spaces are then filled with exudate and fluid, and the development of microvascular thrombi leads to capillary occlusion
2. Proliferative: This stage occurs between the first and third week after the initial insult. Type II pneumocytes, fibroblasts, and myofibroblasts proliferate, resulting in widening of the alveolar septa and conversion of intra-alveolar hemorrhagic exudate into cellular granulation tissue
3. Fibrotic: After 3 weeks from the time of injury, the lungs exhibit remodeling and fibrosis.

The most immediate among the cascade of effects is an increase in alveolar and pulmonary capillary permeability. Protein-rich fluid engulfs the alveolus. Activated neutrophils and macrophages follow, and an inflammatory cascade are initiated. The cascade involves the release of interleukins, tumor necrosis factor, and other inflammatory mediators. Neutrophils release oxidants, leukotrienes, and various proteases.

Massive cell damage, alveolar denudation, and sloughing of cell debris into the lumen of the alveolus are the net result. Additionally, surfactant is remarkably inactivated.

Simultaneously, in the pulmonary capillary bed, endothelial cells swell, platelets aggregate, and a procoagulant cascade arises. This leads to small-vessel thrombosis.

On the clinical level, work of breathing increases secondary to surfactant depletion, alveolar filling, cellular debris within the alveoli, and increased airway resistance. Surfactant loss leads to alveolar collapse because of increased surface tension, which is analogous to the situation observed in premature infants with infant respiratory distress syndrome. As alveoli collapse, closing lung volume capacity rises above the patient's functional residual capacity, further increasing atelectasis and the work of breathing. This is reflected as reduced compliance; that is, additional pressure is required to generate a unit volume.

Q. What is the net effect of all this?

The net effect is impairment in oxygenation. A widened interstitial space between the alveolus and the vascular endothelium decreases oxygen-diffusing capacity. Hypoxia arises as a result of the change described above. Collapsed alveoli result in either low ventilation-perfusion (V/Q) units or a right-to-left pulmonary shunt. The end result is marked venous admixture, the process whereby deoxygenated blood passing through the lungs does not absorb sufficient oxygen and causes a relative desaturation of arterial blood when it mixes with blood that is already oxygenated.

Q. What is the ventilator strategy in ARDS?

The heterogeneous pathology makes the lung particularly susceptible to the volutrauma and barotrauma inherent in the mechanics of conventional ventilation. Any successful ventilatory strategy has to address the balance between the need to optimize alveolar patency and avoid alveolar over-distension and damage.

This has led to the introduction of a more "lung friendly" form of ventilation with small V_Ts, rapid rates, and high positive end-respiratory pressure (PEEP). The rationale of this is that in ARDS the normal lung is essentially small, hence the small V_Ts and the use of a high PEEP serves to increase ventilated lung volume and prevent end-expiratory alveolar collapse. The rapid rates facilitate carbon dioxide clearance with the acceptance that carbon dioxide elimination is not the priority in ARDS.

The approach should be as per the Surviving Sepsis Clinical Practice Guideline and the National Heart, Lung, and Blood Institute's ARDS Network (ARDSNet). The respiratory rate, expiratory time, positive end-expiratory pressure, and FiO_2 are set in as per the ARDSNet protocols. To avoid barotraumas, settings are adjusted to maintain oxygen saturation (SpO_2) of 88–95% and a plateau pressure of 30 cm H_2O or less. Maintaining an arterial pH of 7.30–7.45 is appropriate although patients in some research trials have tolerated permissive hypercapnia and a pH as low as 7.15.

Starting with low V_Ts of 6 mL/kg is superior to starting with traditional V_Ts of 10–15 mL/kg. Similarly, higher positive end-expiratory pressure values (12 cm H_2O or more) are associated with decreased mortality compared with lower values of 5–12 cm H_2O. Conservative fluid therapy (titrated to lower central pressures) has been associated with decreased days on a ventilator and increased days outside the PICU.

Q. What is the benefit of HFOV in ARDS?

High frequency oscillatory ventilation may be regarded as the extreme end of lung protective spectrum. The very small V_Ts (1–3 mL/kg), allow use of a higher end-expiratory lung volume, achieving greater alveolar recruitment while avoiding damage as a result of excessive end-inspiratory lung volumes. The combination of a high continuous distending pressure with minimal pressure changes prevents the damage caused by cyclical alveolar collapse. HFOV also provides a rapid rate (up to 2,400 bpm) and an active expiratory phase, both of which decrease air trapping and maintain normal or near normal carbon dioxide levels. It is for these reasons that HFOV has a well-established position in pediatric and neonatal practice.

Q. What are the gas exchange goals in ARDS?

In terms of determining appropriate gas-exchange goals, it should be stressed that oxygenation and ventilation should have "adequate" rather than "optimal" targets. Permissive hypercapnia and permissive hypoxemia should be employed when clinically indicated, to minimize exposure to toxic ventilatory support. The target PaO_2, SpO_2, and partial pressure of carbon dioxide in arterial blood are likely to differ between patients and within an individual patient over time, based on the degree of ventilatory support the patient requires [i.e., risk of ventilator-induced lung injury (VILI)].

Q. How about an algorithmic approach?

Yes, that should be very much in place. Flowchart 1 shows a general suggested approach to the management of pediatric ARDS.

Initial management should include low-V_T ventilation, optimization of PEEP. If "adequate" oxygenation and ventilation can be obtained with a peak inspiratory pressure less than 30 cm H_2O, a mean airway pressure less than 17 cm H_2O, and an oxygenation index less than 15 cm H_2O, then a suggested approach is to continue with periodic optimization of the delivered V_T and PEEP, along with close cardio-respiratory monitoring. If those ventilation goals cannot be met, consider recruitment maneuvers and/or transitioning to HFOV or airway pressure-release ventilation.

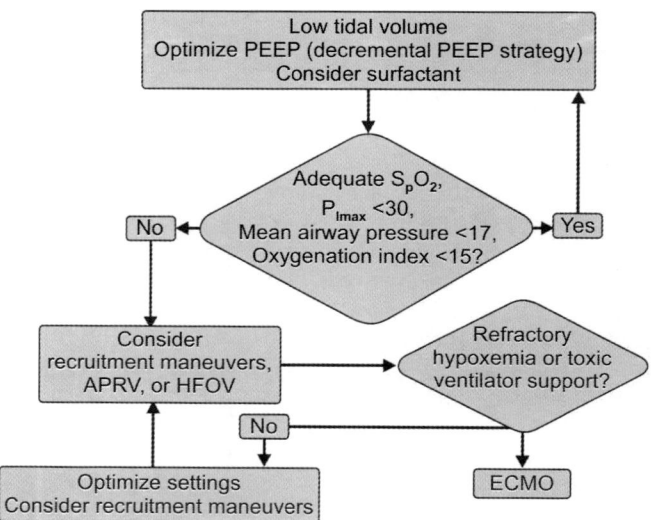

PEEP, positive end-respiratory pressure; SpO_2, oxygen saturation; P_{Imax}, maximum inspiratory pressure; APRV, airway pressure-release ventilation; HFOV, high frequency oscillatory ventilation; ECMO, extracorporeal membrane oxygenation.

Flowchart 1: Proposed algorithm for pediatric acute respiratory distress syndrome

Q. What is the overall strategy to treat ARDS?

Impeccable intensive care is the sheet anchor of ARDS treatment. Early anticipatory management may avoid late complications and poor outcome. It is important to treat the primary cause such as sepsis or pneumonia. Minimizing the risk of multiple organ dysfunction syndrome (MODS) and VILI is essential.

Also important are maintaining nutrition and being cognizant of the risk of numerous complications in critically ill children, including sepsis, fluid overload, inappropriate levels of sedation, and neuromuscular blocking agents.

Though many of the therapies and strategies proposed for ARDS are founded on rational physiologic and pathologic principles, they may not have unequivocal benefits. The contributory factors include an incomplete understanding of the pathophysiology of ARDS, the lack of a standardized diagnostic test, and the heterogeneity of the illness and the patient population.

Additionally, an inability to adequately control for other therapies, specifically ventilation modalities, and the fact that most patients die from MODS or their precipitating illness confound the analysis and interpretation of data from many trials.

Q. What is the effect of prone positioning in ARDS during ventilation?

With the prone position, pulmonary densities redistribute from the dependent lung regions, whereas in the supine position they redistribute to the dependent lung regions. Prone positioning improves V/Q matching and secretion clearance. Dependent lung units are better ventilated in the prone position. The prone position reverses alveolar inflation and ventilation distribution, due to the reverse of hydrostatic pressure overlying the lung parenchyma, reverses the pressure resulting from the weight of the heart and changes in chest wall shape and mechanical properties. On return to the supine position, the alveoli in the dorsal regions may remain open because of PEEP resulting in a persistent response.

Q. Give any role of INO in ARDS?

Inhaled nitric oxide is a selective pulmonary vasodilator with minimal systemic effects. Theoretically, INO selectively increases perfusion of ventilated lung units, reducing V/Q mismatch. For almost two decades, INO has played an essential role in the management of persistent pulmonary hypertension of the newborn. However, its use for pediatric ARDS remains controversial. Despite both pediatric and adult studies finding clear oxygenation improvement with INO, no outcome improvements are found.

Q. How about steroids in ARDS?

The anti-inflammatory and anti-fibrotic properties of corticosteroids suggest that they may have a role in modulating the course of ARDS.

However, the results of numerous trials that have evaluated the role of steroids in the treatment of ARDS have been largely disappointing and complex.

All in all, available evidence argues against the routine use of steroids in ARDS in the wake of their doubtful efficacy and their potential for causing serious adverse effects such as superimposed infection and steroid myopathy.

Q. What are the other nonventilatory strategies for ARDS in children?

Beyond the respiratory management of the pediatric acute lung injury (ALI) or ARDS patient, the clinician must consider fluid management, glucose titration, and transfusion criteria. The care of the pediatric ALI/ARDS patient clearly goes beyond pulmonary support.

Diuretics are frequently administered to pediatric ALI/ARDS patients to manage fluid status. Although no survival difference was found between conservative and liberal fluid-management strategies in adult ALI/ARDS, a conservative fluid approach increased the number of ventilator-free days and intensive care unit-free days, without more adverse effects.

Q. What is the role of nutrition in ARDS?

The importance of providing adequate nutrition early to critically ill children is well established.

Enteral nutrition is superior to and safer than parenteral nutrition and should be used whenever possible.

Despite some evidence that Omega-3 fatty acid supplementation may improve outcomes in adults with ARDS, there is no evidence to support specific dietary modifications in children.

Q. Give any role of NIV in ARDS?

Noninvasive positive pressure ventilation (NIPPV) is frequently applied in patients with clinical and radiographic evidence of lung disease, supplemented with a FiO_2 of greater than 50%.

While indicating the possible use of NIV, the necessity of immediate or early intubation must be categorically excluded before starting to think of NIPPV. The delay in intubation may expose the patient to the risk of cardiac arrest during intubation—if the patient is severely hypoxic and difficult to oxygenate prior to initiate the maneuver—and to the necessity of applying more invasive procedures for treating a worsened pathology. NIPPV can be used early in mild and in early moderate forms of ARDS.

Q. What is the role of extracorporeal membrane oxygenation (ECMO) in ARDS?

Extracorporeal membrane oxygenation can be life-saving for infants and children with refractory hypoxemia due to ARDS. The currently reported overall survival rate for ECMO for pediatric ARDS is 54%. However, recent publications have reported survival rates over 70% in relation to ECMO for pediatric and adult patients with H1N1-influenza-induced ARDS.

In the recent years, the technological advances in extracorporeal life support rival any other in the management of ARDS. These include the introduction of centrifugal pumps, hollow-fiber oxygenators, and improved double-lumen venous cannulas. Centrifugal pumps and hollow-fiber oxygenators facilitate smaller priming volume and shorter pump set-up time.

Q. What is extracorporeal carbon dioxide removal (ECCO$_2$ R) concept?

The ECCO$_2$ R concept, used as an integrated tool with conventional ventilation, is playing a new role in adjusting respiratory acidosis consequent to V_T reduction in a protective ventilation setting. The proposed advantages of ECCO$_2$ R compared to ECMO are the reduction of artificial surface contact, the avoidance of pump-related side effects and technical complications and reduced operating costs. The methodology appears interesting but requires more studies and investigation in the pediatric age.

CONCLUSION

Acute respiratory distress syndrome results from a variety of pulmonary and nonpulmonary insults. The therapy of ARDS is supportive. Low V_T is the only therapy that has consistently shown a mortality benefit and should be implemented in all cases. Mechanical ventilation should be titrated very carefully in order to avoid VILI, and potential MODS.

Acute respiratory distress syndrome is a heterogeneous syndrome that lacks definitive treatment. The cornerstone of management is sound intensive care treatment and early anticipatory ventilation support. A mechanical ventilation strategy aiming at optimal alveolar recruitment, judicious use of PEEP and low V_T remains the mainstay for managing this lung disease. Several treatments have been proposed in rescue settings, but confirmation is needed from large controlled clinical trials before they be recommended for routine care. NIV is suggested with a cautious approach and a strict selection of candidates for treatment. Mild and moderate cases can be efficiently treated by NIV, but this is contraindicated with severe ARDS.

KEY LEARNING POINTS

- Acute respiratory distress syndrome results from a variety of pulmonary and nonpulmonary insults
- The therapy of ARDS is supportive
- Low V_T is the only therapy that has consistently shown a mortality benefit and should be implemented in all cases
- Mechanical ventilation should be titrated very carefully in order to avoid VILI, and potential MODS

SUGGESTED READINGS

1. ARDS Definition Task Force, Ranieri VM, Rubenfeld GD, Thompson BT, Ferguson ND, Caldwell E, et al. Acute respiratory distress syndrome: the Berlin Definition. *JAMA.* 2012;307:2526-2533.
2. ARDS Network. Ventilation with lower tidal volumes as compared with traditional tidal volumes for acute lung injury and the acute respiratory distress syndrome. *N Engl J Med.* 2000;342:1301-1308.
3. Dellinger RP, Levy MM, Carlet JM, Bion J, Parker MM, Jaeschke R, et al. Surviving Sepsis Campaign: international guidelines for management of severe sepsis and septic shock: 2008. *Crit Care Med.* 2008;36:296-327.
4. Gómez-Caro A, Badia JR, Ausin P. Extracorporeal lung assist in severe respiratory failure and ARDS. Current situation and clinical applications. *Arch Bronconeumol.* 2010;46:531-537.
5. Kneyber MCJ, van Heerde M, Markhorst DG. Reflections on pediatric high-frequency oscillatory ventilation from a physiologic perspective. *Respir Care.* 2012;57:1496-1504.
6. Marraro GA, Chen C, Piga MA, Qian Y, Spada C, Genovese U. Acute respiratory distress syndrome in the pediatric age: an update on advanced treatment. *Zhongguo Dang Dai Er Ke Za Zhi.* 2014;16:437-447.
7. Matthay MA, Zemans RL. The acute respiratory distress syndrome: pathogenesis and treatment. *Annu Rev Pathol.* 2011;6:147-163.
8. Santschi M, Jouvet P, Leclerc F, Gauvin F, Newth CJ, Carroll CL, et al. Acute lung injury in children: therapeutic practice and feasibility of international clinical trials. *Pediatr Crit Care Med.* 2010;11:681-689.
9. Valentine SL, Sapru A, Higgerson RA, Spinella PC, Flori HR, Graham DA, et al. Fluid balance in critically ill children with acute lung injury. *Crit Care Med.* 2012;40:2883-2889.

CHAPTER 24

Acute Bronchiolitis

Suraj Gupte, Sahil Pandita, Rita Carswell

INTRODUCTION

Amongst the lower respiratory tract (LRT) infectious diseases in infants and young children, severe bronchiolitis is by and large the most common emergency during winter in particular.

Severe bronchiolitis is characterized by inflammation of bronchioles (often along with bronchi, resulting in dyspnea, usually in infants with significant morbidity and mortality. Coexistence of such conditions as cardiopulmonary disease (congenital heart diseases, chronic lung disease such as asthma or cystic fibrosis), or immunodeficiency is accompanied by enhanced risk of not only severe and prolonged illness but also complications which, if not timely treated, may prove fatal.

CASE 1

A 6-month-old infant, otherwise healthy, was brought to the emergency section with four days' history of running nose, mild cough and slight fever followed by progressively increasing breathlessness.

Physical Examination: Tachypnea with respiratory rate 64/min. Chest (intercostals) retractions; hyper-resonant and wheezy chest; liver just palpable with a span of 5 cm. Except for some dehydration and mild pallor, rest of the physical examination was normal.

Investigations: Hemoglobin 9 g/dL with microcytic hypochromic blood film. Total leukocyte count and differential leukocyte count within normal range.

Chest X-ray (CXR): Hyperinflation with areas of atelectasis.

Treatment: The infant was treated with humidified oxygen, guarded intravenous (IV) fluids and hypertonic (3%) saline nebulization.

Outcome: Response to therapy was gratifying. He was all right by third day of hospitalization and discharged as cured.

CASE REVIEW IN A NUTSHELL

The development of severe respiratory distress with chest retractions preceded by an upper respiratory infection in this 6-month-old infant raised the probability of lower respiratory infection. Since there was no history of either such attack(s) previously or asthma in any family member, diagnosis of asthma was not seriously considered.

The two major diagnoses on the card were pneumonia and bronchiolitis.

The findings of hyper-resonant percussion note suggesting hyperinflated lungs and diffuse wheeze favored the diagnosis of severe bronchiolitis. X-rays showing hyperinflated lungs and areas of atelectasis supported the clinical impression.

Response to simple measures such as humidified oxygen, guarded fluid infusion and nebulization with hypertonic saline lent further support to the clinical diagnosis of severe bronchiolitis.

INTERACTIVE TOPIC REVIEW

Q. What is the epidemiology of bronchitis?

Bronchiolitis, occurring in both epidemic and sporadic forms, develops following spread of infection by direct contact with respiratory secretions.

Globally, most cases of bronchiolitis occur during winter followed by autumn and spring. In India, cases continue to be seen in remaining seasons too though less frequently.

It occurs primarily in the first 2 years of life with peak incidence around 6 months of age.

Q. What is its etiology?

Most often, bronchiolitis is the result of viral infection. The viruses incriminated include:
- Respiratory syncytial virus (RSV)
- Adenoviruses
- Influenza viruses (A and B)
- Parainfluenza viruses
- Herpesvirus
- Enteroviruses.

Q. How about role of bacteria in etiology of bronchitis?

Bacteria such as *Mycoplasma pneumoniae*, *Pneumococcus*, *Streptococcus*, *Haemophilus influenzae*, *Haemophilus pertussis* and even allergy has been incriminated. Convincing evidence in support of this observation is yet to be available.

Q. Outline its pathology and pathophysiology?

Bronchiolitis is characterized by:
- Acute inflammation, edema, and necrosis of epithelial cells lining the bronchioles (accompanied by bronchi as well)
- Increased mucus production
- Narrowing of the small airway (bronchi) lumen.

All of them contribute to obstruction of the small airways. Duration of illness is approximately 2 weeks. Nearly 20% of patients may have symptoms lasting longer than 3 weeks.

As a rule, smaller (bronchioles) airways are predominantly involved. Increased mucus secretion, cell death, and sloughing, followed by a peribronchiolar lymphocytic infiltrate and submucosal edema is produced by infection of bronchiolar respiratory and ciliated epithelial cells. Eventually, the debris and edema produces severe narrowing and obstruction of the bronchioles.

Thereafter, decreased ventilation of portions of the lung causes ventilation or perfusion mismatching; resulting in hypoxia further dynamic narrowing of the bronchioles in expiratory phase produces disproportionate airflow decrease and resultant air trapping. Increased end-expiratory lung volume and decreased lung compliance enhances the work of breathing. Macrophages clear the debris.

Though recovery of pulmonary epithelial cells occurs after 3–4 days, cilia take some two weeks to regenerate.

Q. What are the clinical features of bronchiolitis, both "mild-moderate" and "severe"?

Typically, 4–6 days after the initial onset of symptoms of copious rhinorrhea, the infant develops dyspnea (rapid, shallow breathing), feeding difficulty and prostration. Cough, if present, is usually mild. Fever may be mild to moderate.

If dyspnea is marked, air hunger, flaring of *ala nasi*, chest retractions and cyanosis may be there. Manifestations may worsen to dehydration and respiratory acidosis.

Chest signs include retractions (intercostals, subcostal and suprasternal), hyper-resonant percussion note from emphysema, diminished breath sounds and widespread wheeze with or without some crepitations.

CHAPTER 24: Acute Bronchiolitis

Q. Can there be confusion with other conditions?

Yes, bronchiolitis needs to be differentiated from:
- *Asthma*: Frequent exacerbations
- *Bronchopneumonia*: Coarse crepitations are the dominant finding. Wheeze, if present, only mild
- *Foreign body in the airway*: History of inhalation, localized wheeze, signs of collapse or emphysema
- *Congestive cardiac failure (CCF)*: Fine crepitations with other signs of CCF
- Gastroesophageal reflux
- Congenital anomalies, such as a vascular ring or congenital heart disease.

DIAGNOSIS

A good medical history and physical examination are most important for the diagnosis of bronchiolitis.

Medical history
- Early symptoms are those of a viral upper respiratory tract infection (URI), including mild rhinorrhea, cough, and sometimes low-grade fever
- Older children and many infants do not progress beyond this stage of URI
- For the 40% of infants and young children who progress to LRT involvement, paroxysmal cough and dyspnea develop within 1–2 days.
- Additional common symptoms may be:
    - Increased work of breathing
    - Wheezing
    - Cyanosis
    - Grunting
    - Vomiting (usually post-tussive)
    - Irritability
    - Poor feeding or anorexia.

Physical examination
Following signs are usually encountered:
- Tachypnea (invariably present to variable extent)
- Tachycardia
- Some fever (usually 38–39°C)
- Cyanosis
- Otitis media
- Nasal flaring
- Mild conjunctivitis or pharyngitis
- Intercostal retractions
- Diffuse expiratory wheezing
- Inspiratory crackles
- Apnea, especially, in infants younger than 6 weeks
- Palpable liver and spleen from visceroptosis secondary to hyperinflation of the lungs and consequent depression of the diaphragm.

Q. Give any algorithmic approach to sequence of clinical events in bronchiolitis.

Flowchart 1 shows the sequence of clinical events in bronchiolitis.

Q. Give any clinical scoring system to assess the severity of bronchiolitis?

Clinical scoring systems have been developed to assess the severity of bronchiolitis. One example of clinical scoring system is the respiratory distress assessment instrument. It has undergone validation and reliability measurements. As a result, it has been shown to have good interobserver reliability (Table 1).

Q. What should be the basis of diagnosis of bronchiolitis?

The diagnosis is usually a clinical one and investigations are not generally needed to confirm it. A chest film showing hyperinflated lungs with patches of atelectasis is helpful.

Q. What should be the criteria for hospitalization?

Consider the following if the child is to be admitted:
Admission criteria:
- Apnea
- Requiring oxygen to maintain oxygen saturation more than 92% by pulse oximetry

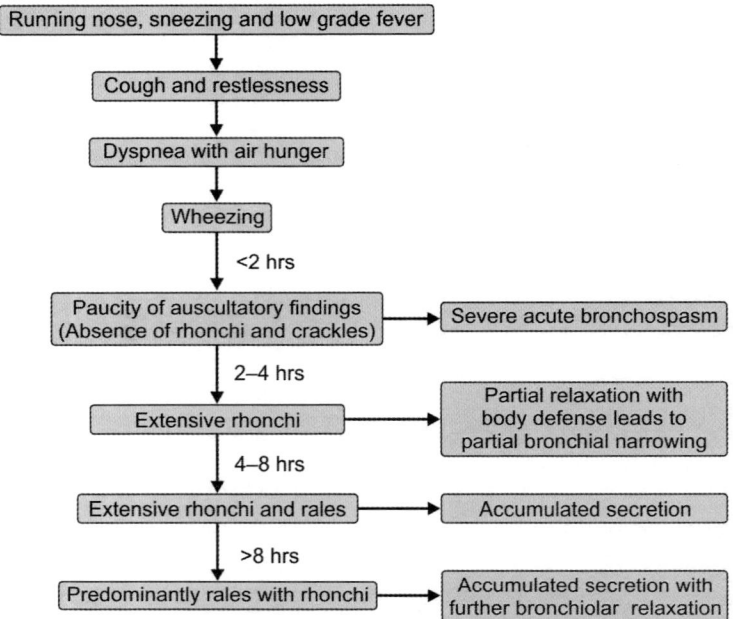

Flowchart 1: Algorithm showing sequence of events during clinical evaluation

TABLE 1: Respiratory distress assessment instrument

	Points					Maximum points
	0	1	2	3	4	
Wheezing						
Expiration	None	End	½	¾	All	4
Inspiration	None	Part	All	–	–	2
Location	None	Segmental: >2–4 lung fields	Diffuse: >3–4 lung fields	–	–	2
Retractions						
Supraclavicular	None	Mild	Moderate	Marked	–	3
Intercostal	None	Mild	Moderate	Marked	–	3
Subcostal	None	Mild	Moderate	Marked	–	3

Score 7–15 (mild), 16–30 (moderate), >30 (severe).

- Requiring support with hydration or nutrition
- CCF.

Lower threshold for admission:
- Pre-existing lung disease, congenital heart disease, neuromuscular weakness, immune-incompetence
- Age less than 6 weeks (corrected)
- Prematurity
- Family anxiety
- Re-attendance.

Q. Give any investigations.

Chest X-ray may reveal:
- Hyperinflation or emphysema
- Patchy infiltrate
- Atelectasis
- Reticular nodular pattern
- Low-lying diaphragm
- Widening of intercostal spaces.
  Arterial blood gas when saturation on pulse-oximetry is less than 92%.

Virologic tests: Rapid antigen detection tests are the most commonly used techniques in the West.

Q. What should be the therapeutic approach in severe bronchiolitis?

Though severe bronchiolitis is an emergency, management is mostly symptomatic and supportive.

Measures include:
- Humidified oxygen inhalation through face mask or head box
- Atmosphere well-saturated with water vapors
- Mild sedation
- Postural drainage and
- IV fluids to combat dehydration.

Q. Do all cases need oxygen?

Humidified oxygen is indicated when oxygen saturation is less than 94% as such or in combination with clinically significant respiratory distress.

Q. What about the bronchodilators?

Bronchodilators are better avoided. Rather than doing any good, they may increase the cardiac output and restlessness.

If opted for, preferred drug is salbutamol or racemic or levo epinephrine by nebulization.

Salbutamol (albuterol) is a selective β-2 agonists that acts by relaxing the pulmonary smooth muscle and, thereby, decreasing airway resistance. Other purative mechanisms are suppression of inflammatory mediators from mast cells, decreased microvascular permeability, and enhanced mucociliary function. Since infants have a paucity of smooth muscle, there is less likely to be benefit from albuterol inhalation.

Understandably, the paucity of smooth muscle in part may account for the very modest benefit noted in patients with bronchiolitis. The peak effect of albuterol is noted within 15 minutes with duration of effect up to 3 hours or 4 hours. The usual dose for young patients with bronchiolitis is 0.02 mL/kg (0.1 mg/kg) to 0.03 mL/kg (0.15 mg/kg) with a minimum of 0.5 mL or a single dose of 0.3 mL/kg (1.5 mg/kg). Hypoxemia has been noticed after albuterol administration, presumably because of the worsening of the ventilation perfusion mismatch. It tends to be short in duration and not of significant clinical concern.

Q. How about steroids?

Though some clinicians believe that early treatment with steroids might shorten the duration of illness, this is not well-founded. In fact, steroids are likely to do more harm than benefit to the infant with bronchiolitis.

Q. Who needs antiviral therapy?

Ribavirin may be considered in the following situations:
- Severely immunocompromised patients who develop laboratory confirmed RSV-associated bronchiolitis, such as children undergoing bone marrow transplantation
- Patients on mechanical ventilation
- Underlying congenital heart disease, cystic fibrosis and other chronic lung diseases, prematurity, very low birth weight (VLBW).

Q. Do any other therapies, including interferon, surfactant, vitamin A, mist therapy, or anticholinergics have any measurable clinical effect?

There is no convincing evidence to support these therapies in bronchiolitis.

Q. What is the role of nebulized epinephrine (adrenaline)?

Addition of adrenaline nebulization may help significantly to reduce the symptoms and the duration of hospital stay in some cases.

Q. What about antibiotic therapy?

It may be given only on the presumption of a causative or superimposed bacterial infection.

Q. What is the role of hypertonic saline nebulization?

It is strongly recommended.

Q. What is the message about bronchodilators, steroids and antibiotics?

The key take-home message is not to routinely prescribe bronchodilators, antibiotics or steroids in bronchiolitis.

Q. What is prognosis and outcome?

- The case fatality rate for bronchiolitis is highest among young infants between 1 month and 3 months of age.
- Former premature infants with birth weights less than 1,500 g have a bronchiolitis mortality rate of 30 per 100,000 live births.

The presence of underlying medical conditions, such as congenital heart disease or chronic lung disease is another important predictor of poor outcome. In these high-risk children, the case fatality rate may be as high as 5%.

Q. What are likely complications?

Short-term:
- Rapidly progressive exhaustion, anoxia and death
- Dehydration, electrolyte imbalance and acid-base imbalance, especially, respiratory acidosis
- CCF
- Bacterial superinfection: Bronchopneumonia, acute otitis media.

Long-term:
- *Bronchiolitis obliterans (BO)*: Obliteration of bronchioles by nodular masses consisting of granulation and fibrotic tissue. Over and above insult to the small airways by viruses (RSV, influenza, parainfluenza, mycoplasma and bacteria (*Haemophilus pertussis*), it may be seen in such inflammatory conditions as juvenile rheumatoid arthritis, systemic lupus erythematosus, scleroderma, Swyer-James syndrome (SJS), and inhalation of toxic fumes (NO_2, NH_3) and following lung and bone marrow transplantation (BO syndrome)
- Hyperlucent lung syndrome (SJS, Macleod syndrome).

Q. What is hyperlucent lung syndrome?

Diminished perfusion and vascular marking of the affected lung, usually following injury to the lung. The most common physical finding is hyper-resonance and small lung with mediastinal shift to the affected side.

CONCLUSION

Severe bronchitis, a common emergency in infants, needs prompt hospitalization. The mainstay of treatment is humidified oxygen along with fluid therapy and adequate nutrition, and prevention of superimposed infection such as pneumonia and heart failure. Use of bronchodilators must be restricted to very ill subjects not responding to usual line of therapy. Steroids need to be withheld. Antiviral drug, ribavirin, is strongly recommended in infants with certain underlying conditions such as cystic fibrosis and immunodeficiency.

KEY LEARNING POINTS

- Severe bronchiolitis is a common pediatric emergency responsible for hospital admissions in infants under the age of 1 year, most commonly affecting 7–12 months old infants
- RSV is the causative pathogen in a vast majority of the cases
- Respiration distress, tachypnea, wheezing, feeding difficulty and chest retractions are the most common clinical features
- As a rule, diagnosis is clinical. CXR does not aid much in diagnosis. Confirmation of diagnosis is possible by antigen testing of nasal or nasopharyngeal aspirates, viral immunofluorescence or polymerase chain reaction
- Humidified oxygen and IV fluids remain the mainstay of treatment
- Bronchodilators and antiviral drugs (ribavirin, oseltamivir) may occasionally be employed in severe cases
- Addition of adrenaline nebulization may help significantly to reduce the symptoms and the duration of hospital stay in some cases.

SUGGESTED READINGS

1. Gupta N, Puliyel A, Manchanda A, Puliyel J. Nebulized hypertonic saline vs epinephrine for bronchiolitis: Proof of concept study of cumulative sum (CUSUM) analysis. *Indian Pediatr.* 2012;49:543-547.
2. Kuzik BA, Al-Qaghi SA, Kent S, Flavin MP, Hopman W, Hotte S, et al. Nebulized hypertonic saline in the treatment of viral bronchiolitis in infants. *J Pediatr.* 2007;151:266-270.
3. Singh D, Gupte S. Pediatric pulmonology. In: Gupte S (Ed). *The Short Textbook of Pediatrics*, 12th edn. New Delhi: Jaypee Brothers Medical Publishers; 2016:321-351.
4. Singh UK, Prasad R, Ram S. Acute bronchiolitis. In: Gupte S, Gupte SB (Eds). *Recent Advances in Pediatrics (Special Vol 21: Neonatal and Pediatric Intensive Care).* New Delhi: Jaypee Brothers Medical Publishers; 2011:387-395.
5. Tal G, Cesar K, Oron A, Houri S, Ballin A, Mandelberg A. Hypertonic saline/epinephrine treatment in hospitalized infants with viral bronchiolitis reduces hospitalization stay: 2 year experience. *Isr Med Assoc J.* 2006;8:169-173.

CHAPTER 25

Pneumonia

Suraj Gupte, Shagufta Khan, Shahid Khan

INTRODUCTION

Pneumonia, inflammation of the lung parenchyma usually from infecting agents, is a leading cause of morbidity and mortality worldwide with predominance in the resource-limited countries. Pneumonia is the single most common cause of under-5 mortality, contributing 19% of all under-5 deaths globally. Nearly, 2 million under-5 deaths occur due to pneumonia; 50% of these are due to the pathogen, *Streptococcus pneumoniae*. Out of the 156 million episodes of clinical pneumonia, 43 million occur in India alone, 8.7% of these being severe and life-threatening. In low, or middle-income countries, pneumonia is responsible for 20% deaths compared to only 4.3% deaths in prosperous countries. Approximately, 50 million new cases of pneumonia occur annually among children younger than 5 years, accounting for 10–20 million hospitalizations as per other estimates.

CASE 1

A child aged 2 years and previously healthy, presented with a 2 days history of high fever (around 40°C) notwithstanding receiving regular antipyretics, cough, and rapid breathing. His vaccination status was up-to-the-mark [including *Haemophilus influenzae* type b (Hib), varicella, hepatitis A, influenza, and typhoid vaccines], except for pneumococcal vaccine.

Examination: Temperature of 39.4°C; pulse 110/min; respiration 56/min; and saturations 92% in air. Chest retractions (intercostal and subcostal) were present. Widespread diffuse crepitations with some rhonchi were present bilaterally.

Provisional diagnosis: Bronchopneumonia.

Investigations: Complete blood picture, hemoglobin 9.2 g/dL; microcytic hypochromic picture, total leukocyte count 12,500/mm^3; differential leukocyte count polys 70%; lymphs 23%; eosinophils 4%; monos 2%; and basophil 1%.

Chest X-ray (CXR): Bilateral diffuse parenchymal opacities both lungs.

Treatment: He was started on intravenous co-amoxiclav along with symptomatic measures including paracetamol. His temperature continued to fluctuate over the next 3 days when he began responding with improvement in cough and breathing, and chest retractions.

He was discharged after 7 days when the CXR showed complete recovery and he was asymptomatic except for a mild cough.

CASE REVIEW IN A NUTSHELL

The presentation of this 2-year-old child with fever, cough, breathlessness, and chest retractions suggested diagnosis of lower respiratory tract infection. Diffuse coarse crepitations along with some rhonchi heard bilaterally suggested diagnosis of broncho-pneumonia. This diagnosis was established radiologically. In view of good chances of the bronchopneumonia being the result of *Streptococcus pneumoniae*, institution of co-amoxiclav was well founded. Amoxicillin also covers Hib infection though that was less likely in this child in view of his having received Hib vaccine on recommended lines.

INTERACTIVE TOPIC REVIEW

Q. What is pneumonia?

The term, pneumonia, refers to infection of the lung parenchyma, which may be primary or secondary to acute bronchitis and/or bronchiolitis complicating an upper respiratory tract infection.

Q. How is pneumonia classified?

Classification of pneumonia is described in box 1.

BOX 1: Classification of pneumonia

I. Etiologic classification
- Bacterial: *Streptococcus pneumoniae* (Pneumococcus), *Staphylococcus, H. influenzae, Escherichia coli, Klebsiella, Hemophilus Pertussis, Mycobacterium tuberculosis*
- Viral: Respiratory syncytial virus, influenza, parainfluenza, adenoviruses, measles, and chickenpox
- Atypical organisms: *Chlamydia, Mycoplasma pneumoniae* spp
- Fungal: *Pneumocystis carinii* (*Pneumocystis jiroveci*), thrush, coccidioidomycosis, histoplasmosis, blastomycosis (usually in immunocompromised subjects)
- Protozoal: *Toxoplasma gondii, Entamoeba histolytica*
- Rickettsial: Typhus + Rocky mountain spotted fever
- Miscellaneous: Aspiration pneumonia (vomitus, amniotic fluid in newborn, drowning, foreign body, chemicals like kerosene oil and liquid paraffin, instilled oil in nose); Loeffler pneumonia; hypostatic pneumonia; ventilator associated pneumonia

II. Anatomic classification
- Bronchopneumonia: Patchy involvement of lungs

Continued

Continued
- Lobar pneumonia: One or more lobes of lung involved
- Interstitial pneumonia/pneumonitis: Alveoli or interstitial tissue between them affected. It is more or less a radiologic diagnosis

III. Classification based on acquisition
- Congenital pneumonia
- Community acquired pneumonia
- Hospital acquired pneumonia

IV. Classification based on chronicity
- Acute pneumonia
- Recurrent pneumonia
- Chronic (persistent) pneumonia

V. World Health Organization classification
- Very severe pneumonia
- Severe pneumonia
- Pneumonia (not severe)
- No pneumonia

Q. What are the definitions of various terms associated with pneumonia?

The definitions of various terms associated with pneumonia are given in box 2.

BOX 2: Certain definitions

- Congenital pneumonia: A pneumonia in which the neonate presents right at birth as a result of hematogenous or ascending infection or aspiration
- Persistent pneumonia: Chronic nonresolving pneumonia in which radiological findings persist for over 1 month
- Recurrent pneumonia: Two or more episodes in 1 year, provided that the earlier episode showed complete resolution with adequate therapy or three or more episodes any time in life
- Community acquired pneumonia: A pneumonia caused by pathogens outside the hospital settings, i.e., in the community per second
- Hospital acquired pneumonia: A pneumonia that develops during hospital stay, at least after 48 hours of admission and not incubating at the time of admission to the facility. It includes ventilator associated pneumonia, postoperative pneumonia, and healthcare associated pneumonia

Q. Is it true that pneumococcal pneumonia accounts for 80–90% of bacterial pneumonias in childhood?

Yes, after 3 years of life, it is responsible for a vast majority of bacterial pneumonias.

Q. What about the relationship between age group and etiological pathogens?

- In neonates and up to 2 months of age: Gram-negative organisms (*E. coli, Klebsiella, Pseudomonas, Proteus*); *Staphylococcus*
- From 2 or 3 months to 3 years: *H. influenzae, S. pneumoniae*; *Staphylococcus* in special situations
- More than 3 years: Invariably pneumococcus
- Staphylococcal pneumonia occurs in neonatal period but may occur at any age in special situations.

Q. What are the predisposing factors for recurrent and chronic (persistent) pneumonia?

Predisposing factors of chronic pneumonia have been described in box 3.

Q. What are the clinical features of pneumonia?

- Most cases have a sudden onset with fever, chills, cough, and breathless. Active movements of alae nasi, grunting respiration, and chest (intercostal) retractions with some cyanosis are alarming manifestations. In some cases, diarrhea, vomiting convulsions, and chest pain (referred to abdomen) may be present
- Chest signs of consolidation include diminished movements of affected side, increased vocal fremitus and resonance, dullness, diminished breath sounds, and bronchial breathing. Crepitations denote beginning of resolution. There is no shifting of mediastinum
- Chest signs of bronchopneumonia include tachypnea, normal or harsh breath sounds, and diffuse harsh crepitations spread all over both lungs
- Chest signs of lobar pneumonia include dullness of percussion note and bronchial breathing over the affecter lobe. With resolution in subsequent days, bronchial breathing gives way to coarse crepitations.

Q. What are World Health Organization recommendations for identifying pneumonia by the health workers?

World Health Organization recommended that very fast breathing, especially in association with cough, difficult breathing, or indrawing of chest must always be considered a reflection of pneumonia, unless proved otherwise. Fever undoubtedly causes elevation in respiratory rate. But, the effect is only weak say 2–3 breaths per 1°C rise above 37°C/min. The cutoff point for high respiratory rate is over 60/min up to 2 months of age, over 50/min between 2 and 12 months, and 40/min between 12 months and 5 years.

Q. In which situations, particular signs and symptoms may not suggest pneumonia though, in fact, it is present?

In debilitated infants and children, despite the presence of extensive pneumonia, signs and symptoms may not be as classical as described above. The diagnosis of pneumonia in such cases is often made following detailed examination and a chest radiograph.

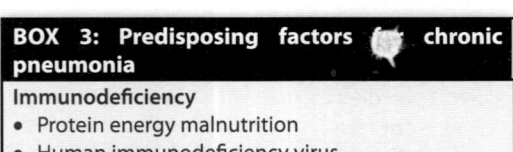

BOX 3: Predisposing factors for chronic pneumonia

Immunodeficiency
- Protein energy malnutrition
- Human immunodeficiency virus

Congenital respiratory malformations
- Tracheoesophageal fistula
- Gastroesophageal reflux

Congenital heart disease
- Ventricular septal defect

Defective clearance of airway secretions
- Cystic fibrosis

Chronic pulmonary diseases
- Tuberculosis
- Bronchiectasis
- Asthma

Q. What are predisposing factors for staphylococcal pneumonia?

Presence of certain predisposing factors (Box 4) should arouse suspicion for staphylococcal pneumonia.

> **BOX 4: Predisposing factors for staphylococcal pneumonia**
> - Infectious diseases of childhood such as measles and chickenpox
> - Staphylococcal infections elsewhere in the body, e.g., skin (furunculosis), throat, etc.
> - Debilitating illnesses, e.g., advanced protein energy malnutrition, cystic fibrosis, malignancies, etc.
> - Hypogammaglobulinemia
> - Immunosuppressive therapy

Q. What are complications of pneumonia?

- Pleural effusion
- Collapse
- Pneumatocele
- Lung abscess
- Bronchiectasis
- Subcutaneous emphysema
- Metastatic spread: Meningitis, septic arthritis, osteomyelitis, etc. of the various types, staphylococcal pneumonia carries the worst prognosis.

Q. What about diagnosis of pneumonia?

- Besides clinical suspicion a CXR (postero-anterior view, ordinarily) is most reliable to detect the type and extent of lesions. Chest X-ray findings suggesting bronchopneumonia include multitude of diffuse patchy consolidations, usually involving both lungs
- Chest X-ray findings suggesting lobar pneumonia (consolidation) include a homogeneous opacity occupying the anatomic area of a lobe without any mediastinal shift, usually involving only one lung
- Detection of pleural effusion, pyopneumothorax, or pneumatoceles (small inflated abscesses) highly favors the diagnosis of staphylococcal pneumonia
- Nonradiopaque foreign bodies may produce multiple abscesses or pneumatoceles, resulting in a radiologic picture simulating that seen in staphylococcal pneumonia. Miliary mottling constitutes another important differential diagnosis.

Recently, lung ultrasonography has been recommended as a more accurate modality for detecting pneumonia in situation where CXR fails to show highly suspected pneumonia.

Q. What conditions need to be borne in mind in case of recurrent or persistent pneumonia?

- Abnormalities of antibody production such as agammaglobulinemia
- Cystic fibrosis
- Cleft palate
- Congenital bronchiectasis
- Immotile cilia syndrome
- Tracheoesophageal fistula
- Gastroesophageal reflux disease
- Increased pulmonary blood flow
- Deficient gag reflex
- Foreign body
- Tuberculosis
- Abnormalities of polymorphonuclear leukocytes
- Neutropenia

Q. What should be therapeutic approach of treatment?

Once the diagnosis of pneumonia is arrived at, it should be decided whether the child needs just outpatient treatment or hospitalization (Box 5). Most children suffering from viral pneumonia have mild illness. They may be treated as outpatients.

Antibiotics in community acquired pneumonia

A specific antibiotic agent is dictated by the anticipated causative agent rather than the anatomic type of pneumonia (Box 6).

> **BOX 5: Indications for hospitalization in pneumonia**
> - Child is sick enough, manifesting features of hypoxia (respiratory distress, cyanosis, restlessness, and seizures)
> - High risk factors
>   - Immunodeficiency
>   - Cystic fibrosis
>   - Congenital heart disease, etc.
> - Poor response to treatment provided as an outpatient

> **BOX 6: Antimicrobials in hospital acquired pneumonia**
> - Pathogen antimicrobial: Gram-negative bacilli aminoglycosides (gentamicin, amikacin, netilmicin)
> - *Klebsiella*: Third generation cephalosporins
> - *Pseudomonas aeroginosa*: Ticarcillin + clavulanic acid, ceftazidime, quinolones
> - *Staphylococcus aureus*: Vancomycin, cloxacillin, quinolones, cefazolin
> - Hospital acquired pneumonias: Here, the recommended antimicrobials again vary with the likely pathogens
> - Response to appropriate antibiotics is as a rule gratifying
> - Poor response should arose the possibility of an underlying pathology that may be congenital or acquired
> - Neonatal pneumonia: Generally speaking, pneumonia in the first week of life is best treated with ampicillin plus an aminoglycoside or cefotaxime; pneumonia after first week may well be nosocomial with vancomycin or a third generation cephalosporin. In case of *Pseudomonas aeruginosa*, ceftazidime or ticarcillin plus an aminoglycoside is a good choice
> - Persistent/recurrent/chronic pneumonia: Therapy is addressed to treatment of superimposed infection plus correction of the underlying condition
> - General measures
>   These comprise:
>   - Good nursing care
>   - Bed rest
>   - Suction
>   - Oxygen
>   - Symptomatic treatment for cough, fever and pain fluid and dietary intake
>   - Treatment of congestive cardiac failure, if present
>   - Physiotherapy, especially breathing exercise during convalescence
>   - Surgical intervention in such children who develop complications like emphysema, tension pneumothorax, (common in *Staphylococcus pneumonia*), etc.

Pneumococcal pneumonia

Penicillin is the drug of choice for pneumococcal pneumonia (*Streptococcus pneumoniae* pneumonia) which is the usual pneumonia encountered in children beyond 1 year of age. In uncomplicated cases, it leads to dramatic response, causing complete resolution in 7–14 days.

In case of penicillin hypersensitivity, amoxicillin or a cephalosporin like cefazolin make an appropriate alternative agent in sensitive strain.

Emergence of multidrug resistant strains of *Streptococcus pneumoniae* (that causes not only pneumonia but also acute otitis media, acute sinusitis, acute bronchitis, etc.) fails to respond to penicillin and other β-lactams and non-β-lactams including cephalosporin. In such a situation, it is advisable to consider use of a β-lactamase inhibitor along with a β-lactam say amoxicillin-clavulanate (co-amoxiclav) or ampicillin-sulbactam for a gratifying outcome.

Staphylococcal pneumonia

A penicillinase-resistant penicillin (cloxacillin) plus ampicillin is the best choice. Alternatively, vancomycin or clindamycin may be employed.

Haemophilus influenzae

Ampicillin and amoxicillin/co-amoxiclav are good enough for mild disease.
For severe illness, choices are:
- Ampicillin plus chloramphenicol or ceftriaxone
- Cefotaxime or ceftriaxone.

Gram-negative organisms

Klebsiella—A combination of cefatoxime or ceftriaxone plus an aminoglycoside (amikacin, netilmicin, gentamicin, etc.) is the therapy of choice.

Pseudomonas pneumonia

Treatment of choice is ceftazidime, piperacillin, or ticarcillin alone or in combination with gentamicin or amikacin.

Pneumocystis carinii (jiroveci) pneumonia (interstitial plasma cell pneumonia)
Cotrimoxazole in very high doses (20 mg/kg/day with reference to trimethoprim).

Thrush pneumonia (pulmonary candidiasis)

Only amphotericin B or 5-fluorocytosine.

Tuberculous pneumonia

Antituberculous therapy (ATT) which is discussed later in the chapter.

Viral pneumonia

- Respiratory syncytial virus: Ribavirin aerosolization
- Influenza virus: Oseltamivir, peramivir

Loeffler pneumonia (Loeffler syndrome)

No antibiotic; only symptomatic treatment.

Mycoplasma pneumoniae (Primary atypical pneumonia)

Erythromycin or tetracyclines in case of grown-up children (>8 years).

Aspiration pneumonia

Use of prophylactic antibiotics is usually recommended.

Needless to say, these recommendations are subject to changes, which may be warranted following receipt of culture and sensitivity report.

Antibiotics in hospital acquired pneumonia

Recommended drugs vary with the likely pathogen(s):
- Gram-negative bacilli: Generally, aminoglycosides (amikacin, netilmicin, and gentamicin)
- *Klebsiella:* Third generation cephalosporin
- *Pseudomonas aeruginosa*: Piperacillin with tazobactam, ticarcillin with clavulanate, ceftazidime, or quinolones
- *S. aureus*: Vancomycin or cloxacillin; quinolones, and cefazolin are good alternatives
- Anaerobes: Metronidazole and clindamycin.

General measures

- Good nursing care
- Bed rest
- Suction to remove secretions from tracheobronchial tree
- Oxygen
- Symptomatic treatment for cough, restlessness, fever, and pain
- Adequate fluid and dietary intake
- Physiotherapy: Breathing exercise during recovery is of value.

Treatment of complications

- Treatment of congestive cardiac failure (CCF), if present
- Surgical intervention may be needed in subjects who have developed complications like empyema or tension pneumothorax, a fairly common occurrence in staphylococcal pneumonia.

Finally, a word of caution. The widespread practice of employing sodium bicarbonate in cases of tachypnea (unless accompanied by documented metabolic acidosis) must be discouraged. Such an administration may prove counterproductive by causing respiratory alkalosis.

Q. How is the prognosis?

Prognosis is generally good following appropriate and in-time treatment.

Q. Is it true that younger children may present with no clinical signs and symptoms of pneumonia?

Yes, in younger children, presentation may mimic a different pathological process and clinical signs on chest auscultation may be absent, leading to a delayed diagnosis. A CXR is of value in such a situation.

Q. When should complication of pleural effusion be suspected?

Pneumonia showing poor response to antibiotics with raised inflammatory markers and a persistent fever should raise the suspicion of a pleural effusion.

Q. What are the four stages of lobar pneumonia?

First stage (congestion)

Occurring within 24 hours of infection, the lung is characterized microscopically by vascular congestion and alveolar edema. Many bacteria and few neutrophils are present.

Second stage (red hepatization)

The stage of red hepatization (2–3 days) is characterized by the presence of many erythrocytes, neutrophils, desquamated epithelial cells, and fibrin within the alveoli.

Third stage (gray hepatization)

In the stage of gray hepatization (2–3 days), the lung is gray-brown to yellow because of fibrinopurulent exudate, disintegration of red cells, and hemosiderin.

Fourth stage (resolution)

Finally comes the stage of resolution, characterized by resorption alveolar exudates, phagocytosis, or coughing out of the residual debris followed by restoration of the architecture of the affected lung lobe. Fibrinous inflammation may extend into the pleural space, causing a rub heard by auscultation. Resolution or organization with pleural adhesions may follow.

Q. What is special about neonatal pneumonia?

Diagnosis of pneumonia in a newborn is usually presumptive, most cases showing bilateral alveolar densities followed by extensive, dense bilateral changes with numerous air bronchograms.

Q. What is differential diagnosis?
- Other causes of lower respiratory tract infection (bronchiolitis, bronchitis)
- Nonradiopaque foreign bodies, which may produce multiple abscesses or pneumatoceles, resulting in a radiologic picture simulating that seen in staphylococcal pneumonia, miliary mottling of hematogenous tuberculosis, and tropical eosinophilia
- Rarely, histoplasmosis and sarcoidosis may also be confused with radiographic picture of staphylococcal pneumonia.

Q. What are the poor prognostic signs?

Poor prognostic signs include:
- Poor nutritional status
- Young age
- Bilateral disease
- Such underlying diseases as cystic fibrosis, immunodeficiency, asthma, and malignancy
- Complications like CCF and respiratory failure.

Very young children who develop pneumonia and survive are at risk for developing lung problems in adulthood, including chronic obstructive pulmonary disease.

Q. What is the best preventive strategy?

In addition to pneumococcal vaccine improved maternal and child healthcare, other health promotional activities in vulnerable areas, health education to sensitize young parents for early recognition of pneumonia and need to consult health providers, are critical for cutting down morbidity and mortality from pneumonia. Ever since 2009, 12th November is being observed as World Pneumonia Day. The goal is to save the lives of millions of children around the world through public education measures about the illness, raising awareness about it among healthcare providers, and advocacy for more funding.

CONCLUSION

Pneumonia, a leading cause of hospitalization and death especially in the resource limited countries, is usually of viral etiology with subtle manifestations and may be treated in the outpatient. Sick children with pneumonia, especially with hypoxic manifestations, need hospitalization. Choice of antibiotic(s) in bacterial pneumonia is dictated by the likely etiologic pathogen, which varies in different age groups and also whether the pneumonia is community acquired or hospital acquired. A pneumonia that persists, despite adequate therapy beyond a month should be labeled "persistent pneumonia"; a radiologically proved pneumonia occurring two times in 1 year or three or more times at any time in life should be considered "recurrent pneumonia". Exclusive breastfeeding for a minimum of 6 months considerably protects the infant from pneumonia and several other infections. Over and above the routine vaccination, immunization with conjugate pneumococcal vaccine can go a long way in preventing pneumococcal pneumonia.

KEY LEARNING POINTS

- Pneumonia, is usually of viral etiology with subtle manifestations, may be treated in the outpatient
- Children with pneumonia with hypoxic manifestations need hospitalization
- At times, radiological pneumonia may occur without clinical signs
- In case of bacterial pneumonia, choice of antibiotic(s) is dictated by the likely etiologic pathogen, which varies in different age groups and also whether the pneumonia is community acquired or hospital acquired
- Though a large majority of the bacterial pneumonias after 6 months of age is secondary to *Streptococcus pneumoniae* infection, pneumonia in a neonate is most likely to be due to Gram-negative pathogens, group B streptococcus, or *Staphylococcus aureus*
- A pneumonia that persists despite adequate therapy after 1 month should be labeled "persistent pneumonia"; a radiologically proved pneumonia occurring at least twice in 1 year or more than 3 times at any time in life should be considered "recurrent pneumonia"
- Exclusive breastfeeding for a minimum of 6 months protects the infant from pneumonia and several other infections

SUGGESTED READINGS

1. American Society of Infectious Diseases. Guidelines for the diagnosis of community-acquired pneumonia in pediatric patients. [online] Available at: http://www.infectiousdiseasenews.com/mobileArticle.aspx?id=78027. Accessed on: 20 June, 2016.
2. Anderson E. Pediatric pneumonia: Issues in diagnostic evaluation. *Pediatr Diagn Therap.* 2010;11:324-332.
3. Bradley J. 2010. Community-acquired pneumonia in infants and children. Presented at: the 23rd Annual Infectious Diseases in Children Symposium; 20-21 November, 2010; New York City. [online] Available at: http://www.infectiousdiseasenews.com/mobileArticle.aspx?id=78027. Accessed on: 22 June, 2016.
4. Centers for Disease Control and Prevention (CDC). Criteria for defining nosocomial pneumonia. [online] Available at: http//www. Cdc.at:gov/ncidod/hip/NNIS/members/pneumonia/final/PneuCriteriaFinal.pdf. Accessed on: 12 December, 2016.
5. Gupte S, Gourinath K. Pneumonia. In: Gupte S, Gupte N (Eds): *Pediatric Infectious Diseases.* Gurgaon (NCR): Macmllan; 2011:324-335.
6. Kalra A, Agarwal S. Hospital acquired pneumonia. In: Gupte S, Sobti P (Eds): *Recent Advances in Pediatrics-18: Hot Topics.* New Delhi: Jaypee Brothers Medical Publishers; 2009:292-299.
7. Vishnu Bhat B, Rathi Sharmila R. Pneumonia. In: Gupte S, Gupte SB, (Eds): *Recent Advances in Pediatrics (Special Vol 21: Neonatal and Pediatric Intensive Care).* New Delhi: Jaypee Brothers Medical Publishers; 2011:397-412.
8. World Health Organization. Top Ten Causes of Death 2008. Geneva: WHO 2008. [online] Available at: http://www.who.int/mediacenter/factsheats/fr310/en/index.html. Accessed on: 12 December, 2016.

Acute Severe Asthma

CHAPTER 26

Abhilasha Singh, Anjul Dayal

INTRODUCTION

Asthma is a disease of the respiratory tract characterized by recurrent and/or chronic episodes of airway inflammation and obstruction (manifested by wheeze or cough, or demonstrated upon pulmonary function testing) and evidence of reversibility of obstruction. Despite advances in the understanding of asthma and development of effective medical interventions to prevent morbidity and improve quality of life, asthma remains a burden in prevalence, healthcare use, and mortality. Prevalence in children continues to show an increasing trend with reported rates between 8.5 and 8.9%. Asthma is most prevalent in children aging 5–14 years.

Asthma is one of the most common chronic diseases in childhood, with increasing prevalence in the past three decades. Severe acute asthma is currently the most common medical emergency in children and is responsible for nearly half a million admissions to the pediatric intensive care unit (PICU) each year.

The terms employed for severe acute asthma exacerbation in the literature include status asthmaticus, near-fatal asthma, sudden asphyxic asthma, and acute fatal asthma. The term, status asthmaticus, refers to an acute asthma exacerbation in which bronchial obstruction is severe and continues to worsen or not improve despite the institution of adequate standard therapy, leading to respiratory failure.

Near-fatal asthma is described as an asthma exacerbation of sudden onset that rapidly progresses to hypercapnia and hypoxemia, leading to respiratory arrest.

A prompt initiation of treatment and continuous monitoring to optimize the therapy helps in better outcome. A number of adjuvant therapies apart from β-agonists and steroids are available and role of noninvasive ventilation (NIV) is increasing being explored in the treatment algorithm of severe asthma.

CASE 1

A 5-year-old girl, a known asthmatic for the past 3 years, presented to the emergency department (ED) with a 2-day history of worsening breathlessness and cough. There was no fever, expectoration, or chest pain. On examination, the patient was conscious and afebrile. She was diaphoretic and could not speak in complete sentences. Pulse rate was 126 beats/min and blood pressure was 90/44 mmHg. Respiratory rate was 70 breaths/min with accessory muscles of respiration in use. Chest auscultation revealed bilateral inspiratory and expiratory wheeze. The remaining physical examination was unremarkable. Oxygen saturation (SpO_2) was 88% by pulse oximetry. Supplemental oxygen, nebulized salbutamol and ipratropium, intravenous (IV) methyl prednisolone, were administered. After 30 minutes of medical treatment, there was no clinical improvement, so the patient was given magnesium sulfate as infusion and she was also started on theophylline infusion. Her arterial blood gas (ABG) showed pH 7.45, partial pressure of oxygen (PaO_2) 90, partial pressure of carbon dioxide ($PaCO_2$) 65, bicarbonate (HCO_3) 26 mEq/L. As there was no improvement, she was started on NIV. An arterial line was placed through the right radial artery. Serum electrolytes, renal and liver function tests, and complete blood counts were normal. On NIV, she had decrease in her wheeze but associated with worsening dyspnea and falling saturation. As the patient was not improving on NIV and was becoming hypoxemic and agitated, she was given ketamine, and oral endotracheal intubation was performed. She was mechanically ventilated with assist or control mode at tidal volumes of 200 mL, rate of 18 and positive end-expiratory pressure (PEEP) of 5 mmH_2O. There was no auto-PEEP and her peak and plateau pressures were within normal limits. She was sedated intermittently with IV midazolam. Other medications and supportive medical care were continued. Arterial blood gases measured after 2 hours of mechanical ventilation were normal [pH 7.48, PaO_2 120, $PaCO_2$ 44, HCO_3 26 mEq/L, fraction of inspired oxygen (FiO_2) 0.3]. She improved with above management and was extubated after 48 hours.

CASE REVIEW IN A NUTSHELL

This child with exacerbation of asthma was breathless and not able to speak in sentences. A prompt treatment with salbutamol, ipratropium, and steroids was started. Arterial blood gas showed hypercapnia. Since that is not the indication for mechanical ventilation, she was started on the adjuvant therapy with magnesium and theophylline. Magnesium sulfate can produce hypotension. Thus, the child was hydrated with saline before starting magnesium. Noninvasive ventilation, a good modality in severe asthma, was started. Worsening of dyspnea with decreasing wheeze is a. ominous sign and denotes life-threatening asthma. Mechanical ventilation, though it should be avoided as far as possible, may be used in life-threatening asthma. Gentle ventilation allowing permissive hypercapnia and avoiding generation of auto PEEP should be goal of mechanical ventilation. The child was intermittently sedated to avoid dyssynchrony. She was monitored very closely in PICU with keeping a close watch on plateau pressure. Mechanical ventilation was managed well and the child was extubated successfully with resolution of the severe spasm.

INTERACTIVE TOPIC REVIEW

Q. What is the pathophysiology of asthma?

Fundamental to the pathophysiology of asthma is are an inflammation and edema of the bronchial mucosa, increased mucus production with airway plugging, and bronchospasm.

All these factors produce increased airway resistance, leading to increased work of breathing. With worsening of the degree of airway obstruction, expiration becomes active and inspiration starts before termination of the previous expiration, resulting in air trapping and hyperinflation.

Ventilation or perfusion mismatch results from areas of obstruction and premature airway closure, leading to hypoxemia.

In a severe asthma exacerbation, the marked changes in lung volume and pleural pressures have a significant impact on cardiopulmonary interactions. Dynamic hyperinflation with progressive increased lung volumes stretches the pulmonary vasculature, increasing pulmonary vascular resistance and right ventricular after load.

The pulmonary vasoconstriction, secondary to hypoxia and acidosis, further contributes to the increase in right ventricular afterload. The high negative pulmonary pressure generated during inspiration in children with a spontaneous breathing, causes an increased left ventricular afterload and decreased cardiac output with exaggerated decrease in systolic blood pressure during inspiration. A fall in systolic blood pressure by more than 10 mmHg during inspiration is termed pulsus paradoxus. The negative intrapleural pressure favors transcapillary fluid edema to the alveolar space.

Q. How to assess the child in emergency department?

Assessing the child in respiratory distress from an acute asthma attack: Effective treatment depends on an accurate and rapid assessment of disease severity upon presentation. Asthma severity is classified according to the presenting features (Table 1).

Clinical assessment needs to focus on the areas detailed in box 1.

Investigations may be needed in certain situations:
- Chest X-ray is usually not needed unless the clinician suspects complications (say, pneumothorax, bacterial pneumonia), the presence of a foreign body or failure to respond to maximized conventional treatment
- Blood gases are not routinely required unless there is no clinical improvement with maximal aggressive therapy. Notably, a normal capillary carbon dioxide level not withstanding persistent respiratory distress points to an impending respiratory failure.

Q. How to monitor such a child admitted in pediatric intensive care unit?

Patients admitted to the PICU require IV access, as well as continuous monitoring of their cardiorespiratory status, including noninvasive blood pressure and SpO_2. Those with respiratory failure requiring mechanical ventilation should undergo the placement of central venous,

TABLE 1: Classification of asthma severity

Moderate	Severe	Impending respiratory failure	Clinical feature	Mild
Might look agitated	Usually agitated	Drowsy or confused	Mental status	Normal
Decreased activity or feeding (infant)	Decreased activity, infant stops feeding	Unable to eat	Activity	Normal activity and exertional dyspnea
Speaks in phrases	Speaks in words	Unable to speak	Speech	Normal
Intercostal and substernal retractions	Significant respiratory distress. Usually all accessory muscles involved, and may display nasal flaring and paradoxical thoraco-abdominal movement	Marked respiratory distress at rest. All accessory muscles involved, including nasal flaring and paradoxical thoraco-abdominal movement	Work of breathing	Minimal intercostal retractions
Loud pan-expiratory and inspiratory wheeze	Wheezes might be audible without stethoscope	The chest is silent (absence of wheeze)	Chest auscultation	Moderate wheeze
91–94%	–	<90%	Oxygen saturation on room air	>94%
60–80%	best <60%	Unable to perform the task	Peak flow vs. personal best	>80%

Note: Definitions are not absolute and can overlap.

> **BOX 1: Clinical assessment**
> - Signs and symptoms of respiratory distress and airway obstruction, including clinical documentation of vital signs. Pulse oximetry should be used in all patients. Pulsed SpO_2 of 92% or less on presentation (before oxygen or bronchodilator treatment) is associated with higher morbidity and greater risk for hospitalization
> - A focused medical history recording previous medications and risk factors for ICU admission and death:
>   - Previous life-threatening events,
>   - Admissions to ICU
>   - Intubation
>   - Deterioration while already on systemic steroids
> - A focused physical examination to estimate the functional severity of airway obstruction, documenting the use of accessory muscles, air entry in both lungs and wheezing, level of alertness, ability to speak in full sentences, and activity level. A silent chest is an ominous sign that there is not enough gas exchange and a warning that respiratory failure is imminent. Mental agitation, drowsiness, and confusion are clinical features of cerebral hypoxemia and should be considered signs of extreme severity
> - When children are able to perform the task, spirometry is an objective measure of airway obstruction. Spirometry is difficult to perform in children younger than 6 years of age and/or during an exacerbation. Peak flow meters may be more readily available but are a less sensitive measure of airway obstruction and may be unreliable, especially in children younger than 10 years of age. Peak flows should be compared to readily available normal values or, if known, the child's "personal best"
>
> ICU, intensive care unit; SpO_2, oxygen saturation

arterial, and urinary bladder catheters. These are often the sickest patients in the PICU and require expert nursing care, monitoring of fluid intake and output, and skin care to prevent decubitus ulcers, as well as frequent clinical examination.

Q. What is the role of oxygen?

Children with severe acute asthma possibly will have ventilation or perfusion mismatch as an effect of mucus plugging and atelectasis, causing hypoxemia. Treatment with β-agonists may aggravate hypoxemia by increasing cardiac output and eliminating the compensatory hypoxic pulmonary vasoconstriction. Oxygen should be used as carrier gas for intermittent or continuous nebulization and to keep SpO_2 above 92%. There is no evidence that oxygen suppresses respiratory drive in children with severe asthma.

Q. What is the role of short-acting inhaled beta-2 agonists?

It is recommended that salbutamol be administered as the drug of choice for rapid reversal of airflow obstruction. Modify therapy based on the early clinical response to treatments. Salbutamol treatments given every 10–20 minutes for a total of 3 doses can be given safely as initial therapy. The dosages are given in table 2.

Q. What is the role of oral or intravenous corticosteroids?

Children who have a moderate-to-severe asthma exacerbation should receive systemic steroids as part of their initial treatment. This medication should be administered as early in the ED visit as feasible. Steroids may reduce the need for hospitalization and the risk of relapse after initial treatment, and may also facilitate an earlier discharge from the hospital. The recommended doses of corticosteroids are listed in table 3. Children with severe asthma or impending respiratory failure should receive IV steroids. The drugs of choice are methylprednisolone and hydrocortisone.

Table 2 presents the drugs with dosage of aerosolized therapy and table 3 recommended steroids with dosage.

Stepwise approach is given in table 4.

TABLE 2: Aerosolized therapies—drugs and dosage recommendations aerosolized therapies

Medication (formulation)	Child dose	Adolescent dose	Notes
Inhaled short-acting β-2-agonists			
Salbutamol			
Nebulizer solution (2.5 mg/3mL, 5 mg/mL)	2.5–5 mg every 20 min for 3 doses, then 2.5–5 mg every 1–4 h as needed 0.5 mg/kg/h by continuous nebulization <30 kg: 2.5 mg ≥30 kg: 5 mg	2.5–5 mg every 20 min for 3 doses, then 2.5–10 mg every 1–4 h as needed, or 10–15 mg/h continuously	For optimal delivery, dilute aerosols to minimum of 3 mL NS at gas flow of 6–8 L/min. Use large volume nebulizers for continuous administration. May mix with ipratropium nebulizer solution
MDI (90 μg/puff)	6 puffs (range: 4–8 puffs) every 20 min for 3 doses, then every 1–4 h as needed	6 puffs (range: 4–8 puffs) every 20 min up to 4 h, then every 1–4 h as needed	In mild-to-moderate exacerbations, is as effective as nebulized therapy with appropriate administration technique. Add mask in children unable to manage an MDI device
Levosalbutamol Nebulizer solution (0.31 mg/3 mL, 0.63 mg/3 mL, 1.25 mg/0.5mL, 1.25 mg/3 mL)	0.075 mg/kg (minimum dose 1.25 mg) every 20 min for 3 doses, then 0.075-0.15 mg/kg (not to exceed 2.5 mg) every 1-4 h as needed	1.25– 2.5 mg every 20 min for 3 doses, then 1.25–5 mg every 1-4 h as needed	
MDI (45 μg/puff)	See salbutamol MDI dose above	See salbutamol MDI dose Above	
Anticholinergics in combination with short-acting β-2 agonist			
Ipratropium bromide		Not necessary as first-line therapy in children with mild exacerbations	
Nebulizer solution (500 μg/2.5mL)	500 μg with first 3 doses of albuterol, (250 μg may be used where available) not to exceed 1,500 μg in the first hour of treatment	500 μg with first 3 doses of albuterol, not to exceed 1,500 μg in the first hour of treatment	Add to short-acting β-2 agonist therapy for children with moderate and severe exacerbations
MDI (18 μg/puff)	4-8 puffs every 20 min as needed up to 3 h	8 puffs every 20 min as needed up to 3 h	
Ipratropium bromide with salbutamol		May mix ipratropium bromide in same nebulizer with salbutamol	
Nebulizer solution (Each 3 mL vial contains 0.5 mg ipratropium bromide and 2.5 mg albuterol)	1.5 mL every 20 min for 3 doses	3 mL every 20 min for 3 doses	Ipratropium is not necessary as first-line therapy in children with mild exacerbations

NS, normal saline; MDI, metered-dose inhaler.

CHAPTER 26: Acute Severe Asthma

TABLE 3: Corticosteroids–drugs with dosage recommendations

Medication	Dosage	Notes
Prednisone Prednisolone Methylprednisolone (sodium succinate)	1 mg/kg once daily (maximum 60 mg/day) for a total of 5 days	Dosages in excess of 1 mg/kg of prednisone or prednisolone have been associated with adverse behavioral effects in children, whereas 1 mg/kg provides equivalent pulmonary benefit with decreased adverse effects
	IV methylprednisolone: 1–2 mg/kg/dose (maximum 60 mg q.6 h) IV hydrocortisone: 5–7 mg/kg (maximum 400 mg q.6 h)	
Dexamethasone	Oral: 0.6 mg/kg once daily (max 16 mg/dose) for 1–2 days Intramuscular (dexamethasone sodium phosphate): 0.6 mg/kg single dose (max 15 mg)	

No advantage has been found for higher dose corticosteroids in severe asthma exacerbations.
There is no advantage for IV administration over oral therapy, provided gastrointestinal function is intact.
Therapy following a hospitalization or ED visit is typically 5 days, but may last from 3–10 days. Studies indicate there is no need to taper the systemic corticosteroid dose when given up to 10 days.
Any previous IV doses may be considered as part of the total steroid dose.

IV, intravenous; ED, emergency department.

TABLE 4: Stepwise approach to severe asthma

Therapeutic modality	Remarks
Salbutamol, ipratropium, steroids	These medications should be ordered for all patients admitted to the pediatric intensive care unit
Continuous salbutamol	0.5–1 mg/kg/h. If <20 kg, give 10–20 mg/h; 20–30 kg, give 10–30 mg/h, >30 kg, give 15–45 mg/h
IV Magnesium	25–50 mg/kg/dose (maximum 2 g) infused over 20–30 min. Follow by continuous infusion of 15–25 mg/kg/h. Mg level ≈ 4 mg/dL Monitor for hypotension
IV Terbutaline	Loading dose of 10 µg/kg over 10 min followed by 0.4 µg/kg/min Increase by 0.4 µg/kg/min every 15 min. Range 0.1–10 µg/kg/min (average dose is 4 µg/kg/min)
IV Theophylline	Loading dose of 5 mg/kg over 20 min followed by continuous infusion of 0.5–1 mg/kg/h. Check serum theophylline concentration 30 min after the end of the loading dose. Target theophylline concentration is 10–20 mg/L
Noninvasive ventilation	Consider bilevel positive airway pressure to unload work of breathing. Inspiratory positive airway pressure:10; expiratory positive airways pressure: 5
IV Ketamine	1 mg/kg/h for sedation. Bronchodilatory properties. Increase airway secretions
Ventilation	Try to avoid neuromuscular blockade. Permissive hypercapnia. Pressure control/pressure-regulated volume control/pressure support ventilation Monitor peak to plateau pressure difference

IV, intravenous.

Q. How does ipratropium work?

Ipratropium bromide, a quaternary ammonium atropine derivative, produces bronchodilatation by inhibition of cholinergic-mediated bronchospasm, occurring without the inhibition of mucociliary clearance. It is an important adjunct in the treatment of moderate-to-severe asthma exacerbation.

Nebulized ipratropium, in 0.25–0.50 mg doses, can be used every 20 minutes during the first hour, followed by the same dose range every 6 hours. Systemic effects are usually minimal; nevertheless, mydriasis and blurred vision have been reported.

Q. Can magnesium sulfate be used in severe asthma?

Magnesium, a calcium antagonist, causes smooth muscle relaxation as a result of the inhibition of calcium uptake.

Dose in severe acute asthma is 25–50 mg/kg/dose (maximum 2 g), infused for 20–30 minutes. A larger loading dose of magnesium sulfate may be more effective since it achieves serum magnesium concentrations between 3 and 5 mg/dL.

Q. Is there a role of "Helium-Oxygen Mixture (Heliox)"?

Helium is a low density gas, when used in a mixture with oxygen, it reduces turbulent airflow, enhancing laminar flow and in consequence reducing airflow resistance. As of now, there is only a limited evidence for the routine use of helium-oxygen mixtures in acute asthma.

Q. What is the role of ketamine?

Ketamine, a noncompetitive N-methyl-D-aspartate receptor antagonist, is used routinely as an anesthetic, analgesic, and sedative. Despite the current lack of high level evidence, it has shown beneficial clinical effect in children with acute asthma. In critically ill children with asthma, a loading dose of ketamine (2 mg/kg) followed by continuous infusions (20–60 µg/kg/min) significantly improves the PaO_2/FiO_2 ratio, the dynamic compliance and $PaCO_2$, and peak inspiratory pressures in mechanically ventilated patients.

Q. Can noninvasive ventilation be used in severe asthma?

Noninvasive positive pressure ventilation (NPPV) also called as bilevel positive airway pressure in addition to conventional therapy showed clinical improvement and correction of gas exchange abnormalities in children with severe asthma. Noninvasive positive pressure ventilation is well-tolerated in children, including patients as young as 1 year. However, understrict monitoring is required with the use of a small dose of benzodiazepines with or without a low dose ketamine infusion or dexmedetomidine. Typically recommended settings include an inspiratory positive airway pressure of 10 cmH$_2$O, an expiratory positive airway pressure of 5 cmH$_2$O, with or without a low back-up ventilation rate. In patients with severe asthma, a low level of continuous positive airway pressure may reduce the premature airway closure point, reducing intrinsic end expiratory pressure and subsequently, the inspiratory workload.

In addition, the use of NPPV may well improve the delivery of aerosolized salbutamol to poorly ventilated areas.

Q. What is the role of endotracheal intubation and ventilation for impending respiratory failure in asthma?

A group of children with status asthmaticus who fail to maintain their work of breathing require intubation. Box 2 lists the indications of intubation.

BOX 2: Indications of endotracheal intubation
- Altered mentation
- Decreasing respiratory effort
- Poor perfusion

The most experienced incubator in the team needs to be entrusted the procedure. A cuffed endotracheal tube should be used if available to allow for adequate ventilator pressures. Preparation for intubation should include multiple backup plans in the event that rapid sequence induction fails. Patient should be pre-oxygenated with a nonrebreather or, if tolerated, positive pressure ventilation.

On successful intubation, it is important to maintain a careful balance between providing enough pressure to oxygenate the patient but not so much as to cause barotrauma or prevent venous return and impair cardiac output.

Optimizing oxygenation and pulmonary pressures at the expense of hypercapnia are important. Mechanical ventilation modes that allow for pressure-regulated support and long expiratory times should be used to adequately balance these needs. Peri- and post-intubation is a high risk time for cardiac arrest. Deterioration of blood pressure or oxygenation should prompt an immediate assessment for sources utilizing the DOPE mnemonic (D, dislodgment; O, obstruction; P, pneumothorax; E, equipment malfunction).

Severe obstructive shock may follow hyperinflation which may get extracorporeal membrane oxygenation (ECMO) worsened acutely after intubation and positive pressure ventilation. Compression of the chest immediately after intubation may help deflate the lungs somewhat to reduce this pressure. In patients who continue to have poor oxygenation and/or hemodynamics despite aggressive ventilator strategies, aggressive airway clearance with bronchoscopy, inhaled volatile anesthetics, or even ECMO may be needed.

CONCLUSION

Early recognition of severe asthma from the patients' appearance, work of breathing, and breath is mandatory for good therapeutic response. A planned approach with multiple tiers of medications and clear endpoints can help direct the management of these patients. First-line therapy involves prompt administration of inhaled β-agonists and anti-cholinergics with systemic steroids. Second-line therapy comprising magnesium sulfate may be added quickly to nonresponders, in addition to continuous β-agonist nebulization. Third-line agent is indicated in refractory status asthmaticus. Patients in severe respiratory distress who can tolerate a mask may benefit from NPPV. The decision to intubate an asthmatic must be based on clinical judgment, though the decision can be aided by hypercarbia or hypoxia on a blood gas.

KEY LEARNING POINTS

- Careful assessment and stepwise approach is the key for management of severe asthma
- Adjuvant therapy, like magnesium sulfate, theophylline, and ketamine, are good management modalities in severe asthma
- Noninvasive ventilation has revolutionized the management of patients. Its advantages include improved patient comfort and reduced need for sedation
- Intubation and mechanical ventilation, the last resort in therapy, require close monitoring to avoid complications like pneumothorax and auto positive end-expiratory pressure

SUGGESTED READINGS

1. Baker AK, Carroll CL. High-Dose magnesium Infusions for acute Severe asthma in children: If a Little Is Good, Is More Even Better? *Pediatr Crit Care Med.* 2016;17:177-178.
2. Cook J, Saglani S. Pathogenesis and prevention strategies of severe asthma exacerbations in children. *Curr Opin Pulm Med.* 2016;22:25-31.
3. Dunn R, Szefler SJ. *Ann Am Thorac Soc.* 2016;13:S103-104.
4. Hakimeh D, Tripodi S. Recent advances on diagnosis and management of childhood asthma and food allergies. *Ital J Pediatr.* 2013.27;39:80-84.
5. Hedlin G, Konradsen J, Bush A. An update on pediatric asthma. *Eur Respir Rev.* 2012;21:175-185.
6. Hendaus MA, Jomha FA, Alhammadi AH. Is ketamine a lifesaving agent in childhood acute severe asthma? *Ther Clin Risk Manag.* 2016;12:273-279.
7. Memon BN, Parkash A, Ahmed Khan KM, Gowa MA, Bai C. Response to nebulized salbutamol versus combination with ipratropium bromide in children with acute severe asthma. *J Pak Med Assoc.* 2016;66:324-326.
8. Nieva IFF, Anand KJS. Severe Acute Asthma Exacerbation in Children: A Stepwise Approach for Escalating Therapy in a Pediatric Intensive Care Unit. *Pediatr Pharmacol Ther.* 2013;18:88-104.

SECTION 6
Cardiology

CHAPTER 27

Malignant Hypertension

Dinesh Chirla, Rakshay Shetty

INTRODUCTION

A commonly encountered and important clinical problem hypertension can be secondary to a multitude of causes. Malignant hypertension is defined as acutely elevated blood pressures associated with end-organ damage, typically involving the brain, heart, eyes, and the kidney. Papilledema is required to diagnose malignant hypertension. As the symptoms and signs can mimic many other common pediatric clinical diagnoses, it is important to evaluate the child carefully and thoroughly.

Inadequately treated malignant hypertension can cause significant morbidity and mortality. The current preferred terminology in vogue for malignant hypertension is hypertensive emergency or crisis.

CASE 1

A previously healthy, well-nourished, 4-year-old boy presented to the emergency room (ER) with an episode of generalized tonic-clonic seizure. He had complained about headache a day prior to the seizure. Mother noticed dark-colored urine for a couple of days, but she presumed it was secondary to poor water intake and urinary concentration. There was history of upper respiratory tract infection 2 weeks ago. He was born to nonconsanguineous parents and never had any major health issues earlier.

On examination in the ER, he was in the postictal state. His perfusion was adequate and he did not require any airway support. General physical examination was normal. Vital signs were stable except the blood pressure, which was 190/140 mmHg in the left upper limb. Four-limb blood pressure was checked which did not show any differential hypertension. Cardiovascular examination showed normal heart sounds and no murmurs. Abdomen was soft and there were no palpable masses.

On neurological examination, he was in postictal state, but there was no evidence of any focal deficits or meningeal signs. Fundus examination showed bilateral papilledema.

He was admitted in the intensive care unit and was started on continuous monitoring. Initial laboratory tests were sent and he was started on intravenous sodium nitroprusside infusion. Blood counts were normal and there was no evidence of microangiopathy on peripheral smear.

- Urinalysis showed hematuria and 3+ proteinuria
- Renal function tests showed elevated urea and creatinine
- Serum electrolytes were normal
- Urine protein creatinine ratio showed non-nephrotic range proteinuria
- Complement 3 level was low and antistreptolysin O titer was positive
- Liver function tests were normal, except for hypoalbuminemia

- Ultrasound abdomen showed grade 1 renal parenchymal changes in structurally normal kidneys
- Two-dimensional echocardiography did not show any evidence of coarctation of aorta. There was no concentric left ventricular hypertrophy. Neuroimaging was normal
- A presumptive diagnosis of acute glomerulonephritis (AGN) was made
- Renal biopsy showed crescentic glomerulonephritis
  He received two sessions of hemodialysis and treated with intravenous pulse methyl prednisolone followed by oral prednisolone. He received intravenous sodium nitroprusside infusion for 2 days, which was subsequently changed to oral labetalol and amlodipine.

CASE REVIEW IN A NUTSHELL

This 4-year-old child presented with generalized tonic-clonic seizures, which were controlled with intravenous lorazepam. The seizure episode turned out to be secondary to very high blood pressure (190/140 mmHg) which was accompanied by papilledema. The presence of edema and high-colored urine supported by laboratory findings and a preceding upper respiratory tract infection a couple of weeks back pointed to the underlying problem as AGN. In the investigations, presence of 3+ proteinuria appeared to be somewhat unusual for poststreptococcal AGN. Renal biopsy provided answer to this aberration. It showed crescentic glomerulonephritis.

On the therapeutic front, high blood pressure was brought down gradually employing intravenous sodium nitroprusside infusion, which is considered to be a good choice in renovascular hypertension. Subsequently, oral labetalol and amlodipine may be employed as was done in this case.

Most cases of poststreptococcal AGN usually need only supportive therapy. This, being a case of crescentic glomerulonephritis, he was treated with intravenous pulse methyl prednisolone followed by oral prednisolone. Two sessions of hemodialysis were also administered.

INTERACTIVE TOPIC REVIEW

Q. How is malignant hypertension defined?

Malignant hypertension is defined as average systolic blood pressure (SBP) or diastolic blood pressure (DBP) more than 5 mmHg higher than the 99th percentile for age and sex, associated with signs and symptoms of end-organ involvement (heart, brain, eyes, and kidneys) (Table 1).

Q. What are the causes of malignant hypertension?

Malignant hypertension can complicate any of the umpteen numbers of conditions causing hypertension (Box 1). Less effective blood pressure control based on outpatient SBP measurement is known to be an independent risk factor for hypertensive crisis.

Q. What are the features of malignant hypertension?

Hypertensive emergencies are by definition associated with end-organ damage. The various manifestations are given in table 2.

TABLE 1: Stages of hypertension

Stage	Criteria
Prehypertension	Average SBP or DBP 90–95th percentile
Stage 1 hypertension	Average SBP or DBP 95–99th percentile + 5 mmHg
Stage 2 hypertension	Average SBP or DBP >99th percentile + 5 mmHg
Hypertensive urgency	Associated with symptoms like nausea, headache and blurred vision
Hypertensive emergency	Associated with symptoms and end-organ involvement like encephalopathy or pulmonary edema

SBP systolic blood pressure; DBP, diastolic blood pressure.

BOX 1: Causes of malignant hypertension

Cardiac
- Coarctation of aorta

Renal
- Acute glomerulonephritis
- Dysplastic kidneys
- Posterior urethral valves with obstructive uropathy
- Chronic kidney disease
- Renal artery/vein thrombosis
- Hemolytic uremic syndrome
- Lupus nephritis

Endocrine
- Hyperthyroidism
- Cushing's disease
- Some forms of congenital adrenal hyperplasia
- Hyperaldosteronism

Malignancies
- Pheochromocytoma
- Neuroblastoma

Central nervous system
- Raised intracranial pressure

Miscellaneous
- Autoimmune diseases

Drugs
- Steroids
- Amphetamines
- Cocaine
- Calcineurin inhibitors

Q. How should a child with malignant hypertension be approached clinically?

Since malignant hypertension is a medical emergency, evaluation of the child for the etiology of the hypertension and management of blood pressures should proceed simultaneously. Detailed family history, history of renal, cardiac, or endocrine diseases, and drug history should be obtained. Physical examination should concentrate on measuring four-limb blood pressure, looking for stigmata of endocrinopathies like Cushing's disease and thyrotoxicosis, auscultation for renal bruit, focused neurological examination, detailed cardiovascular examination, and a fundus examination to look for end-organ involvement. It is important to use an appropriately sized cuff for blood pressure measurements and in children with malignant hypertension, invasive arterial blood pressure measurement will be beneficial.

Q. How should this child be investigated?

Investigative approach to malignant hypertension are given in boxes 2–4.

Q. How should the child be managed?

Any child with malignant hypertension requires admission and there is no role for ambulatory

TABLE 2: Manifestations of hypertensive emergencies

System	Manifestations
Central nervous system	Cerebral infarction, hemorrhage, encephalopathy, posterior reversible encephalopathy syndrome
Cardiovascular system	Congestive cardiac failure, pulmonary edema
Eyes	Papilledema, retinal hemorrhages, retinopathy, loss of vision, acute ischemic optic neuropathy
Kidneys	Renal failure

BOX 2: Investigative approach to malignant hypertension: Initial investigations for delineating the etiology

- Complete blood picture
- Blood glucose
- Blood gas analysis
- Blood urea, serum creatinine, serum calcium, phosphorus, uric acid, and serum electrolytes
- Complete urine examination and urine culture
- Ultrasound of kidney, ureter, and bladder for renal anomalies
- Chest X-ray for pulmonary edema
- Renal Dopplers for renovascular hypertension
- Two-dimensional echocardiography to rule out coarctation of aorta and left ventricular hypertrophy
- Antistreptolysin O titer, complement 3 levels

> **BOX 4: Investigative approach to malignant hypertension: Tests to detect end-organ damage**
> - Chest radiograph for pulmonary edema
> - Electrocardiograph, two-directional two-dimensional echocardiography
> - Neuroimaging for encephalopathy

> **BOX 3: Investigative approach to malignant hypertension: Additional investigations for hypertensive crisis**
> - 8 AM serum cortisol levels
> - 24-h urinary cortisol
> - Dexamethasone suppression test if elevated cortisol
> - Thyroid function test
> - 24-h urinary catecholamines and vanillylmandelic acid levels
> - Plasma renin activity and aldosterone
> - Adrenal imaging if required

management. The child should be managed in an intensive care unit with continuous monitoring. Parenteral antihypertensives should be instituted promptly. However, aggressive and overzealous reduction of blood pressures to normal ranges may cause sudden hypoperfusion of end-organs, hence blood pressure reduction should be graded and controlled. Arterial blood pressure monitoring is ideal. The goal should be to reduce not more than 25% of initial blood pressures over the first 8 hours of treatment and to gradually normalize over the next 24–48 hours. Hypertensive urgencies may be managed with oral or parenteral antihypertensives with typical duration of blood pressure normalization of 24 hours. A recent Cochrane review concluded there is no randomized controlled trial (RCT) evidence demonstrating that antihypertensive drugs reduce mortality or morbidity in patients with hypertensive emergencies and there is insufficient RCT evidence to determine which drug or drug class is most effective in reducing mortality and morbidity.

There is growing evidence that the renin-angiotensin system plays a key role in the pathogenesis of hypertensive crises. Recent studies have shown that oxidative stress and factors affecting endothelial function are also important. There has been a lot of research on the immunologic and genetic basis of hypertension. The drug therapy of hypertensive emergency has also witnessed tremendous changes in parallel with the recent advances in pathogenesis. Detailed pathogenetic mechanisms of hypertensive crises are beyond the scope of this chapter.

- Nicardipine and labetalol are the first line intravenous antihypertensive agents used in pediatric hypertensive crises. Esmolol is less frequently used. Nicardipine is a second-generation dihydropyridine calcium channel blocker, which causes vasodilatation. There is now a vast experience with intravenous nicardipine, which has become a viable alternative to sodium nitroprusside in children. Patients treated with nicardipine are more likely to reach the physician-specified SBP target range within 30 minutes than those treated with labetalol. In a recent design simulation, Peacock et al. showed that the rate of clinically relevant blood pressure drop within 30 minutes of initiation in the nicardipine group would be 61% versus 14–19%, with more than 20% heart rate (HR) decrease, for labetalol
- Labetalol is an α- and β-blocker. It is contraindicated in children with bronchial asthma or heart disease. It causes vaso-dilatation due to α-blockade. Children with ischemic brain injury are prone to develop severe hypotension when on labetalol and hence caution is required
- Sodium nitroprusside is a venous as well as arterial vasodilator. It thus reduces both preload and afterload and hence beneficial for cardiac failure secondary to severe hypertension. It has been the drug of choice for many years for acute hypertension. It is known to cause tachyphylaxis and cyanide toxicity with prolonged use and has slowly fallen out of favor. The role currently is limited to situations where other agents are not available or suitable. Hydralazine is a direct arterial smooth muscle vasodilator. Though

there are no published RCTs, hydralazine has been used as an alternative to labetalol
- Clevidipine butyrate, an ultrashort-acting calcium channel antagonist, has been evaluated in managing perioperative hypertension and has been found to be safe and effective. Because it is prepared in a lipid solution, it is contraindicated in those with egg and soy allergy as well as those with lipid disorders
- Isradipine, an orally administered second generation dihydropyridine calcium channel blocker, has been used for treatment of acute hypertension in hospitalized pediatric patients
- Fenoldopam is a selective dopamine D_1 receptor agonist, which has been tried in the management of pediatric acute hypertension. It has been shown to cause significant reduction in blood pressure, but side effects like tachycardia and flushing have been noted
- Phentolamine is specifically used in hypertension secondary to catecholamine excess. Clonidine is a centrally acting α_2 adrenergic agonist. It is minimally removed by hemodialysis and is useful in hypertension secondary to renal failure. Intravenous furosemide infusion or bolus dose can be given in children with volume overload
- Oral or sublingual nifedipine, which was extensively used in the past for acute pediatric hypertension, is no longer recommended for management of hypertensive crisis, in view of reports of sudden and severe hypotension in adult patients with nifedipine use (Table 3)

Blood pressure normative data in boys is presented in table 4.

TABLE 3: Recommended pharmacotherapy for malignant hypertension

Drug	Dose	Onset of action	Common adverse effects
Nicardipine	• 0.5–1 µg/kg/min, and can be titrated up every 15–30 min, with a maximum dose of 4 µg/kg/min	• 1–2 min	• Hypotension, tachycardia, flushing, and palpitations
Sodium nitroprusside	• 0.5–10 µg/kg/min	• 1–2 min	• Cyanide toxicity, metabolic acidosis, methemoglobinemia, tachycardia, altered mental status
Labetalol	• IV 0.2 mg/kg over 2 min, if no response in 5–10 min, increase to 0.4–1.0 mg/kg (maximum bolus dose 20 mg) or continuous intravenous infusion 0.4–1.0 mg/kg/h (maximum dose 3 mg/kg/h)	• 5 min	• Airway reactivity • Bradycardia • Urinary retention
Furosemide	• IV 1–5 mg/kg/dose 6 hourly or continuous IV infusion 0.1–1.0 mg/kg/h	• 2–5 min	• Dyselectrolytemia
Hydralazine	• 0.1–0.3 mg/kg (maximum 10 mg) slow IV over 3–5 min • Can repeat every 4–6 h or continuous infusion 4–6 µg/kg/min (maximum 300 µg/min)	• 10–20 min	• Tachycardia • Severe headache • Fluid retention • Raised intracranial pressure

IV, intravenous.

CHAPTER 27: Malignant Hypertension

TABLE 4: Boys 1-17 years old: clinic blood pressure normative data, by age and height percentiles

Age years	BP percentile	SBP mmHg Percentile of height							DBP mmHg Percentile of height						
		5th	10th	25th	50th	75th	90th	95th	5th	10th	25th	50th	75th	90th	95th
1	50th	80	81	83	85	87	88	89	34	35	36	37	38	39	39
	90th	94	95	97	99	100	102	103	49	50	51	52	53	53	54
	95th	98	99	101	103	104	105	105	54	54	55	56	57	58	58
	99th	105	106	108	110	112	113	114	61	62	63	64	65	66	66
2	50th	84	85	87	88	90	92	92	39	40	41	42	43	44	44
	90th	97	99	100	102	104	105	106	54	55	56	57	58	58	59
	95th	101	102	104	106	108	109	110	59	59	60	61	62	63	63
	99th	109	110	111	113	115	117	117	66	67	68	69	70	71	71
3	50th	86	87	89	91	93	94	95	44	44	45	46	47	48	48
	90th	100	101	103	105	107	108	109	59	59	60	61	62	63	63
	95th	104	105	107	109	110	112	113	63	63	64	65	66	67	67
	99th	111	112	114	116	118	119	120	71	71	72	73	74	75	75
4	50th	88	89	91	93	95	96	97	47	48	49	50	51	51	52
	90th	102	103	106	107	109	110	111	62	63	64	65	66	66	67
	95th	106	107	109	111	112	114	115	66	67	68	69	70	71	71
	99th	113	114	116	118	120	121	122	74	75	76	77	78	78	79
5	50th	90	91	93	95	96	98	98	50	51	52	53	54	55	55
	90th	104	105	106	108	110	111	112	65	66	67	68	69	69	70
	95th	108	109	110	112	114	115	116	69	70	71	72	73	74	74
	99th	115	116	118	120	121	123	123	77	78	79	80	81	81	82
6	50th	91	92	95	96	98	99	100	53	53	54	55	56	57	57
	90th	105	106	108	110	111	113	113	68	68	69	70	71	72	72
	95th	109	110	112	114	115	117	117	72	72	73	74	75	76	76
	99th	116	117	119	121	123	124	125	80	80	81	82	83	84	84
7	50th	92	94	95	97	99	100	101	55	55	56	57	58	59	59
	90th	106	107	109	111	113	114	115	70	70	71	72	73	74	74
	95th	110	111	113	115	117	118	119	74	74	75	76	77	78	78
	99th	117	118	120	122	124	125	126	82	82	83	84	85	86	86
8	50th	94	95	97	99	100	102	102	56	57	58	59	60	60	61
	90th	107	109	110	112	114	115	116	71	72	72	73	74	75	76
	95th	111	112	114	116	118	119	120	75	76	77	78	79	79	80
	90th	119	120	122	123	125	127	127	83	84	85	86	87	87	88
9	50th	95	96	98	100	102	103	104	57	58	59	60	61	61	62
	90th	109	110	112	114	115	117	118	72	73	74	75	76	76	77
	95th	113	114	116	118	119	121	121	76	77	78	79	80	81	81
	99th	120	121	123	125	127	128	129	84	85	86	87	88	88	89

Continued

SECTION 6: Cardiology

Continued

Age years	BP percentile	SBP mmHg Percentile of height							DBP mmHg Percentile of height						
		5th	10th	25th	50th	75th	90th	95th	5th	10th	25th	50th	75th	90th	95th
10	50th	97	98	100	102	103	105	106	58	59	60	61	61	62	63
	90th	111	112	114	115	117	119	119	73	73	74	75	76	77	78
	95th	115	116	117	119	121	122	123	77	78	79	80	81	81	82
	99th	122	123	125	127	128	130	130	85	86	86	88	88	89	90
11	50th	99	100	102	104	105	107	107	59	59	60	61	61	62	63
	90th	113	114	115	117	119	120	121	74	74	75	76	77	78	78
	95th	117	118	119	121	123	124	125	78	78	79	80	81	82	82
	99th	124	125	127	129	130	132	132	86	86	87	88	89	90	90
12	50th	101	102	104	106	108	109	110	59	60	61	62	63	63	64
	90th	115	116	118	120	121	123	123	74	75	75	76	77	78	79
	95th	119	120	122	123	125	127	127	78	79	80	81	82	82	83
	99th	126	127	129	131	133	134	135	86	87	88	89	90	90	91
13	50th	104	105	106	108	110	111	112	60	60	61	62	63	64	64
	90th	117	118	120	122	124	125	126	75	75	76	77	78	79	79
	95th	121	122	124	126	128	129	130	79	79	80	81	82	83	83
	99th	128	130	131	133	135	136	137	87	87	88	89	90	91	91
14	50th	106	107	109	111	113	114	115	60	61	62	63	64	65	65
	90th	120	121	23	125	126	128	128	75	76	77	78	79	79	80
	95th	124	125	127	128	130	132	132	80	80	81	82	83	84	84
	99th	131	132	134	136	138	139	140	87	88	89	90	91	92	92
15	50th	109	110	112	113	115	117	117	61	62	63	64	65	66	66
	90th	122	124	125	127	129	130	131	76	77	78	79	80	80	81
	95th	126	127	129	131	133	134	135	81	81	82	83	84	85	85
	99th	134	135	136	138	140	142	142	88	89	90	91	92	93	93
16	50th	111	112	114	116	118	119	120	63	63	64	65	66	67	67
	90th	125	126	128	130	131	133	134	78	78	79	80	81	82	82
	95th	129	130	132	134	135	137	137	82	83	83	84	85	86	87
	99th	136	137	139	141	142	144	145	90	90	91	92	93	94	94
17	50th	114	115	116	118	120	121	122	65	66	66	67	68	69	70
	90th	127	128	130	132	134	135	136	80	80	81	82	83	84	84
	95th	131	132	134	136	138	139	140	81	85	86	87	87	88	89
	99th	139	140	141	143	145	146	147	92	93	93	94	95	96	97

BP, blood pressure; SBP, systolic blood pressure; diastolic blood pressure.
For research purposes, the SDs propvide allowance for computing BP Z score and percentiles for boys with height percentiles (i.e., the 5th, 10th, 25th, 50th, 75th, 90th, and 95th percentiles). These height percentiles must be converted to height Zscores given by: 5% = −1.645; 10% = −1.28; 25% = −0.68; 50% = 0; 75% = 0.68; 90% = 1.645, and then computed.

Source: 4th task force pediatrics 2004; 114(2 suppl):555.

CONCLUSION

Pediatric acute hypertension has seen lot of advances over the last two decades both in its pathophysiology and management. Yet, early recognition, appropriate, aggressive but cautious management of blood pressure remains the cornerstone for successful outcomes.

KEY LEARNING POINTS

- Malignant hypertension is an acutely elevated blood pressures associated with end-organ damage, typically involving the brain, heart, eyes, and the kidney
- Papilledema is required to diagnose malignant hypertension
- As the symptoms and signs can mimic many other common pediatric clinical diagnoses, it is important to evaluate the child carefully and thoroughly
- Left inadequately treated, malignant hypertension may cause significant morbidity and mortality
- Early recognition, appropriate, aggressive but cautious management of blood pressure remains the cornerstone for successful outcomes

SUGGESTED READINGS

1. Flynn JT, Tullus K. Severe hypertension in children and adolescents: pathophysiology and treatment. *Pediatr Nephrol.* 2009;24:1101-12.
2. Kurnutala LN, Soghomonyan S, Bergese SD. Perioperative acute hypertension—role of Clevidipine butyrate. *Front Pharmacol.* 2014;5:197.
3. Miyashita Y, Peterson D, Rees JM, Flynn JT. Isradipine for treatment of acute hypertension in hospitalized children and adolescents. *J Clin Hypertens (Greenwich).* 2010;12:850-855.
4. Peacock WF, Varon J, Baumann BM, Borczuk P, Cannon CM, Chandra A, et al. CLUE: a randomized comparative effectiveness trial of IV nicardipine versus labetalol use in the emergency department. *Crit Care.* 2011;15:R157.
5. Rodriguez MA, Kumar SK, De Caro M. *Hypertensive crisis. Cardiol Rev.* 2010;18:102-107.
6. Rodrigo R, González J, Paoletto F. The role of oxidative stress in the pathophysiology of hypertension. *Hypertens Res.* 2011;34:431-440.
7. Takahashi H, Yoshika M, Komiyama Y, Nishimura M. The central mechanism underlying hypertension: a review of the roles of sodium ions, epithelial sodium channels, the renin-angiotensin-aldosterone system, oxidative stress and endogenous digitalis in the brain. *Hypertens Res.* 2011;34:1147-1160.
8. Webb TN, Shatat IF, Miyashita Y. Therapy of acute hypertension in hospitalized children and adolescents. *Curr Hypertens Rep.* 2014;16:425.

Acute Severe Hypertension

CHAPTER
28

VR Veeturi, Satya Prasad

INTRODUCTION

According to the fourth report of the National High Blood Pressure Education Program Working Group on high blood pressure in children and adolescents, the definition of hypertension in children, unlike in adults, need to be statistical rather than function. Children with blood pressure between 95th percentile and 99th percentile plus 5 mmHg are categorized as stage 1 hypertension; those with blood pressure above 99th percentile plus 5 mmHg as stage 2 hypertension. Stage 1 hypertension, provided that it is asymptomatic and without target organ damage, allows time for evaluation before embarking on therapy. However, stage 2 hypertension is a call for more prompt evaluation and antihypertensive drug treatment.

Severe hypertension, including both hypertensive emergency and urgency, in pediatric practice is predominantly secondary to an underlying disease process though now primary essential hypertension in association with obesity too is on the increase in children. The greatest risk in untreated severe hypertension lies in end-organ damage. Adequate evaluation and prompt pharmacotherapy are, therefore, important.

CASE 1

A 7-year-old boy presented with headache, palpitations, periorbital puffiness, reduced urine output, and drowsiness of 3 days duration with a preceding history of sore throat about a fortnight back.
Physical examination: Well-nourished and well-built with a weight of 24 kg and height 116 cm; disoriented in time and space; pulse rate 110/min; respiratory rate 30/min; periorbital edema ++; pedal edema +; blood pressure 130/90 mmHg.
Investigations: Hemoglobin 10.8 g/dL, normocytic normochromic picture; serum proteins 6.2 (albumin 4.1, globulin 2.1) g/dL, blood urea nitrogen (BUN) 48; urine: numerous red blood cells, pus cells 4–6/hpf; normal biochemistry.
Diagnosis: Poststreptococcal acute glomerulonephritis with secondary critical hypertension.
Treatment given: Nifedipine 0.25 mg/kg/dose orally every 6 hours along with supportive measures.
Outcome: Both systolic and diastolic blood pressure was lowered but too much more than the desired level within 20 minutes. Eventually, the child was put on labetalol infusion.

CASE REVIEW IN A NUTSHELL

The clinical profile of this 7-year-old boy developing periorbital and pedal edema following an attack of sore throat (in all probability strep throat is consistent with acute glomerulonephritis). Headache and change in sensorium point to probability of coexisting hypertension, which was substantiated by documented high blood pressure of 145/100 mmHg. Results of such laboratory tests as urine microscopy showing hematuria and elevated BUN support the clinical impression. Normal serum protein and absence of albuminuria exclude any chance of nephrotic syndrome.

Diagnosis of severe hypertension ["hypertensive emergency" on account of involvement of central nervous system (CNS)] rather than sheer "hypertensive crisis" was well founded. This warranted lowering of the blood pressure by 10% in first hour and 25% in first 8 hours and rest of 75% in next 24–36 hours. In this context, it would have been better using an alternative drug such a labetalol rather than nifedipine, which is known to achieve a major fall in a very short time. A very quick lowering of blood pressure is not quite desirable in view of the likelihood of complication of cerebral ischemia.

INTERACTIVE TOPIC REVIEW

Q. What is hypertension?

Hypertension is defined as the blood pressure of 95th percentile or more with reference to the age, sex, and height recorded on at least 3 occasions. Normal blood pressure in children is related to the age and sex and hence one has to refer to the nomograms charts for normal blood pressure values.

According to National High Blood Pressure Education Program Working Group on high blood pressure in children and adolescents, blood pressure between 90th and 95th percentiles should be labeled as "prehypertension" or "borderline" high blood pressure. One has to watch for hypertension when the blood pressure is persistently about 90th percentile.
- Stage 1 hypertension: 95th–99th percentile + 5 mmHg
- Stage 2 hypertension: 95th percentile +5 mmHg
 Blood pressure measurement up to 90th percentile is considered normal.

Q. What is white-coat hypertension?

By the term, white-coat hypertension is meant a clinical condition in which the patient has blood pressure levels that are above the 95th percentile when measured in a physician's office or clinic, whereas the patient's average blood pressure is below the 90th percentile outside of a clinical setting.

Q. What is severe hypertension?

Severe hypertension or hypertensive crisis includes both hypertensive urgency and hypertensive emergency.

A hypertensive emergency is defined as highly raised blood pressure (>95th percentile) with involvement of target organs (Box 1).

BOX 1: Broad manifestations of target organs involvement in hypertensive emergency

- Central nervous system
  - Encephalopathy
  - Stroke
  - Intracranial hemorrhage
- Cardiovascular system
  - Heart failure
  - Ischemic heart disease
  - Pulmonary edema
  - Aortic dissection
- Renal
  - Proteinuria
  - Hematuria
  - Pyuria
- Ocular
  - Blindness

Unlike hypertensive emergency, in hypertensive urgency, blood pressure is very high but end-organ damage is not there.

Q. Is the differentiating feature between hypertensive emergency and urgency in any way important?

Of course it is. In hypertensive emergency, it is mandatory to bring down very high blood pressure immediately to safeguard against further end-organ insult and dysfunction.

In case of hypertensive urgency, immediate reduction is not required. Blood pressure can be brought down slowly over a somewhat longer period of time.

Q. What is an appropriate way of measuring blood pressure in children?

An accurate measurement of blood pressure is important and it requires due attention to the comfort of the child, proper skills and techniques of blood pressure measurement. For correct measurement of blood pressure selection of appropriate sized cuffs are important in children. The age appropriate cuff sizes are, infants—2.5 cm, 1-12 months—5 cm, 1-8 years—9 cm, and older children 12.5 cm. Systolic pressure is indicated by appearance of Korotkoff sound and the diastolic pressure is ideally noted when the sounds are muffled. However, if it is not possible to appreciate the change in the intensity of the sounds, disappearance of the sounds may be recorded as diastolic blood pressure. In children, blood pressure is measured by palpatory method (the appearance of radial pulsation while deflating the cuff is systolic blood pressure) and auscultatory method.

In infants, the methods are flush method, oscillometry, and Doppler methods. The procedure of flush method of blood pressure recording in infants is as follows:
- To start with, the infant must be quiet and comfortable. You may give him a pacifier or a feeder
- Then the cuff (2.5-3 cm size so that it covers the two-thirds of the limb) is applied. It is, however, not inflated. An elastic crape bandage or a rubber band, about 2.5 cm wide, is applied round the forearm distal to the cuff
- Now the cuff is inflated to around 200 mmHg. At this stage, the crape bandage or band is speedily removed. As the cuff is gradually deflated, a flush appears in the forearm. At this point, the pressure is noted. This is the mean blood pressure of the infant. The method cannot be repeated for the next 15 minutes
- Electronic transducer (ultrasound) and oscillometry are far more sophisticated facilities.

Q. What is ambulatory blood pressure monitoring?

Ambulatory blood pressure monitoring (ABPM) is a procedure in which a special portable blood pressure device worn by the patient records blood pressure over a specified period, usually 24 hours. Ambulatory blood pressure monitoring is very useful in the evaluation of hypertension in children. By frequent measurement and recording of blood pressure, ABPM enables computation of the mean blood pressure during the day, night, and over 24 hours as well as various measures to determine the degree to which blood pressure exceeds the upper limit of normal over a given time period, the so-called "blood pressure load". It is especially helpful in the evaluation of white-coat hypertension, as well as the risk for hypertensive organ injury, apparent drug resistance, and hypotensive symptoms with antihypertensive drugs. Ambulatory blood pressure monitoring is also useful for evaluating patients for whom more information on blood pressure patterns is needed, such as those with episodic hypertension, chronic kidney disease, diabetes, and autonomic dysfunction.

Q. What are the causes of hypertension in children?

In 90% of children, hypertension is secondary. Among them, renal causes account for about 75% of cases. Hypertension without any known underlying disease (essential hypertension) accounts for only 5-10% of cases in children. However, these patients will have family history, obesity, excess salt intake, stress, and other reasons. Most often, it is recognized in adolescents.

Secondary hypertension in children includes the causes of both transient and chronic hypertension. Most importantly, the cause of hypertension varies with age. Boxes 2 and 3 list the causes of hypertension in children.

CHAPTER 28: Acute Severe Hypertension

> **BOX 2: Causes of transient hypertension in children**
> - Common causes
>   - Acute poststreptococcal glomerulonephritis
>   - Hemolytic uremic syndrome
>   - Anaphylactoid purpura
>   - Postrenal transplant/urological surgery
>   - Hypervolemia administration
>   - Renal trauma
> - Others
>   - Increased intracranial pressure
>   - Guillain–Barré syndrome
>   - Poliomyelitis
>   - Hypernatremia
>   - Corticosteroids/contraceptive
>   - Familial dysautonomia
>   - Postcoarctation repair

> **BOX 3: Causes of chronic hypertension in children**
> - Renal
>   - Chronic glomerulonephritis
>   - Chronic pyelonephritis
>   - Hydronephrosis
>   - Vesicoureteral reflux nephropathy
>   - Malformations of kidney (dysplastic, polycystic, segmental hypoplasia, multicystic kidney)
>   - Renal tumors
> - Vascular/renovascular
>   - Coarctation of aorta
>   - Umbilical artery catheterization
>   - Renal artery stenosis
>   - Renal vein thrombosis
>   - Renal arteritis with or without aortitis
> - Endocrine disorders
>   - Congenital adrenal hyperplasia (11B-hydroxylase and 17-hydroxylase defect)
>   - Cushing syndrome
>   - Pheochromocytoma
>   - Neuroblastoma
>   - Primary aldosteronism
> - Other causes
>   - Intracranial mass
>   - Hemorrhage
>   - Essential hypertension

Q. What are the usual clinical features of hypertension?

Clinical features of hypertension depend upon the underlying cause and severity of hypertension. Most of the patients with mild hypertension and borderline hypertension and adolescents with essential hypertension may remain asymptomatic. Hypertension is recognized in them during routine medical examinations. Especially in essential hypertension, the blood pressure is only slightly elevated with diastolic pressure at or slightly above the 95th percentile for the age.

The usual symptoms attributed to hypertension are headache, nausea, vomiting, dizziness, and irritability.

Q. Clinically, when should severe hypertension be suspected?

- With severe hypertension, patient may develop hypertension crisis and hypertensive encephalopathy. Patients may have altered sensorium, visual disturbances, persistent vomiting, seizures, cranial nerve palsies, and other neurologic deficits
- Heart failure, though uncommon in children, can develop. More than the symptoms of hypertension, the clinical features of the underlying causes of hypertension are common in children. These symptoms are of help in proper diagnosis
- Renal or renovascular disorders present with such symptoms as polyuria, edema, and decreased urine output
- In pheochromocytoma, episodes of palpitation, sweating, and flushing are common. Cushing syndrome is usually characterized by obesity, buffalo hump, hirsutism, and abdominal striates.

Similarly, features of other diseases may be present.

Q. What are the ophthalmoscopic findings in hypertensive retinopathy?

Hypertensive retinopathy will show specific changes (Box 4).

BOX 4: Grading of fundoscopic finding in hypertension	
Grade I:	Copper-wire appearance of arterioles which assume shape of broad yellow lines
Grade II:	Thickened arterioles without visible blood column nip the veins.
Grade III:	Hemorrhages and exudates. Considerable narrowed arterioles with a diameter, which is only one-fourth of that of veins, appear as broad white silver lines. Blood column is not visible. Dilatation of vein distal to the artery is apparent.
Grade IV:	Papilledema on top of changes seen in grade 3 retinopathy

Clinically, it is useful to separate mild (grades I and II) from severe retinopathy (grades III and IV). Prognosis is different in these categories. The presence of exudates and hemorrhages significantly influence the improvement.

Q. What about diagnosis?

- The first and foremost thing in the diagnosis of hypertension is proper recording of the blood pressure. Several recordings are important before labeling a child as suffering from hypertension
- Appropriate sized cuffs, appropriate method of recording, and comfort of the child during blood pressure recording are important
- Mild blood pressure and borderline elevation requires close follow-up and repeated measurements. Other associated features help in finding the etiology.

Q. What is the role of investigations?

Only after confirming hypertension, investigations should be planned. No need to do battery of investigations in all children. Start with investigation for common cause(s) and consider advanced investigations later to confirm the diagnosis.

Initial investigations for hypertension include hemogram, urine analysis, urinary electrolytes, blood urea, nitrogen, serum creatinine, chest X-ray echocardiography, and electrocardiography. In select cases, renal imaging studies, urinary catecholamines, angiography, renal biopsy, plasma renin activity, renal scintiscan, etc. may be done depending on the merits of the cases.

Urine analysis: One of the most important screening test and should be done in all cases. Proteinuria, hyaline, and granular casts characterize chronic glomerulonephritis. Leucocytes and granular casts indicate pyelonephritis. Hematuria, beside glomerulonephritis, is indicative of many other renal disorders. A 24 hours urinary protein analysis may be required.

Urine culture: As urinary tract infection, either isolated or in association with reflux or obstructive nephropathy is the important cause of hypertension, urine culture should be considered in all cases.

Hemogram: Required as a supportive investigation for the diagnosis of pyelonephritis, hemolytic uremic syndrome, etc.

Renal function tests: Raised blood urea and creatinine are observed in renal disorders. Decreased creatinine clearance suggests diminished glomerular filtration.

Serum electrolytes: Abnormalities in electrolytes are observed in disorders like renal and endocrine causes.

Urinary electrolyte: Helps in diagnosing renal disease including renal tubular disorders.

Plasma renin activity: Increased plasma renin suggests renal or renovascular disorder.

Urinary catecholamines: They are elevated in pheochromocytoma

Imaging studies: Chest X-ray is useful in the diagnosis of cardiovascular causes like coarctation of aorta. Similarly, electrocardiography and echocardiography help in identifying coarctation of aorta and helpful in assessing cardiac response to the elevated blood pressure.

Renal ultrasonography is a useful non-invasive tool. It helps in evaluating renal parenchyma, diagnosis of hydronephrosis, renal mass and suprarenal masses.

Renal radionuclide scan: It helps in distinguishing variations in renal perfusion.

Renogram: Rate of uptake and disappearance of I132-labeled Hippuran helps in identification of renovascular disorders.

Renal angiography: It demonstrates lesions in the main arteries or the segmental branches. Doppler ultrasonography may demonstrate arterial and venous blood flow.

Other tests may be done as and when indicated.

Q. What are the goals of treatment in severe hypertension?

Main goal is to bring down very high blood pressure in a way that end-organ damage via hypoperfusion does not occur or is halted. This means that too rapid reduction should not be attempted else there may occur cerebral infarction. In order to attain a good balance between reducing blood pressure and safeguarding from end-organ hypoperfusion, antihypertensive drugs with rapid onset and rapid offset are needed. At the same time, provision of the continuous blood pressure monitoring employing invasive arterial lines should be in place.

Q. What are salient details of drugs recommended in severe hypertension?

These are listed along with their dosage and special comments in table 1.

Q. What should be the actual therapeutic approach?

Acute severe hypertension (hypertensive crisis), an emergency, needs aggressive, well-monitored intravenous antihypertensive medication

TABLE 1: Antihypertensive drugs for severe hypertension

Drug	Dosage	Special comments
Sodium nitroprusside	• 0.5–10 µg/kg/min in 5% dextrose	• Since it may cause cyanide toxicity, cyanide levels should be monitored when used for >72 h and in renal failure, else coadminister with sodium thiosulfate
Labetalol	• IV bolus: 0.20–1.0 mg/dose q5–10 min (maximum 40 mg) • IV infusion: 0.25–3.0 mg/kg/h	• ADRs include pallor, abdominal discomfort, diarrhea, bradycardia, hypotension (orthostatic) • Avoid in overt heart failure and bronchial asthma
Nicardipine	• IV bolus: 30 µg/kg (maximum 2) mg/dose q15 min • IV infusion: 0.5–4.0 µg/kg/min (maximum 5 mg/h)	• ADRs include reflex tachycardia, flushing, nausea, headache, raised ICP, phlebitis
Clonidine	• 0.05–0.1 mg/dose PO; may repeat qhr to a maximum of 0.8 mg total dose	• ADRs include dryness of mouth and drowsiness (somnolence)
Minoxidil	• 0.1–0.2 mg/kg/dose	• Very powerful, long-acting oral direct vasodilator
Nitroglycerine	• 1–3 µg/kg/min	• ADRs include headache, tachycardia, methemoglobinemia
Phentolamine	• 0.1–0.2 mg/kg; may be repeated q2–4 h	• Abdominal discomfort, reflex tachycardia
Hydralazine	• 0.2–0.6 mg/kg/dose IV, IM	• If given as IV bolus, it should be every 4 h
Esmolol	• IV infusion (preferably constant) 100–500 µg/kg/min	• ADRs include profound bradycardia
Nifedipine	• 0.2–0.5 (maximum 10) mg/kg PO q4–6 hourly	• ADRs include sudden fall in BP (excessive), peripheral edema

IV, intravenous; IM, intramuscular; ADRs, adverse drug reactions; ICP, intracranial pressure; PO, per os.

(Table 1). The aim is to reduce the blood pressure by up to 25% in the first 8 hours; out of this, 10% reduction should be in the first hour. The remaining 75% reduction needs to be achieved gradually in the next 36–48 hours. Cerebral ischemia may occur in case of too rapid reduction in blood pressure.

The child needs admission in pediatric intensive care unit (PICU) and stabilization of airway, breathing, and circulation (ABC), if required.

The drugs of choice are:
- Intravenous labetalol
- Sodium nitroprusside or
- Sublingual nifedipine.

Start with intravenous labetalol or sodium nitroprusside infusion and titrate the rate of infusion depending upon the response. While patient is on high dose infusion, sudden profound hypotension can develop. Understandably, very close monitoring and titration of the drug is required.

In the event of the child developing hypotension, stop the infusion and then decide depending upon the blood pressure levels whether to continue or not and also consider using alternative drugs.

Sublingual nifedipine has very short duration of action and is not an ideal drug in hypertensive crisis. However, as and when labetalol or sodium nitroprusside is not available, nifedipine (preferably oral rather than sublingual) can be tried cautiously.

Alternatively, intravenous hydralazine, or diazoxide may be used.

Once the blood pressure levels are reduced and remained stable for some time, start on oral antihypertensive drugs in place of the parenteral drug.

Q. Which is a better route if nifedipine is to be used: oral or sublingual?

Oral route should be preferred over sublingual route for administration of nifedipine.

Q. Is the pharmacotherapy of hypertensive crisis in pheochromocytoma in any way different?

Hypertensive crisis due to pheochromocytoma requires use of α-adrenergic blocking agents like phentolamine 1–2 mg intravenously. Its beneficial effect starts in about a minute. Propranolol should be added only after starting α-adrenergic blockers. Otherwise, it may cause rebound hypertension.

Q. Any algorithmic approach to management?

Figure 1 provides an algorithmic stepped-care approach to antihypertensive treatment.

Q. What is the eventual course and prognosis?

Poorly controlled hypertension predisposes to many hypertension-related problems including stroke and ischemic heart disease.

Adolescents detected to have essential hypertension are likely to continue to have hypertension as adults. In cases of secondary hypertension, the prognosis is dependent on the underlying course and its natural course. The prognosis of surgically connected coarctation is variable. The prognosis in cases of chronic renal disease depends upon the response to dialysis and transplant. Neonates who develop hypertension due to umbilical artery catheterization have favorable outcome with most of them improving.

CONCLUSION

The sheet anchor of therapeutic approach to acute severe hypertension (both hypertensive urgency and emergency) is to protect against damage or further damage to end organs. Treatment has to be prompt. Rather than immediately bringing down the blood pressure to normal, it should be achieved in decrements:

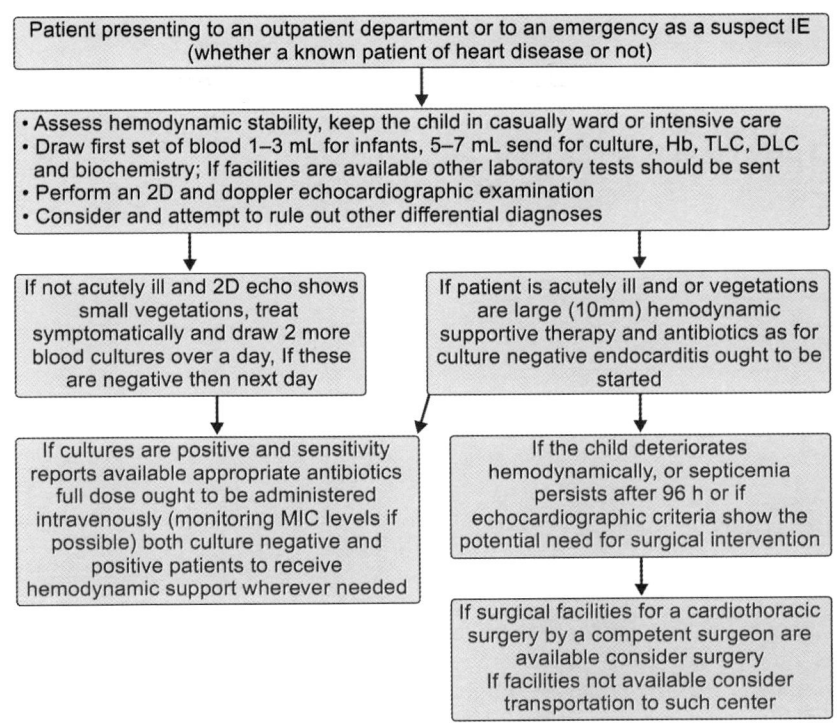

Figure 1: Algorithmic stepped-care approach to pharmacotherapy in pediatric hypertension

10% in first hour, 25% in first 6–8 hours, and rest subsequently (36–48 h) in hypertensive emergency. In hypertensive urgency, decrease can be achieved relatively slowly.

KEY LEARNING POINTS

- Aim of treatment of severe hypertension (both hypertensive urgency and emergency) is to protect against damage/further damage to target organs
- A careful balance between lowering of blood pressure and safeguarding from hypoperfusion of target organs is needed
- Treatment has to be prompt
- Rather than immediately bringing down the blood pressure to normal, it should be achieved in decrements; 10% in first hour, 25% in first 6–8 hours, and rest subsequently (36–48 h) in hypertensive emergency
- In hypertensive urgency, decrease can be achieved relatively slowly
- Attention should also be directed to supportive measures, treatment of underlying disease (say acute glomerulonephritis) and requisite lifestyle change

SUGGESTED READINGS

1. Dayal A, Bahe A. Hypertensive emergencies. In: Gupte S, Gupte SB, Gupte M (Eds): *Recent Advances in Pediatrics-23: Hot Topics*. New Delhi: Jaypee Brothers Medical Publishers; 2015:440-456.
2. Robinson KA, Robinson R. Pediatric hypertension: A-Z. London: Smith & Smith; 2012.
3. Sinclair E. Severe Hypertension. Philadelphia: Academicia 2013.
4. Taylor RE. Hypertensive emergency and crisis. *Br J Pediatr Emergence*. 2013;7:45-56.

CHAPTER 29

Congestive Heart Failure

Anjul Dayal, Abhilasha Singh

INTRODUCTION

The term congestive heart failure (CHF) refers to a clinical state of systemic and pulmonary congestion resulting from inability of the heart to pump as much blood as required for the adequate metabolism of the body. The clinical picture of CHF results from a combination of "relatively low output" and compensatory responses to increase it.

Congestive cardiac failure (CCF) usually results either from an excessive volume or pressure overload on normal myocardium (left to right shunts, aortic stenosis), or from primary myocardial abnormality (myocarditis, cardiomyopathy). Arrhythmias, pericardial diseases and combination of various factors can also result in CHF. The resultant decrease in cardiac output triggers a host of physiological responses aimed at restoring perfusion of the vital organs. Important among these are renal retention of fluid, renin-angiotensin mediated vasoconstriction, and sympathetic overactivity. Excessive fluid retention increases the cardiac output by increasing the end diastolic volume (preload), but also results in symptoms of pulmonary and systemic congestion.

In the pediatric age group, the underlying abnormality is often a large left to right intracardiac shunt, most commonly a ventricular septal defect (VSD), or an obstructive lesion, such as an aortic coarctation.

CASE 1

A 3-month-old male baby presented to the emergency room with the chief complaints of lethargy, poor feeding, and respiratory distress. He was well before 5 days prior to admission, when he developed a febrile illness with cough, rhinorrhea, and poor feeding with vomiting. He subsequently developed progressive respiratory distress. His parents report that he sweats a lot over the forehead when feeding.

Ante natal and post natal history was unremarkable.

Examination: He was febrile, and tachypneic (respiratory rate 72/min), tachycardiac (heart rate 160/min), blood pressure 92/68 mmHg. Oxygen saturation at room air was 99%. He was pale, lethargic, and with mild to moderate subcostal and intercostal retractions. His lungs had scattered crackles with slightly decreased aeration in the left lower lobe. The precordium was slightly active. His heart was of regular rate and rhythm, with a grade II/VI holosystolic murmur at the mid-lower-left sternal border with radiation to the cardiac apex. The S1 is normal and the S2 is prominent. An S4 gallop is noted at the cardiac apex. His abdomen was soft, nondistended and nontender. The liver edge was palpable 3–4 cm below the right costal margin. There were no palpable masses or splenomegaly. His extremities were cool, with peripheral pulses were felt but feeble with no radial-femoral delay. The capillary refill was 4–5 seconds (delayed).

Investigations: Chest X-ray (CXR) showed moderate cardiomegaly with a moderate degree of pulmonary edema. There were no pleural effusions.

A 12-lead electrocardiogram showed a sinus tachycardia, normal PR and QTc intervals, and a left axis deviation.

> An echocardiogram revealed a large perimembranous VSD with nonrestrictive left to right shunting. All cardiac chambers were dilated. Left ventricular contractility was at the lower range of normal. There was no pericardial effusion.
> Treatment: He was loaded with digoxin, and also started on diuretics and afterload reduction. His symptoms improved and he was discharged on higher caloric density formula and anti-failure treatment.
> He was referred for surgical correction of the VSD at 6 months of age.

CASE REVIEW IN A NUTSHELL

This child was brought with features suggestive of acute decompensation of heart failure. Child was treated with supportive treatment initially. Child was also investigated for the possibility of myocarditis and pulmonary edema. Child was started on digoxin and diuretic therapy. Acute treatment consists of management of pulmonary edema, management of respiratory distress, and mechanical ventilation in severe cases to reduce the work of breathing. In severe acute cases initially vasoactive agents like inotropes and inodilators are required. Management of nutrition is an important aspect of treatment which is often forgotten. Surgical treatment of underlying lesion is important to prevent recurrent episodes of heart failure. This child had underlying VSD as the surgically correctable lesion which is been planned to be operated after the acute episode is over.

INTERACTIVE TOPIC REVIEW

Q. What are the causes of congestive heart failure according to age?

Congestive heart failure in the fetus

The etiologic conditions in the fetus include:
- Supraventricular tachycardia
- Severe bradycardia due to complete heart block
- Anemia
- Severe tricuspid regurgitation due to Ebstein's anomaly of the tricuspid valve
- Mitral regurgitation from atrioventricular (AV) canal defect
- Myocarditis.

Most of these are recognized by fetal echocardiography.

Severe CHF in the fetus produces hydrops fetalis with ascites, pleural and pericardial effusions and anasarca. Digoxin or sympathomimetics to the mother may be helpful in cases of fetal tachyarrhythmia or complete heart block, respectively.

Congestive heart failure on first day of life

It is noteworthy that most structural heart defects do not cause CHF within hours of birth. In fact, myocardial dysfunction secondary to asphyxia, hypoglycemia, hypocalcemia, or sepsis is usually responsible for CHF within first 24 hours of birth.

Also, tricuspid regurgitation secondary to hypoxia induced papillary muscle dysfunction or Ebstein's anomaly of the valve may cause CCF on first day. This improves as the pulmonary artery pressure falls over the next few days.

Congestive heart failure in first week of life

Serious cardiac disorders (potentially curable but carrying a high mortality), if left untreated, often present with CHF in the first week of life. The closure of the ductus arteriosus is often the precipitating event.

It is important to check the peripheral pulses and oxygen saturation in both the upper and lower extremities. A lower saturation in the lower limbs means right to left ductal shunting and occurs due to pulmonary hypertension, coarctation of aorta or aortic arch interruption.

Interestingly, an atrial septal defect (ASD) or VSD does not lead to CHF in the first 2 weeks of life. Therefore, an additional cause must be sought (e.g., coarctation of aorta or total anomalous pulmonary venous connection).

Premature infants have a poor myocardial reserve and a patent ductus arteriosus (PDA) may result in CHF in the first week in them.

Adrenal insufficiency due to enzyme deficiencies or neonatal thyrotoxicosis could present with CHF in the first few days of life.

Congestive heart failure beyond second week of life

The most frequent cause of CHF around 6–8 weeks of life is a VSD. This is because the volume of the left to right shunt increases as the pulmonary resistance falls. Other left to right shunts like PDA present similarly.

Left coronary artery arising from the pulmonary artery, a rare disease in this age group merits separate mention, since it is curable and often missed.

Congestive heart failure beyond infancy

Onset of CHF beyond infancy is unusual in patients with congenital heart disease and suggests a complicating factor like valvular regurgitation, infective endocarditis, myocarditis, and anemia. Uncommonly, worsening of aortic or pulmonary stenosis may cause CHF in childhood. Acquired diseases are common cause of CHF in children.

Q. What is the functional category of heart failure?

Heart failure can be classified into four functional categories.

Category 1

Volume overload: Large left to right shunts, valvular insufficiency, or systemic arteriovenous fistulae.

Category 2

Pressure overload: Outflow or inflow obstruction.

Category 3

Disorders affecting the inotropic state: Myocarditis, electrolyte disturbances, hypoxia, acidosis, various cardiomyopathies, coronary artery lesions, endocrine or metabolic derangements, septic shock, toxic shock.

Category 4

Alterations in the chronotropic state: Supraventricular or ventricular tachycardia and complete heart block.

Q. What is the pathophysiology of congestive heart failure?

Several neurohormonal and biochemical derangements occur, perpetuating symptomatology and leading to chronic heart failure.

Changes in calcium handling occur within the myocardium secondary to impairment of sarcoplasmic reticulum function, anaerobic metabolism, and developing acidosis. The fall in cardiac output and changes in regional circulation accompanying heart failure leads to an activation of the renin-angiotensin-aldosterone system and the sympathetic nervous system. Activation of these systems can lead to direct myocardial toxicity, peripheral vasoconstriction, and increased renal sodium and water reabsorption. Cardiac β-receptors are down-regulated causing a reduced inotropic response to β-adrenergic stimulation. Myocardial remodeling including hypertrophy, cell injury, and fibrosis, interferes with normal myocyte function and increases vulnerability to cardiac arrhythmias.

Q. What are the clinical features of congestive heart failure?

- Signs and symptoms of impaired myocardial performance:
  - Cardiomegaly: Represents ventricular hypertrophy and/or dilatation
  - Tachycardia: Mediated by an increased adrenergic drive. This is the body's attempt to improve cardiac output and oxygen delivery
  - Gallop rhythm: Represents either increased flow across the AV valves in the presence of a large left to right shunt, or rapid filling of a noncompliant ventricle
  - Atrioventricular valve regurgitation: Due to ventricular dilatation, decreased ventricular contractility, and at times infarction of papillary muscles
  - Decreased or increased arterial pulsations depending on the lesion leading to heart failure. Extremities are usually cool, with weak peripheral pulses secondary to systemic vasoconstriction. Arterial

pulses may be bounding with lesions causing a large diastolic runoff as seen with large arteriovenous fistulas, PDA, or an aortopulmonary window (other aortopulmonary communication)
  ○ Growth failure: A consequence of decreased systemic perfusion and raised energy requirements
  ○ Diaphoresis (especially with feeding): Represents increased adrenergic activity
- Signs and symptoms of pulmonary congestion:
  ○ Tachypnea: Secondary to interstitial and bronchiolar edema
  ○ Wheezing: Due to external compression on airways, e.g., from an enlarged left atrium
  ○ Rales: Implies the process is severe, with involvement of the alveolar spaces
  ○ Mild cyanosis: Secondary to impaired gas exchange (pulmonary edema)
  ○ Dyspnea
  ○ Orthopnea
  ○ Persistent cough
- Signs and symptoms of systemic venous congestion:
  ○ Hepatomegaly: This may be associated with a mild elevation in the bilirubin level and liver function tests
  ○ Jugular venous distention: Seen only in older children and adolescents
  ○ Peripheral edema: Facial edema is most common in infants and children. Extremity edema may be seen in older children and adolescents. Ascites is usually only seen in older age groups with very advanced heart failure.

Q. Mention the laboratory investigations required in congestive heart failure?

Chest X-ray is one of the more useful studies in the initial assessment of a patient with suspected heart failure. This allows evaluation of heart size and contour, pulmonary vascularity, presence of pleural effusions, abdominal, and cardiac situs (i.e., whether situs inversus or dextrocardia is present), aortic arch sidedness (occasionally, since the X-ray sign of a right or double aortic arch is very subtle), and lung expansion.

Electrocardiogram is most useful in instances where heart failure is secondary to an arrhythmia, anomalous coronary artery, or myocarditis. In fact, it is useful in all patients with heart failure to assess for structural anomalies, cardiac function, and cardiac chamber sizes. Since filling chamber enlargement is one of the initial abnormalities in heart failure, the earliest sign of heart failure will be cardiomegaly (before pulmonary edema) on CXR, and the earliest sign of heart failure on an echocardiogram will be enlargement of the filling chambers (left atrium for left sided heart failure, right atrium for right sided heart failure) and/or decreased ventricular contractility.

Arterial blood gas (in very ill patients), serum electrolytes (including calcium and magnesium levels), and a complete blood count are additional investigations of value.

Q. What are the therapeutic options for congestive heart failure?

Major goals in the treatment of CHF include relief of pulmonary and systemic venous congestion, improvement of myocardial performance, and reversal of the underlying disease process. Historically, digoxin has been one of the most widely used pharmacologic agents in the treatment of heart failure in infants and children.

Additional inotropic agents used in the treatment of acute heart failure include:
- Dopamine
- Dobutamine
- Phosphodiesterase inhibitors (milrinone and amrinone).

Diuretic therapy is an integral part of the treatment of children with CHF. Three most commonly utilized classes of diuretics include:
1. Loop diuretics (furosemide)
2. Potassium sparing diuretics (spironolactone)
3. Thiazide diuretics (hydrochlorothiazide).

Among the benefits of diuretic therapy, there are improvements in systemic, pulmonary, and venous congestion.

Spironolactone may exert additional beneficial effects by attenuating the development of aldosterone-induced myocardial fibrosis and catecholamine release.

Q. Are there any adverse effects of diuretic therapy?

Of course, potential complications of diuretic therapy include:
- Volume contraction
- Electrolyte abnormalities (hyponatremia, hypo- or hyperkalemia, hypochloremia), and
- Metabolic alkalosis or acidosis.

Hence, electrolyte balance should be carefully monitored, especially during aggressive diuresis, as the failing myocardium is more sensitive to arrhythmias induced by electrolyte dyscrasias.

Q. Any advances in the management?

"Afterload reduction" is one of the newer concepts in this respect. Relaxation of arteriolar smooth muscle helps to decrease the systemic vascular resistance and augment cardiac output.

Venodilatation exerts its effect on preload by increasing venous capacitance, thus lowering filling pressures.

The angiotensin-converting enzyme (ACE) inhibitors decrease systemic vascular resistance and have a favorable effect on the body's neurohormonal response to heart failure and cardiac remodeling. They are thought to have beneficial hemodynamic effects in patients with decreased systemic ventricular contractility, and those patients with large left to right shunts.

The phosphodiesterase inhibitor milrinone is often used in the intensive care setting of acute, new onset systemic ventricle dysfunction (e.g., myocarditis), and in the immediate postoperative setting following cardiopulmonary bypass (ischemia-reperfusion injury).

The dosage of oral medicationsis presented in table 1.

Treatment of chronic heart failure with the use of β-blockers is now an accepted practice. Step wise treatment is detailed in table 2. The beneficial effects are thought to be derived from the reversal of myocardial dysfunction occurring secondary to sympathetic activation and down-regulation of β-adrenergic receptors, coronary artery vasodilatation, and possible anti-oxidant effects.

Additional nonpharmacologic therapeutic measures include:
- Elevation of the head and shoulders to 30–45 degrees
- Bed rest
- Dietary changes (higher caloric intake, and a low sodium diet in older children and adolescents)
- Packed red blood cell transfusion
- Iron supplementation
- Administration of supplemental oxygen

TABLE 1: Dosage of oral medications

Digoxin	10 µg/kg/day (in two divided doses for children <years)
Furosemide	1–4 mg/kg/day (1–2 doses)
Spironolactone	2–4 mg/kg/day (2 doses)
Captopril	Neonates: (0.4–1.6 mg/kg/day) in 3 divided doses Infants and children: 0.5–4 mg/kg/day in 3 divided doses
Enalapril	0.1–0.5 mg/kg/day (2 doses)—avoid in neonates
Losartan	0.5 mg/kg/day once daily
Metroprolol	0.1–0.2 mg/kg/dose (2 doses) and increases to 1 mg/kg/dose or maximally tolerated dose over weeks or months
Carvedilol	0.05 mg/kg/dose (twice daily) and increase to 0.4–0.5 mg/kg/dose (twice daily) or maximally tolerated dose

TABLE 2: Stepwise treatment protocol for congestive heart failure

Step 1	In acute decompensation: Bed rest, propped up position, humidified oxygen, and volume restriction
Step 2	Start digoxin (not in acute decompensation). Assess reversible and precipitating causes. Assess need for surgical or interventional procedures
Step 3	Add ACE inhibitors. In case of ACE inhibitor induced intractable cough, shift over to ARB. Switch to nitrates if ACE Inhibitor or ARB is not tolerated
Step 4	Add carvedilol in compensated heart failure especially with tachycardia
Step 6	Cardiac surgery or transplant. Ventricular assist device as a bridge to transplant.

ACE, angiotensin-converting enzyme; ARB, angiotensin-receptor blocker.

Oxygen is a pulmonary vasodilator. In known large left to right shunt lesions, its administration decreases pulmonary vascular resistance, increases the degree of left to right shunting, and worsens the degree of pulmonary edema. Prostaglandins E1 infusion is essential in infants, especially within 1 week of life with duct dependent lesion.

Q. What is the role of surgery in treatment of congestive heart failure?

In patients with heart failure, the treatment plan should ultimately deal with the underlying condition. This may include surgical repair of a shunt lesion or valvular anomaly, interventional cardiac procedures, radiofrequency ablation, or cardiac transplantation.

Repair of congenital heart defects with large left to right shunts (VSD, ASD, AV canal), or those with valvular abnormalities carry a very low surgical mortality. Patients with cardiomyopathies or hypoplastic left heart syndrome will occasionally require a heart transplant as a last resort and ventricular assist device as a bridge to cardiac transplant.

Q. What is the management of acute decompensation (pulmonary edema)?

For acute pulmonary edema, several treatment methods are used. To treat acute pulmonary edema, the hydrostatic force pushing the fluid out into the alveolar space can be reduced by reducing back pressure (preload and afterload reduction) by the following therapeutic measures: diuresis, vasodilation (increases vascular capacitance), and augmenting contractility (reduces back pressure). The most important parameter to increase the pressure within the alveolus to counterbalance the excessive hydrostatic pressure to reverse pulmonary edema is the positive end-expiratory pressure.

CONCLUSION

Despite the diverse etiologies of heart failure in the pediatric population, the presentation of heart failure represents a common constellation of symptoms, signs, and physical findings. Physical findings include rales and peripheral edema. The long-term treatment of CHF in children includes digoxin, diuretics and afterload reduction with ACE inhibitors. Angiotensin converting enzyme inhibitors are increasingly valuable in maintaining cardiac function long term. Beta-blockers have been increasingly used in children, and may have a role in the treatment of patients with idiopathic dilated cardiomyopathy. Surgical treatment, such as partial vectriculectomy, ventricular assist device, and cardiac transplant has been a new lease of life to children with intractable heart failure.

KEY LEARNING POINTS

- Heart failure in children can be due to varied etiology
- Onset of symptoms gives insight to the probable etiology
- Stepwise management of cardiac failure is the best approach for the treatment
- Cardiac surgery, especially cardiac transplant, is being increasingly used in pediatric population.

SUGGESTED READINGS

1. Braunwald E. The management of heart failure: the past, the present, and the future. *Circ Heart Fail*. 2008;1:58-62.
2. Chaturvedi V, Saxena A. Heart failure in Children. *Indian J Pediatr*. 2009;76:195-205.
3. Chioncel O, Ambrosy AP, Bubenek S, Filipescu D, Vinereanu D, Petris A, et al. Epidemiology, pathophysiology, and in-hospital management of pulmonary edema: data from the Romanian Acute Heart Failure Syndromes registry. *J Cardiovasc Med (Hagerstown)*. 2016;17:92-104.
4. Frobel AK, Hulpke-Wette M, Schmidt KG, Läer S. Beta-blockers for congestive heart failure in children. *Cochrane Database Syst Rev*. 2009:CD007037.
5. Hsu DT, Pearson GD. Heart failure in children: part II: diagnosis, treatment, and future directions. *Circ Heart Fail*. 2009;2:490-498.
6. Lindle KA, Dinh K, Moffett BS, Kyle WB, Montgomery NM, Denfield SD, et al. Angiotensin-converting enzyme inhibitor nephrotoxicity in neonates with cardiac disease. *Pediatr Cardiol*. 2014;35:499-506.
7. Massin MM, Astadicko I, Dessy H. Epidemiology of heart failure in a tertiary pediatric center. *Clin Cardiol*. 2008;31:388-391.
8. Thomas TO, Chandrakasan S, O'Brien M, Jefferies JL, Ryan TD, Wilmot I, et al. The use of a Berlin Heart EXCOR LVAD in a child receiving chemotherapy for Castleman's disease. *Pediatr Transplant*. 2015;19:E15-8.

SECTION 7
Infectious Diseases

CHAPTER

Severe Dengue

30

Anupam Bahe, Anjul Dayal

INTRODUCTION

Dengue or "breakbone fever" has gradually evolved as one of the important causes of febrile illness in the tropical and subtropical region. It may be caused by any one of the four serologically-related but antigenically distinct dengue virus serotypes (DENV 1, 2, 3, or 4). The primary vector for viral transmission is the *Aedes aegypti* (Linnaeus) mosquito. Despite the inadequate surveillance of cases from the underdeveloped tropical countries, the average number being reported per year has increased drastically.

Dengue disease is a rapidly increasing public health priority with a global distribution. Resource-poor countries are particularly vulnerable to transmission of dengue disease and it is present in urban and suburban areas in the America, Eastern Mediterranean, Western Pacific, South-East Asia, and mainly rural areas in Africa. A host of factors including the relentless urbanization with poor hygiene, dilapidated health systems to increasing international travel fuel the spread of this disease geographically and increase the disease burden of tropics significantly. This disease has been found to have profound effect on multiple organ systems.

CASE 1

A 7-year-old boy presented with breathlessness, periorbital puffiness, decreased urine output, and drowsiness of 3 days duration. He had a preceding history of fever, body ache 7 days prior to admission. He was given oral paracetamol four times a day. However, he was afebrile since last 2 days. Well-nourished and well-built with a weight of 25 kg and height of 118 cm, febrile (102°F) drowsy, pulse 82/min, respiratory rate 44/min presented with periorbital puffiness and pedal edema. Extremities were cold, peripheral pulses were feeble, capillary filling time (CFT) >3 s, blood pressure (BP) 78/66 mmHg. On examination, icterus was present; liver was palpable 5 cm below costal margin, liver span was 12 cm, there was no splenomegaly. On auscultation, air entry was decreased on right side and few scattered crepitations were present over interscapular and infraxillary area, bronchial breath sounds were heard at interscapular region. His Glasgow coma scale (GCS) was 12/15.

Investigations: Hemoglobin (Hb) 11 g/dL, hematocrit 42, normocytic normochromic picture, total leukocyte count 4,800 (N25L70, platelet count 20,000/cm^3), serum bilirubin 2.0 (total)/0.3 (indirect)/1.7 (direct), serum glutamic pyruvic transaminase (SGPT) 125, serum glutamic oxaloacetic transaminase (SGOT) 77, alkaline phosphatase 225, serum ammonia 189, serum creatinine 0.7, serum proteins 6.2 (albumin 4.0, globulin 2.1), and X-ray chest showed right-sided pleural effusion. Ultrasound of abdomen showed minimal hepatomegaly and free-fluid in abdominal cavity. His nonstructural protein-1 (NS1) antigen test and immunoglobulin M (IgM) for dengue were positive.

Diagnosis: Severe dengue

Treatment given: Fluids which were titrated to hematocrit and to maintain urine output of 0.5–1 mL/kg/h, intravenous dobutamine, later started on tablet Lasilactone.

Investigations done: His hematocrit was monitored and intravenous fluids were titrated accordingly, platelet counts monitored for drop below 5,000/cm^3, two-dimensional echocardiography was done.

Outcome: The child improved with intravenous fluids, later injection dobutamine was started. On day, 3 he was started on tablet lasilactone for 2 days. He was subsequently discharged on day 5.

CASE REVIEW IN A NUTSHELL

The child presented with features of severe dengue with compensated shock and acute hepatitis. He was treated with intravenous bolus and was started on maintenance fluids and the fluids were titrated according to his hematocrit and urine output. He was subsequently started on dobutamine in view of persisting shock. His hemodynamics improved and his intravenous fluids were gradually tapered and stopped. His hepatitis improved over the period of 3 days.

Once the diagnosis of dengue fever is established, the treatment is usually based on the intravascular fluid management and in this case, fluid was started and optimized according to hematocrit and urine output. Shock in dengue is associated with narrow pulse pressure and thus in view of persisting shock, a vasoactive agent, dobutamine, was started. Dobutamine is inotropic agent with vasodilatory action.

Usually hepatitis in case of dengue is self-resolving and does not require any special management. Laboratory features of hepatitis improved with resolution of shock. Child presented with low platelet count.

Since there were no clinical features of bleeding, no blood products were transfused. However, complete blood picture was repeated for evaluating hematocrit to titrate the ongoing fluid management.

INTERACTIVE TOPIC REVIEW

Q. What is the case definition of dengue?

The case definition of dengue case has evolved over last 2 decades. According to the World Health Organization (WHO) 1997 classification, dengue has been traditionally classified into dengue fever (DF), dengue hemorrhagic fever (DHF), and dengue shock syndrome (DSS).

Dengue fever: Fever and at least two features such as ocular pain, headache, muscle or joint pains, cutaneous rash, bleeding manifestations, and reduced leukocyte count.

Dengue hemorrhagic fever: Fever, thrombocytopenia ($\leq 100 \times 10^9$/L), bleeding manifestations, and evidence of plasma leakage.

Dengue shock syndrome: Dengue hemorrhagic fever with tachycardia or low pulse pressure (<20 mmHg) or hypotension (systolic BP <90 mmHg).

Q. In which way has the 1997 World Health Organization classification been modified?

The 2009 modification of categorization by WHO includes dengue with or without warning signs or severe dengue (Fig. 1).

Dengue: Fever and two of these: nausea, vomiting, skin rash, bodyache, leukopenia, or any warning sign.

Warning signs include pain in the abdominal or presence of tenderness, persistent vomiting, clinical evidence of fluid accumulation like effusions and ascites, bleeding, liver enlargement, or rise in hematocrit ($\geq 20\%$) with rapid reduction in platelet count (<50,000/mm^3).

Severe dengue: Evidence of severe plasma leakage, bleeding, and organ impairment. Organ impairment includes hepatic involvement in form of transaminases elevated beyond 1,000 IU/L and central nervous system

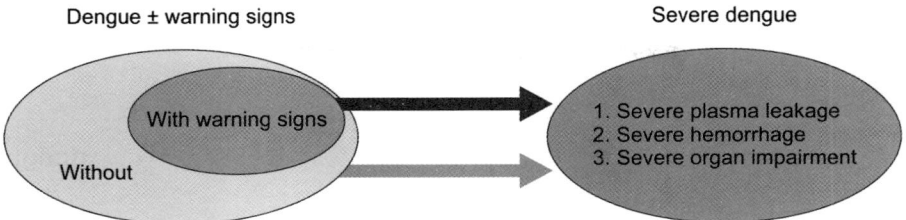

Figure 1: Possible spectrum of dengue fever as per World Health Organization

Criteria for dengue ± warning signs

Probable dengue
Live in/travel to dengue endemic area.
Fever and 2 of the following criteria:
- Nausea, vomiting
- Rash
- Aches and pains
- Tourniquet test positive
- Leukopenia
- Any warning sign

Laboratory-confirmed dengue
Importent when no sign of plasma leakage

Warning signs*
- Abdominal pain or tenderness
- Persistent vomiting
- Clinical fluid accumulation
- Mucosal bleed
- Lethargy, restlessness
- Liver enlargement >2 cm
- Laboratory: increase in HCT concurrent with rapid decrease in platelet

(*Requiring strict observation and medical intervention)

Criteria for severe dengue

Severe plasma leakage
Leading to:
- Shock (DSS)
- Fluid accumulation with respiratory distress

Severe bleeding
As evaluated by clinician

Severe organ involvement
- Liver: AST or ALT ≥1,000
- CNS: Impaired consciousness
- Heart and other organs

HCT, hematocrit; DSS, dengue shock syndrome; AST, aspartate aminotransferase; ALT, alanine transaminase; CNS, central nervous system.

manifestations like alteration in sensorium or cardiac or other organ involvement.

In essence it is a continuum of the same disease process varying in severity

Q. In spite of the recent categorization, why do the majority of the studies widely use the more popular dengue fever, dengue hemorrhagic fever, and dengue shock syndrome classification for a case definition? Is it justified?

Studies have demonstrated overlap between case definitions of DF, DHF, and DSS, supporting the concept of dengue as a continuous spectrum of disease rather than distinct entities. Indeed, the term DHF is considered to place undue emphasis on hemorrhage when plasma leakage leading to shock is a more significant warning sign. Manifestations of severe dengue include organ failure, but this was not included in the 1997 case definitions.

The 2009 classification into severity levels is considered to be more sensitive in capturing severe disease than the 1997 guidelines, with observed sensitivities of up to 92% and 39%, respectively. A multicenter study across 18 countries demonstrated that approximately 14% of cases could not be classified using the DF or DHF or DSS classification, even when strict DHF criteria were not applied, compared with only 1.6% with the revised system. The new classification is particularly useful with respect to triage and management of dengue, reporting during surveillance and for endpoint measurements in dengue clinical trials.

Furthermore, research on the revised 2009 classification system is necessary in order to optimize dengue case definitions. There is a need for more precise definition of warning signs to enable optimal triaging for more accurate identification of patients who require hospitalization as opposed to those who can be treated as outpatients.

Q. What are the stages of dengue fever?

Following an incubation period, the illness begins abruptly, going through three phases
1. Febrile phase: Presents with either mild fever only or a more incapacitating disease. This latter presentation is characterized by the sudden onset of high fever, severe headache, retro-orbital pain, myalgia, arthralgia and rash with symptoms occurring predominantly in the early febrile stage.
2. Critical phase: The skin is flushed with the appearance of a petechial rash. This usually occurs around the time of defervescence, typically on days 3–7, and is associated with capillary leakage and hemorrhage.
3. Recovery phase: There is a resolution of capillary leak and improvement in shock. The urine output improves and fluid requirement decreases rapidly.

Q. At times, a patient with severe dengue may well be afebrile. What could be the explanation for this?

As pointed out earlier, the dengue illness passes through three phases: (i) febrile, (ii) critical, and (iii) recovery.

After a period of 3–7 days incubation, the natural course runs in form of fever lasting for 2–7 days, and subsequently a critical phase may occur during defervescence starting from 3–7 days of the illness when plasma leakage dominates the clinical picture. Those surviving this phase of plasma leakage would eventually recover. More severe disease is associated with higher viral load.

Q. What are the risk factors for severe dengue? Can we accurately predict during the febrile period which patient is likely to progress to severe dengue?

It is very difficult to predict the subset of patients who will progress from nonsevere to severe illness. Similarly, it can be difficult to differentiate DHF from DF and other viral diseases, e.g., typhoid fever, particularly during the acute phase of the illness (Fig. 2).

Q. Why does the patient have jaundice? What are the mechanisms of liver function derangements in dengue fever? How do you interpret the results of liver function tests in dengue fever? Does the patient have hepatitis?

The most commonly involved vital organ involved in dengue is liver. The spectrum of

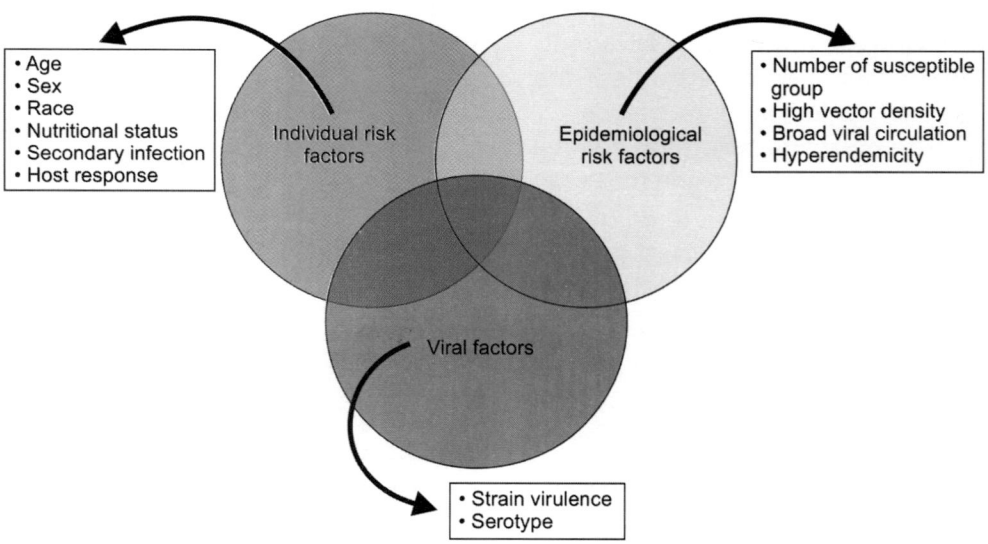

Figure 2: Risk factors for severe dengue

involvement includes asymptomatic elevation of hepatic transaminases to occurrence of severe manifestation in form of acute liver failure (ALF).

The prime targets for DENV infection are hepatocytes and Kupffer cells. The various pathways involved in this apoptotic process include viral cytopathy, hypoxic mitochondrial dysfunction, the immune response, and accelerated endoplasmic reticular stress. Expression of DENV-induced tumor necrosis factor-related apoptosis-inducing ligand (TRAIL) and tumor necrosis factor (TNF)-α and Fas signaling have also been implicated in this process. The pathogenesis of hepatic injury in dengue is believed to be primarily a T-cell mediated process involving interaction between antibodies and the endothelium and a concomitant cytokine storm often labeled as cytokine "Tsunami," and host factors like genetic polymorphisms. Dengue infection induces a cytokine storm and concentrations of cytokines like interleukin (IL)-2, IL-6, TNF-α, and interferon (IFN)-γ reach peak levels in the initial 3d. Interleukin-4, 5, and 10 contribute to later in the course of disease.

Dengue-related hepatic involvement of the liver is suggested in the form of liver enlargement and elevated transaminases.

Manifestations such as abdominal pain and anorexia are significantly more common in DF than in DHF. Hepatomegaly is present in both DF and DHF but more common in DF. The most common abnormality detected is the raised transaminase levels. Raised aspartate aminotransferase (AST) levels are more common than raised alanine transaminase (ALT) levels in the majority of patients. The elevation in AST is more than ALT, more during the first week of infection, with a tendency to decrease to normal levels within three weeks. The AST released from damaged myocytes could explain the higher levels of AST than those of ALT in patients with dengue fever at an earlier stage. The increased AST to ALT ratio is useful for differential diagnosis from acute hepatitis caused by the hepatitis A, B, or C viruses where it is rarely observed.

Median AST and ALT values are to be higher for severe forms of dengue than for uncomplicated dengue fever.

Factors predicting liver damage are bleeding, secondary infection, thrombocytopenia, high-blood concentration, female sex, and younger age. Coagulation abnormalities occur in some subjects. Increasing bleeding episodes have been found with increasing AST or ALT levels. Generally, liver synthetic function in terms of coagulation factor production are well-compensated.

Q. Is it safe to use paracetamol for fever control in dengue fever?

Acute liver failure due to paracetamol overdose may be due to either a single large overdose or cumulative multiple overdoses. The latter is being increasingly recognized as an important cause of ALF due to paracetamol overdose. Mild-to-moderate hepatitis is well-known in dengue. However the metabolism of paracetamol is also reduced in patients with hepatitis.

World Health Organization guidelines discourage the use of other nonsteroidal anti-inflammatory drugs (NSAIDs), such as ibuprofen or antipyretics, in DF.

Interestingly, dengue has also been implicated as the cause of worsening of chronic liver disease, i.e., being the acute component of acute on chronic liver failure (ACLF).

Q. What are the other modalities of treating liver dysfunction in dengue fever?

In the management of patients with dengue with ALF, besides supportive measures, specific measures have also been tried with success.

Infusion of N-acetyl cysteine (NAC), use of molecular adsorbent recirculating system (MARS), and liver transplantation are the other modalities.

Liver transplantation becomes a difficult proposition in lieu of hemodynamic compromise, bleeding, and organ impairment seen during dengue infection.

However, the cornerstone of management remains optimization of fluids, targeting optimal tissue perfusion and avoidance of hepatotoxic drugs.

Finally, hepatic involvement is more often severe in children compared to adults. Management is primarily supportive and the outcome is usually good.

Q. Can dengue present as multiple organ dysfunction syndrome?

Yes, it can. With DENV infection, high level of viremia is associated with involvement of different organs (liver, brain, kidney, heart, lungs, hematopoietic) in the severe form of the disease.

Q. What about the laboratory diagnosis of dengue?

Isolation of viruses can take 7–10 days. Serological tests are generally the tests of choice to diagnose acute flavivirus infections, with most utilizing IgM capture enzyme-linked immunosorbent assay (ELISA) formats. More than 90% of the subjects are IgM positive by the 4th day of illness but positive IgM antibody may also be due to infection up to 3 months earlier.

Commercial kits for the measurement of antibodies include the ELISA kits, a dipstick, and a rapid dot-blot assay.

Q. What should be the criteria to make a choice in testing?

The choice of a test depends on the availability of facilities and human resources and, also, the time of sampling (Fig. 3).

Q. What are the salient details about the NS1 test?

The NS1 protein is a 50 kDa (353 or 354 amino acids) glycoprotein which has a high amino acid and nucleotide homology among flaviviruses. NS1 is synthesized by all flaviviruses and is secreted from infected mammalian cells. The presence of secreted NS1 (sNS1) in the blood stream stimulates a strong humoral response. NS1 does not form part of the virion but is released from the DENV-infected cells. Preliminary studies have shown that this nonstructural glycoprotein is involved in viral RNA replication, and it has been found in acute-phase blood samples of patients with primary or secondary DENV infections. NS1 antigen can be detected with

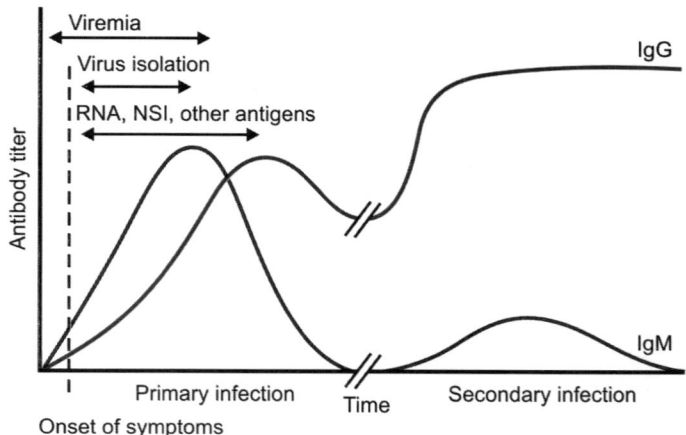

RNA, ribonucleic acid; NS1, nonstructural protein 1.

Figure 3: Major diagnostic markers for dengue infection

good sensitivity (71-100%) till day 3 of fever, whereas IgM has a sensitivity of 0-50% at this time. On day 4 of illness, both the tests have a comparative sensitivity. Beyond day 4, IgM antibody detection is superior to NS1. Later, combining this assay with IgM and or IgG detection may, therefore, be necessary for confidence in diagnosing DENV infection.

Q. What is the management strategy of patients with compensated shock?

The algorithm for management of patients with compensated shock is depicted in flowchart 1.

Q. Is it possible to differentiate septic shock from dengue shock early in the course of illness?

Though dengue shock syndrome is a distinct entity from septic shock with some overlapping features but it is difficult to differentiate them early during the course of illness. Also both entities can be concomitantly present in the same patient.

The severe dengue patients are significantly less likely to have systemic inflammatory response syndrome, be tachycardic, and have a narrower pulse pressure at admission when compared with septic shock patients. Mental status is better preserved, and spontaneous clinical bleeding is more common in children with DSS compared with those in septic shock. These likely results are due to predominantly vasodilatory state in septic shock versus vasoconstrictory state that is the initial response in DSS.

Q. What is the management strategy of patients with decompensated shock?

The algorithm for management of patients with decompensated shock is depicted in flowchart 2.

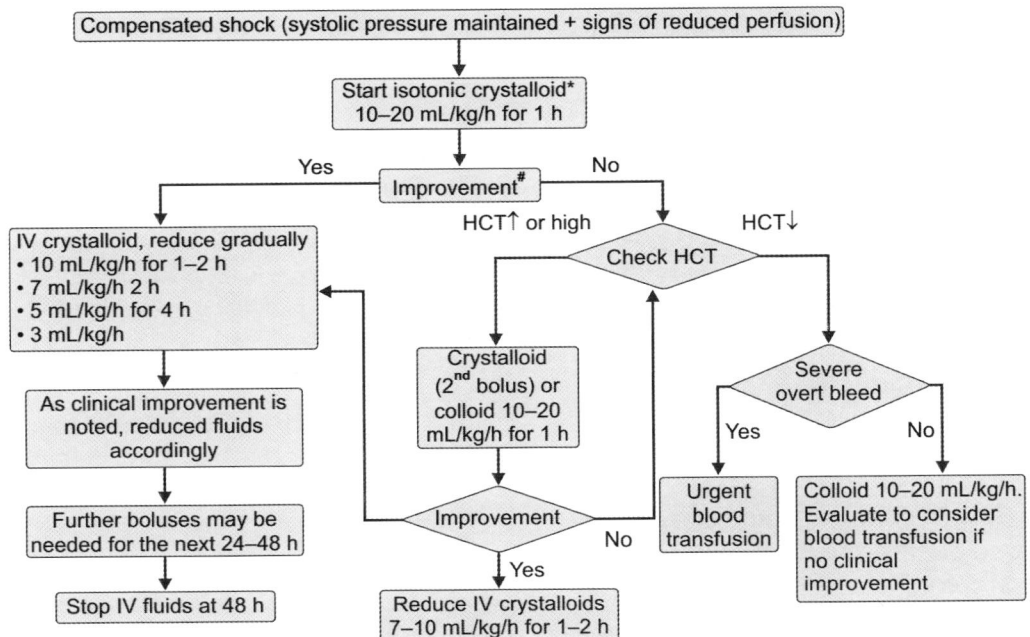

IV, intravenous; HCT, hematocrit; ↑, increase; ↓, decrease.
*Colloid is preferable if the patient has already received previous boluses of crystalloid.
#Reassess the patient's clinical condition, vital signs, pulse volume, capillary refill time and temperature of extremities.

Flowchart 1: Algorithmic approach to management strategy of patients with compensated shock

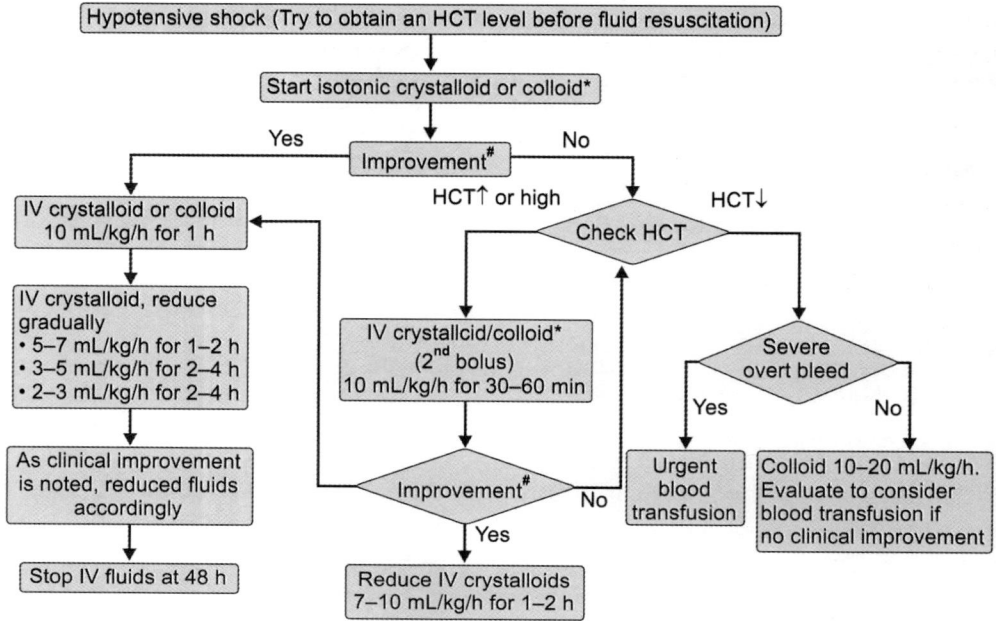

IV, intravenous; HCT, hematocrit; ↑, increase; ↓, decrease.
*Colloid is preferable if the patient has already received previous boluses of crystalloid.
#Reassess the patient's clinical condition, vital signs, pulse volume, capillary refill time and temperature of extremities.
Flowchart 2: Algorithmic approach for management of patients with decompensated shock

Q. What are the parameters used for hemodynamic assessment?

Seven parameters are monitored:
- Mental status
- Heart rate
- Blood pressure
- Respiratory rate
- Capillary time
- Peripheral pulses
- Extremities (warm or cold) (Table 1).

Q. How frequently should complete blood picture and what parameters be monitored?

The white blood cells (WBC) count may be normal with predominant neutrophils in the early febrile phase. Thereafter, there is a fall in the WBC count and neutrophils towards end of febrile phase. Leukopenia (WBC <5,000 cells/cm³) usually precedes thrombocytopenia or rising hematocrit and is helpful in predicting the critical phase of plasma leakage. A sudden rise in hematocrit is usually observed at least 48 hours prior to or simultaneously with drop in platelet count (Fig. 4).

Hemoconcentration may be demonstrated by an increasing level of hematocrit in spite of adequate hydration. Hemoconcentration or rising hematocrit is objective evidence of plasma leakage. Hematocrit should be monitored every 2 hours and thereafter 4 hours..

The patient's baseline hematocrit on the first 3 days of illness is a useful reference point. The sequential changes in the hematocrit are the most useful guide to decision-making about fluid therapy. Random hematocrit levels are not meaningful for interpretation of the real-time clinical situation.

CHAPTER 30: Severe Dengue

TABLE 1: Parameters used for hemodynamic monitoring

Parameters	Stable condition	Compensated shock	Hypotensive shock
Sensorium	Clear and lucid	Clear and lucid (shock can be missed if you do not touch the patient)	Change of mental status (restless and combative)
Capillary refill time	Brisk (<2 s)	Prolonged (>2 s)	Very prolonged, mottled skin
Extremities	Warm and pink	Cool peripheries	Cold and clammy
Peripheral pulse	Good volume	Weak and therapy	Feeble or absent
Heart rate	Normal for age	Tachycardia	Severe tachycardia with bradycardia in the late shock
Blood pressure	Normal for age, normal pulse pressure for age	Normal systolic pressure but rising diastolic pressure. Narrowing pulse pressure. Postural hypotension	Narrowed pulse pressure (<20 mmHg), hypotension (see definition below), unrecordable blood pressure, metabolic acidosis
Respiratory rate	Normal for age	Tachypnea	Hyperpnea, Kussmaul breathing

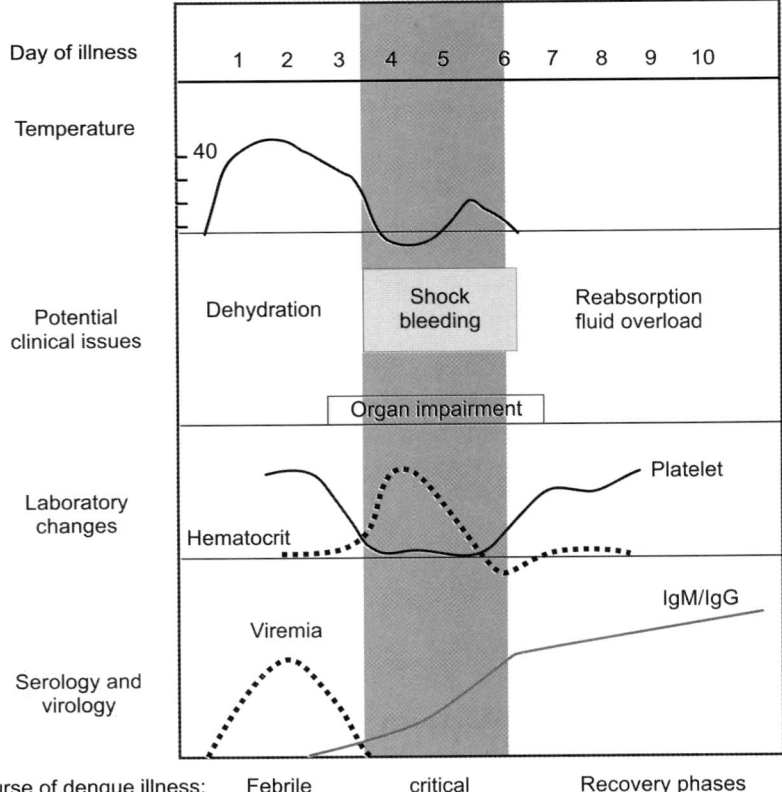

IgM, immunoglobulin M; IgG, immunoglobulin M.

Figure 4: The course of dengue illness

Note: Temperature is given in degrees Celsius (°C).

Q. What is the management strategy of patients with increasing hematocrit?

A rising or persistently high-hematocrit together with unstable vital signs (such as narrowed pulse pressure) indicates active plasma leakage and the need for a further bolus of fluid replacement. However, a rising or persistently high hematocrit together with stable hemodynamic status and adequate urine output does not require extra intravenous fluid. In the latter case, close monitoring is needed and mostly hematocrit will start to fall within the next 24 hours as plasma leakage stops.

Q. What is the management strategy of patients with decreasing hematocrit?

Major hemorrhage is indicated by a fall in hematocrit together with unstable vital signs (narrowed pulse pressure, tachycardia, metabolic acidosis, and poor urine output).

In the event of a severe hemorrhage, urgent blood transfusion should be given. If there is no clinical sign of bleeding, then a further bolus of 10–20 mL/kg of colloid should be given, followed by repeat clinical assessment and hematocrit level determination plus a review to consider blood transfusion. Concealed bleeding may take several hours to become apparent and the patient's hematocrit will continue to decrease without achieving hemodynamic stability.

On the contrary, a decrease in hematocrit together with stable hemodynamic status and adequate urine output indicates hemodilution and/or reabsorption of extravasated fluids In this case intravenous fluids must be discontinued immediately to avoid pulmonary edema.

Q. What are indications for transfusion of blood products?

Blood transfusion is lifesaving and should be given as soon as severe bleeding is suspected or recognized.

> **BOX 1: Situations predicting severe bleeding**
> - Persistent and/or severe overt bleeding in the presence of unstable hemodynamic status, regardless of the hematocrit level
> - Decrease in hematocrit after boluses of fluid resuscitation together with unstable hemodynamic status
> - Refractory shock that fails to respond to consecutive fluid resuscitation of 40–60 mL/kg
> - Hypotensive shock with inappropriately low or normal hematocrit
> - Persistent or worsening metabolic acidosis in patients with a well-maintained systolic blood pressure, especially in those with severe abdominal tenderness and distension

The existence of severe bleeding should be considered in certain situations (Box 1).

Q. Any other guideline for blood transfusion in dengue?

Blood transfusion is life-saving and should be given as soon as severe bleeding is suspected or recognized.

However, blood transfusion must be given with caution because of the risk of fluid overload. Also do not wait for the hematocrit to drop too low before deciding on blood transfusion. A hematocrit of <30% as a trigger for blood transfusion, as recommended in the Surviving Sepsis Campaign Guideline, is not applicable to dengue.

CONCLUSION

All patients with severe dengue should be admitted to a hospital. Judicious intravenous fluid resuscitation is the essential and usually sole intervention required. The crystalloid solution should be isotonic and the volume just sufficient to maintain an effective circulation during the period of plasma leakage. Plasma losses should be replaced immediately and rapidly with isotonic crystalloid solution.

In case of hypotensive shock, colloid solution is preferred. Continue replacement of further plasma losses to maintain effective circulation for 24–48 hours.

> **KEY LEARNING POINTS**
>
> ☞ Recognize the critical period which begins with defervescence and lasts for 24–48 hours. Patients may rapidly deteriorate during this period
> ☞ Recognize and treat early shock. Early shock is characterized by narrowing pulse pressure, increasing heart rate, and delayed capillary refill or cool extremities
> ☞ Use only the minimum amount of intravenous fluid to keep the patient well-perfused. Decrease intravenous fluid rate as hemodynamic status improves or urine output increases
> ☞ Do not transfuse platelets until there is clinical bleed or need for an invasive procedure. Platelet transfusions do not decrease the risk of severe bleeding and may instead lead to fluid overload and prolonged hospitalization.

SUGGESTED READINGS

1. Kyle JL, Harris E. Global spread and persistence of dengue. *Annu Rev Microbiol.* 2008;62:71-92.
2. Chowell G, Torre CA, Munayco-Ee C, Suárez-OL, López-CR, Hyman JM. Spatial and temporal dynamics of dengue fever in Peru: 1994-2006. *Epidemiol Infect.* 2008;136:1667-1677.
3. Freedman DO, Weld LH, Kozarsky PE, Fisk T, Robins R, von Sonnenburg F. Spectrum of disease and relation to place of exposure among ill returned travelers. *N Engl J Med.* 2006; 354:119-130.
4. Gubler DJ. Cities spawn epidemic dengue viruses. *Nat Med.* 2004;10:129-130.
5. Gupte S, Shaik FA, Green J, Singh UK. Dengue. In: Gupte S, Gupte N (Eds): *Pediatric Infectious Diseases.* Gurgaon: Macmillan; 2012:181-202.
6. Halstead SB. Dengue. *Lancet.* 2007;370:1644-1652.
7. Statler J, Mammen M, Lyons A, Sun W. Sonographic findings of healthy volunteers infected with dengue virus. *J Clin Ultrasound.* 2008;36:413-417.
8. Wilder SA, Gubler DJ. Geographic expansion of dengue: the impact of international travel. *Med Clin North Am.* 2008;92:1377-1390.
9. World Health Organization. Handbook of clinical management of Dengue. WHO Library Cataloguing-in-Publication Data 2012. Geneva: WHO 2012.

CHAPTER 31

Cerebral Malaria

Anjul Dayal, Abhilasha Singh

INTRODUCTION

Malaria is the most important of the parasitic diseases of humans and its neurological complication, cerebral malaria is arguably one of the most common nontraumatic encephalopathies in the world. Malaria affects about 5% of the world's population at any time and causes somewhere between 0.5 and 2.5 million deaths each year. Infection rates have remained high despite public health measures. That is due to the rise of strains resistant to the available antimalarial medicines, and to social factors (migration, deforestation, irrigation, occupation of areas without programs for vector eradication).

Though there are four species of human malaria, *Plasmodium falciparum* causes nearly all the deaths and neurological complications. Severe malaria occurs predominantly in patients with little or no background immunity, i.e., children growing up in endemic areas, or travellers or migrants who come from areas without malaria, but are exposed to malaria later in life.

Manifestations of severe malaria differ depending on the age of the patient and previous exposure. In the first 2 years of life, severe anemia is a common presenting feature of cerebral malaria. In older children, seizure in cerebral malaria is the commonest mode of presentation. Metabolic acidosis, mainly a lactic acidosis, is common at all ages. Severe malaria is a multisystem disease, and the outcome often depends on the degree of vital organ dysfunction.

CASE 1

A 4-year-old boy was admitted to the emergency outpatient clinic with intractable seizures for the previous hour. He was febrile on arrival and was severely dehydrated.

His Glasgow Coma Score (GCS) on presentation was: EMV (eye, motor and verbal responses) score 11, plantar response bilaterally was extensor, and pupils were reacting normally bilaterally. Abdominal examination showed liver 2 cm palpable below costal margin and spleen 6 cm palpable.

He was immediately resuscitated with fluid bolus followed by supplemental oxygen and airway management. He was given lorazepam followed by fosphenytoin for control of seizures.

Blood analysis was suggestive of anemia (hemoglobin: 9.8 g/dL), total leukocyte count of 4,100 with platelets of 1.2 L. C-reactive protein was 12.20 mg/L. A blood smear revealed the presence of *P. falciparum* ring forms with a parasitemia level of 6%. Rapid antigenic tests were positive for *P. falciparum*.

Other investigation showed serum sodium 130.6 mmol/L, albumin 2.8 g/dL, elevated lactate dehydrogenase (1,043 U/L). Liver parameters and creatinine were normal. There was arterial hypoxemia, hyperlactatemia (5.46 mmol/L), and metabolic acidosis.

CHAPTER 31: Cerebral Malaria

His cerebrospinal fluid and electroencephalogram (EEG) findings were normal. He was started on supportive therapy and intravenous artesunate in the recommended dose. Repeat blood smear after 2 days showed clearance of the parasite. He was discharged in a clinically stable condition and advised primaquine single dose to prevent recrudescence and relapse. Follow-up after 1 month showed no residual neurological deficit.

CASE REVIEW IN A NUTSHELL

This child was admitted with seizures and fever with falciparum malaria positive. The status epilepticus is one of the common presentations of cerebral malaria. The prompt treatment of seizures with short-acting benzodiazepines and anticonvulsants and supportive care as management of airway, maintaining of adequate intravascular volume and correction of electrolyte imbalance help in initial stabilization of the child. The definitive treatment is treatment of malaria with antimalarial medications. Such a child should be managed in pediatric intensive care unit with constant monitoring. The management of increased intracranial pressure with osmotic diuretics and hypertonic saline is another main aspect of treatment. Decrease in parasitic index is the indicator of improvement.

INTERACTIVE TOPIC REVIEW

Q. What is the definition of cerebral malaria?

Cerebral malaria, the most common cause of nontraumatic encephalopathy in the world, is defined as a deep level of unconsciousness in the presence of a *P. falciparum* asexual parasitemia, after the correction of hypoglycemia and exclusion of other encephalopathies, especially bacterial meningitis and locally prevalent viral encephalitides.

Q. What are the features of severe malaria?

Definition of severe falciparum malaria: One or more of the criteria written in the box below

BOX 1: Features of severe malaria
- Cerebral malaria (unarousable coma)
- Severe normocytic anemia (hemoglobin <5 g/dL)
- Renal failure (serum creatinine >3 mg/100 mL)
- Pulmonary edema
- Hypoglycemia (<60 mg/100 mL)
- Circulatory collapse/shock (systolic blood pressure less than 50 mmHg in children below 5 years)
- Spontaneous bleeding/disseminated intravascular coagulopathy
- Repeated generalized convulsions
- Acidemia
- Macroscopic hemoglobinuria
- Other manifestations:
  - Impaired consciousness but arousable
  - Prostration, extreme weakness (inability to stand or sit)
  - Hyperparasitemia (>5% red blood cells infected)
  - Jaundice (total serum bilirubin >3 mg/dL)
  - Hyperpyrexia (axillary temperature >39.5 °C)

(Box 1) in the presence of asexual parasitemia define severe falciparum malaria.

Q. What is the antimalarial chemotherapy of severe and complicated malaria?

Ideally, antimalarial drug should be given initially by intravenous infusion, which should be replaced by oral administration as soon as condition permits (Tables 1 and 2).

National Anti-Malaria Program (NAMP)'s drug policy in all cases of severe malaria is either intravenous quinine or parenteral artemisinin derivatives to be given irrespective of chloroquine-resistance status. A single dose of primaquine (0.75 mg/kg) is to be given for gametocytocidal action irrespective of the drug given.

Q. Which one to use: quinine or artemisinin?

Artemisinin is the most rapidly acting of all known antimalarial drugs. They often produce a 10,000-fold reduction of parasites per asexual cycle. They have the broadest time window of antimalarial effects from ring

TABLE 1: Drug and dosage of antimalarial in complicated and severe malaria according to National Anti-Malaria Program (NAMP)

Drug	Dosage
Quinine salt	• 20 mg salt/kg (loading dose) diluted in 10 mL/kg of glucose containing isotonic fluid/kg by infusion over 4 hours • Then, 12 hours after the start of loading dose give a maintenance dose of 10 mg salt/kg over 2 hours. This maintenance dose should be repeated every 8 hours, calculated from beginning of previous infusion, until the patient can swallow • When patient can swallow, start quinine tablets, 10 mg salt /kg 8 hourly to complete a 7-day course of treatment (including both parenteral and oral) • If controlled IV infusion cannot be administered, then quinine salt can be given in the same dosages by IM injection in the anterior thigh (not in buttock). The dose of quinine should be divided between two sites, half the dose in each anterior thigh. If possible IM quinine should be diluted in normal saline to a concentration of 60–100 mg salt/mL (quinine is usually available as 300 mg salt/mL).

- Loading dose of quinine should not be used if the patient has received quinine, quinidine, or mefloquine within the preceding 12 hours. Alternatively, loading dose can be administered as 7 mg salt/kg by IV infusion pump over 30 minutes, followed immediately by 10 mg salt/kg diluted in 10 mL isotonic fluid/kg by IV infusion over 4 hours
- Quinine should not be given by bolus or push injection
- If there is no clinical improvement after 48 hours of parenteral therapy, the maintenance dose of quinine should be reduced by one-third to half, i.e., 5–7 mg salt/kg
- Quinine should not be given subcutaneously as this may cause skin necrosis.

IM, intramuscular; IV, intravenous.

TABLE 2: Alternative drugs rather than quinine in severe malaria

Drug	Dosage
Artesunate	2.4 mg/kg IV (loading dose), followed by 1.2 mg/kg at 12 and 24 hours, then 1.2 mg/kg daily for 6 days. If the patient is able to swallow, then the daily dose can be given orally or Artemether 3.2 mg/kg (loading dose) IM, followed by 1.6 mg/kg daily for 6 days. If the patient is able to swallow, then the daily dose can be given orally

- Artesunate, 60 mg per ampoule is dissolved in 0.6 mL of 5% sodium bicarbonate diluted to 3–5 mL with 5% dextrose and given immediately by IV bolus (push injection)
- Artemether is dispensed in 1 mL ampoule containing 80 mg of artemether in peanut oil
- At the end of the therapy, a single dose of sulfadoxine-pyrimethamine as 25 mg/kg of sulfadoxine and 1.25 mg/kg of pyrimethamine or mefloquine 25 mg/kg (divided into two doses of 15 mg/kg and 10 mg/kg 4–6 h apart) is to be given

forms to early schizonts. Thus, they can stop parasite maturation, particularly from the less pathogenic circulating ring stages to the more pathogenic cytoadherent stages.

However, artemisinin should be used when rate-controlled intravenous infusion of quinine is not possible; patients have contraindications to quinine use and evidence of inadequate response or resistance to quinine noted. Simultaneous use of quinine and artemisinin is not indicated as it may be harmful and there is no added advantage.

CHAPTER 31: Cerebral Malaria

Q. What are the pathological features of cerebral malaria?

The histopathological hallmark of cerebral malaria is engorgement of cerebral capillaries and venules with parasitized red blood cells (PRBCs) and nonparasitized red blood cells (NPRBCs).

The cut brain is slate grey with petechial hemorrhages. The endothelium does not demonstrate microscopical damage, but immunohistochemical staining suggests endothelial activation and disruption of the blood-brain barrier.

Q. What are the factors influencing development of severe malaria?

Several factors impact a patient's risk of developing severe malaria, particularly the species of malaria parasite and the patient's immune status, the latter depending on previous exposure to malaria.

P. falciparum is the most virulent of the plasmodia. Complications of *P. falciparum* infection are the result of cytokine release and of the parasite's unique ability to cause PRBCs to adhere to vascular endothelium and cause red blood cell (RBC) sequestration, altered blood flow, and ischemia.

Immune status of the patient also greatly affects the manifestations of malaria. In populations originating from areas of constant, high-intensity malaria transmission, most mortality occurs among younger children, as a result of severe anemia. In the same populations, infected adults and older children may have minimal symptoms or may be asymptomatic.

Q. What is sequestration?

The sequestration of RBCs containing mature forms of the parasite (trophozoites and meronts) in the microvasculature is thought to cause the major complications of falciparum malaria, particularly cerebral malaria. This process varies considerably between organs (the brain is particularly affected) and at a microvascular level varies between vessels. The sequestration of PRBCs in the relatively hypoxic venous beds allows optimal parasite growth and prevents the PRBCs from being destroyed by the spleen. It is the sequestered parasite that cause pathology in severe malaria, and prognosis is related to sequestered biomass. The peripheral blood parasite count is a relatively poor predictor of the size of this biomass.

Q. What is cytoadherence?

Sequestration is thought to be a specific interaction between PRBCs and the vascular endothelium (cytoadherence). This phenomenon seems to be mediated by plasmodium-derived proteins on the surface of PRBCs and modified erythrocyte cell wall proteins and ligands on endothelial cells. The adhesion of the PRBCs reduces the microvascular blood flow, which may explain organ and tissue dysfunction such as coma. The metabolically active sequestered parasites may compete with host tissues for substrates—for instance, glucose—and also produce toxins that interfere with host tissue metabolism.

Cytoadherence begins when the parasites produce visible malaria pigment (usually becoming visible under light microscopy around 16 h), which is maximal at the late stages. Cytoadherence occurs predominately in capillaries and venules, as it is overcome by large shear stresses encountered on the arterial side. Freshly isolated PRBCs capable of cytoadherence have electron dense "knobs" protruding from their surfaces, composed of proteins derived from the parasite, notably the adhesion *P. falciparum* erythrocyte membrane protein-1 (PfEMP-1). These families of large proteins (200–350 kDa) which are expressed on the exterior of PRBCs vary antigenically with time in cloned parasites. This programmed variation allows the parasites to evade host immune responses. These proteins have adhesive properties and are primarily responsible for cytoadherence.

A family of more than 150 highly variable ("*var*") genes encode PfEMP-1, which can bind to several candidate endothelial receptors.

Q. What is rosetting?

The adherence of NPRBCs to PRBCs (rosetting) and PRBCs to PRBCs (agglutination) has also been implicated in the pathogenesis of cerebral malaria, although most clinical studies have failed to show an association. In rosetting, the *var* genes seem to be responsible for the ligands and this intererythrocytic interaction is pH and heparin sensitive.

Q. How does red cell deformability influence severity of cerebral malaria?

As the parasite grows within the RBCs, the erythrocyte becomes less deformable which may contribute to the RBC destruction and impair the microcirculatory flow. The reduction in red cell deformability not only occurs in PRBC, but also in the NPRBC. The NPRBCs have to undergo considerable deformation as they squeeze through the sequestered microcirculation. Red cell deformity measured at low shear rates encountered in capillaries and venules, proved the most powerful prognostic indicator of severe malaria, although not associated with the syndrome of cerebral malaria itself.

Q. What are the diagnostic modalities available for detection of malaria?

Diagnostic techniques

Diagnostic tests for malaria include standard thick and thin blood smears, rapid antigen detection tests, polymerase chain reaction (PCR), and antibody tests. Thick and thin blood smears remain the most widely available and used tests. Thick blood smears test for the presence or absence of parasites, and thin blood smears allow speciation and quantification. The sensitivity and specificity of blood smears vary greatly and are influenced by
- Laboratory skill
- Timing and quality of smear collection, and
- Level of parasitemia.

Most skilled laboratory personnel can detect parasite levels as low as approximately 50 parasites/µL of blood. One set of negative thick and thin blood smears is never sufficient to exclude malaria, even when prepared by the most skilled hands, but three sets of negative blood smears are generally considered sufficient, although additional smears may be necessary in some cases.

Many rapid antigen tests are available. Most of these tests differentiate between *P. falciparum* and nonfalciparum infections through the detection of histidine-rich proteins and/or parasite lactate dehydrogenase. Polymerase chain reaction tests are at least as sensitive and specific as the traditional blood smear and can detect parasite levels of less than or equal to 1 parasite/µL. The use of PCR is clinically limited because the test may continue to be positive for more than 1 week after treatment because of persistence of antigen in the serum. Currently, PCR is used mainly to confirm positive blood smears and is valuable in identification of malaria species, particularly when the results of smears are not definitive or there is a mixed infection.

Q. What are the clinical features of cerebral malaria?

Clinical features

Cerebral malaria is a diffuse encephalopathy in which focal neurological signs are relatively unusual. Cerebral malaria presents usually with a 1–4 day history of fever and convulsions. Focal motor and generalized tonic-clonic convulsions are the most common clinically detected seizures, but subtle or subclinical seizures detected with EEG are also common. Seizures are associated with a poor outcome, particularly prolonged seizures. Between seizures, the EEG shows bilateral diffuse slowing of the brain waves, often asymmetric (not inevitably associated with clinical signs).

Compared with adults, children have a higher incidence of seizures. There may be passive resistance to neck flexion, but of a lesser degree to the "meningism" associated with meningitis.

Cerebral malaria is often accompanied by multisystem dysfunction. Hence, an assessment of the degree of anemia, jaundice and, most importantly, the presence of acidotic (Kussmaul's breathing) breathing is important.

Prognosis of cerebral malaria worsens considerably with coexistent renal failure, severe jaundice, or metabolic acidosis. The metabolic acidosis is caused by either an acute renal failure, or a lactic acidosis, or a combination of both. Acute pulmonary edema may occur. Rarely, patients with severe malaria have disseminated intravascular coagulation and evidence of bleeding, usually from the upper gastrointestinal tract but sometimes in the skin.

Pulse is usually rapid and full with a low or normal blood pressure. The peripheries are well-perfused, although shock may occur and is often terminal.

Hypoglycemia is common in severe malaria, occurring in about 20% of children with cerebral malaria. Restoration of normoglycemia, however, is often not associated with a change in the level of consciousness.

On direct ophthalmoscopy, retinal hemorrhages are found in about 15% of patients. These are boat, or flames-shaped and sometimes resemble Roth spots with a pale center. Papilledema is very unusual and even if present, develops at a later stage. The pupillary reactions are usually normal and the range of eye movements full, although gaze is dysconjugate. Sixth nerve palsies may occur rarely. The corneal reflexes are usually present although in very deep coma, they may be lost. The remainder of the cranial nerve examination is usually normal.

Opening cerebrospinal fluid pressures are raised in children with cerebral malaria and there is evidence of brain swelling on computed tomography scan in most of the children.

The most likely cause of raised intracranial pressure in cerebral malaria is an increase in cerebral blood volume, particularly during the initial stages and in those children with moderate degrees of intracranial hypertension. Cerebral blood volume could be increased by the sequestration of PRBCs in the vascular compartment, either acting as a diffuse space occupying lesion or obstructing venous outflow. An increased cerebral blood flow could be caused by other features of cerebral malaria, such as seizures, hyperthermia, and anemia.

Q. What are the treatment modalities for cerebral malaria?

The management of cerebral malaria is similar to that of any seriously ill unconscious patient. Impairment of consciousness, convulsions, and other neurological features should raise the possibility of cerebral malaria in any child who might possibly have been exposed to this infection during the previous year. Complications of cerebral malaria, such as convulsions, hypoglycemia, and hyperpyrexia, should be prevented or detected and treated early.

Intensive care with rehydration and thereafter careful fluid balance management are necessary to navigate the narrow divide between underhydration and worsening renal impairment and lactic acidosis, and overhydration and pulmonary edema. Children are less likely to develop pulmonary edema and more likely than adults to be hypovolemic and underperfused. Many require rapid restoration of an adequate circulating blood volume.

Initial hypoglycemia should be treated with a rapid infusion of 25% (for infants and small children) or 50% dextrose. To prevent and monitor for hyperinsulinemic hypoglycemia, administration of a 5 or 10% dextrose solution should be started when treatment with quinine derivatives is initiated, and blood glucose levels should be tested frequently. Quinine-induced hypoglycemia may develop several days after the beginning of treatment.

Hypovolemia and shock must be managed with intravenous crystalloids or colloids, and vasoactive agents to maintain mean arterial pressure. This maintains cerebral perfusion pressure and decreases increased intracranial pressure.

Severe anemia may necessitate blood transfusion. Blood transfusion is indicated when the packed cell volume falls below 20%, and may be beneficial above this threshold. Unwarranted blood transfusions may increase the chances of acute respiratory distress syndrome, hence judicious approach for blood transfusion should be used.

Seizures may be acutely treated with benzodiazepines (midazolam or lorazepam). In case of prolonged seizures or status epilepticus, algorithmic approach for management is required. This includes management of airway, injectable anticonvulsants like phenytoin/fosphenytoin, phenobarbitone, or sodium valproate.

In the event of development of renal failure, adjustment of drug doses is necessary.

As a rule, multiple smears with parasite quantification should be done to monitor therapeutic success.

Very high levels of parasitemia or failure to respond to treatment may indicate primary drug failure/resistance. Therapy should be adjusted and exchange transfusion considered in such situations.

Exact criteria for initiating therapy are unclear. Some authorities have suggested that exchange transfusion may be beneficial for any severely ill patient with parasitemia of more than 15% or for any patient with parasitemia of 5–15% who has signs of poor prognosis.

Specific parenteral antimalarial treatment is the only intervention that unequivocally affects the outcome of cerebral malaria. Resistance has meant that chloroquine can no longer be relied on in most tropical countries. The dosage and duration of quinine or artesunate have been detailed earlier in the chapter.

Clinical trials do not demonstrate efficacy for other ancillary treatments, including anticytokine agents, chelation agents, corticosteroids, mannitol, dextran, heparin, and malaria hyperimmunoglobulin.

Q. What are the neurological sequelae?

Neurological sequelae are associated with protracted seizures, prolonged and deep coma, hypoglycemia, and severe anemia. Some neurological deficits are transient (for example, ataxia), whereas others (hemiparesis and cortical blindness), often improve over months, complete resolution may not occur.

Children with severe neurological sequelae (spastic tetraparesis, vegetative states) usually die within a few months of discharge.

More subtle deficits—for example, cognitive difficulties, and language and behavioral problems—are increasingly recognized.

CONCLUSION

Cerebral malaria, a common problem in endemic areas, should be considered in any patient with impairment of consciousness. Urgent treatment with appropriate antimalarial drugs is required. Prognosis often depends on the management of other complications—for example, renal failure, acidosis. Therapies that interfere with underlying pathophysiological processes, for example, reduced red cell deformability and cytoadherence, require further investigation. Further research on the pathogenesis of coma and neurological damage is required to develop other ancillary treatments.

KEY LEARNING POINTS

- Cerebral malaria is a severe and potentially fatal disease if not treated appropriately in a tertiary cares setting
- Though *P. falciparum* is the usual causative pathogen, even *P. vivax* can also cause falciparum malaria
- Specific parenteral antimalarial treatment is the only intervention that unequivocally affects the outcome of cerebral malaria.

SUGGESTED READINGS

1. Boivin MJ, Bangirana P, Byarugaba J, Opoka RO, Idro R, Jurek AM, et al. Cognitive impairment after cerebral malaria in children: a prospective study. *Pediatrics*. 2007;119:e360-e366.
2. Duque V, Seixas D, Ventura C, Cunha S, Silvestre AM. Plasmodium falciparum malaria, bilateral sixth cranial nerve palsy and delayed cerebellar ataxia. *J Infect Dev Ctries*. 2012;6:290-294.
3. Okoromah CA, Afolabi BB. Mannitol and other osmotic diuretics as adjuncts for treating cerebral malaria. *Cochrane Database Syst Rev*. 2004;(4):CD004615.
4. Pino P, Taoufiq Z, Nitcheu J, Vouldoukis I, Mazier D. Blood-brain barrier breakdown during cerebral malaria: suicide or murder? *Thromb Haemost*. 2005;94:336-340.
5. Taylor TE, Fu WJ, Carr RA, Whitten RO, Mueller JS, Fosiko NG, et al. Differentiating the pathologies of cerebral malaria by postmortem parasite counts. *Nat Med*. 2004;10:143-145.
6. Tripathy R, Parida S, Das L, Mishra DP, Tripathy D, Das MC, et al. Clinical manifestations and predictors of severe malaria In Indian children. *Pediatrics*. 2007;120:e454-e460.
7. Turner L, Lavstsen T, Berger SS, Wang CW, Petersen JE, Avril M, et al. Severe malaria is associated with parasite binding to endothelial protein C receptor. *Nature*. 2013;498:502-505.

CHAPTER 32

Influenza

Suraj Gupte, R Kumar, Anthony Block

INTRODUCTION

Though pandemic influenza usually occurs thrice in a century, seasonal influenza occurs year after year. Usually, it is a benign respiratory illness that settles in around a week. In some children with risk factors (say, underlying immunodeficiency/immunosuppression, cystic fibrosis, congenital heart disease, diabetes, etc.), it may cause complications that may prove fatal. With the increasing resistance to the M2 inhibitors, neuraminidase inhibitors such as oseltamivir and zanamivir are only specific drugs that are currently recommended.

Nonpharmacological approaches, which usually are the only course available, are important in management.

Prophylaxis lies in influenza vaccine which is recommended after the age of 6 months.

CASE 1

History: A 17-year-old girl, a known case of well-controlled diabetes type 1 on insulin, woke up one morning with running nose and sneezing. Her parents, believing she had developed common cold, instilled otrivin nasal drops in her nose, made her swallow a tablet of a decongestant + antipyretic (sinarest) and bundled her to school. Within a couple of hours, she was back home with high fever and persistent cough. At school, she had vomited twice and was administered a tablet of metoclopramide (perinorm) and oral rehydration salts (ORS).

By the evening, her condition further deteriorated with worsening of cough, fatigability, and shortness of breath.

Her immunization status was good, except for influenza vaccine.

Physical Examination: Clinical workup showed that she had a temperature of 104°F and was moderately dehydrated, with cold, clammy, and sweaty skin. Other findings included running nose, congested throat, tachypnea (rate 26/min), tachycardia (rate 110/min), bilateral coarse crepitations and low blood pressure (105/60 mmHg).

Investigations:
- Hemoglobin: 12.5 g/100 mL
- Total leukocyte count: 15,000/mm^3
- Differential leukocyte count: Polymorphonuclear neutrophils—50%, lymphocytes—46%, monocytes—2%, eosinophils—2%
- Chest X-ray: Interstitial pneumonitis
- Rapid influenza antigen test (RIAT): Positive for influenza type A.

Treatment Given and Response: Over and above routine insulin, after admission to the hospital, she was started on intravenous fluids and symptomatic and supportive treatment along with high-dose amoxycillin. Subsequently, she was also administered injectable trivalent influenza vaccine. Oseltamivir, 75 mg twice a day for 5 days, too was given.

She responded to this treatment and was discharged after a week. At the time of discharge, she continued to have some cough and bodily weakness.

CASE REVIEW IN A NUTSHELL

This adolescent girl presented with coryza followed by high fever, chills, rigors, headache, and bodily pains and vomiting and chest signs of pneumonia. Chest X-ray showed evidence of interstitial pneumonia. All these manifestation could be from influenza or some other viral infection. The positivity of the RIAT for influenza established the diagnosis. Pneumonia in influenza may be viral or superimposed bacterial in etiology. In this case, since it was present very early in illness and was interstitial radiologically, in all probability it was of viral origin.

Diabetes is a high risk factor for influenza complications. This child was, therefore, rightly given influenza vaccine and oseltamivir along with high dose amoxicillin on top of insulin which she was already taking for his diabetes type 1.

Response to this treatment was gratifying. She recovered in a week's time.

INTERACTIVE TOPIC REVIEW

Q. What are types of influenza virus?

Influenza viruses belong to the family, orthomyxoviridae. Type A and type B are the principle influenza viruses that cause seasonal influenza. Type C may cause an inapparent or asymptomatic illness. Since it usually remains unnoticed, it is virtually of no clinical significance.

Q. What is the pathophysiology?

After the influenza virus invades the host's cells, replication occurs in various steps (Fig. 1). It terminates with maturity of the virus.

The mature virus buds off from the cell in a sphere of host phospholipid membrane, acquiring hemagglutinin, and neuraminidase with the membrane coat. A noteworthy point is that the virus adheres to the host cell through hemagglutinin. Once the neuraminidase of the mature viruses has cleaved sialic acid residues from the host cell, the mature virus detaches. Following the release of the new influenza virus, the host cell undergoes death.

Q. What are different means of transmission and spread?

Influenza has the potential for rapid spread, often involving large populations.

Influenza spreads in the following three main ways:

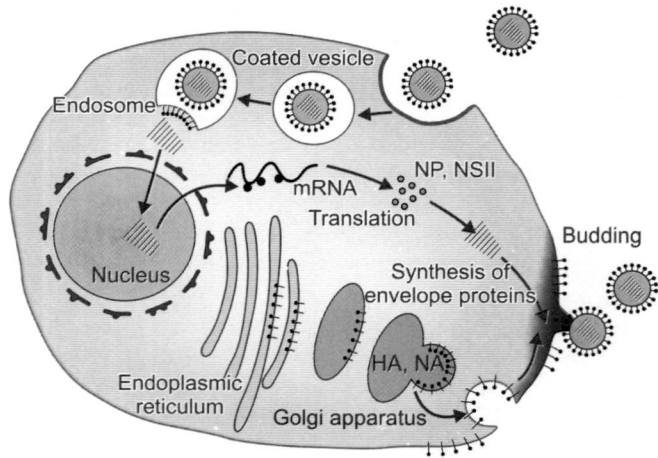

NP; nucleoprotein; NS1, nonstructural protein; HA, hemagglutinin; NA, neuraminidase.
Figure 1: Influenza virus replication. Note the various steps of replication of the virus

1. Direct transmission: Here, an infected subject sneezes mucus directly into the eyes, nose, or mouth of another subject
2. Airborne (aerosol) transmission: Here, an infected subject produces aerosols (by coughing, sneezing, or spitting) that another subject inhales. Some droplets, being very small are easy to inhale. Though a single sneeze releases up to 40,000 droplets, a sheer one droplet is good enough to cause an infection. A close contact (up to 1–2 meters) is needed for transmission. The majority of the droplets, being quite large, quickly settle out of air. The low humidity and lack of ultraviolet radiation from sunlight in winter facilitates survival of the virus. Hence, seasonal influenza usually in November to April period of the year
3. Direct contact: Hand-to-eye, hand-to-nose, or hand-to-mouth transmission either from the contaminated surfaces or direct personal contact such as a handshake
4. Fomites: Here, transmission/spread occurs through handling of fomites such as toys, garments, handkerchiefs, door knobs, currency notes, etc.

Q. What is viral shedding?

The term, "viral shedding", denotes the time during which a person may be infectious to the other person. It is an important feature at the onset of symptoms or just before the onset of illness (0–24 h). Viral shedding continues for 5–10 days. Young children may shed virus longer, placing others at risk for contracting infection with the virus.

Classically, it begins a day prior to appearance of manifestations. Then, the virus is usually released over the next 5–7 days. A small proportion of subjects may shed the virus for a longer period. Children shed virus for as long as 2 weeks after infection. They are supposed to be more infectious than the adults. Between second day and third day after contracting infection, the subject is most infective (contagious). More the viral shedding higher is the fever.

Influenza virus is capable of survival outside the body and transmitted by contaminated surfaces like toys, currency notes, door-knobs, light switches and other household items.

Q. What's the duration of survival of influenza virus in different situations?

Duration of survival of influenza virus in various situations is as follows:
- Hard, nonporous surfaces (plastic, metal): 1–2 days
- Dry paper tissues: 15 minutes
- Skin: 5 minutes
- Mucus on currency notes: Up to 17 days.

Avian influenza viruses, when frozen, can survive indefinitely. Heating to 56°C for a minimum of 60 minutes and acidic pH (<7) inactivate them.

Q. What are other epidemiological aspects of influenza?

Influenza is a disease of the relatively colder months (October to March) of the year. The portal of entry is the upper airway. Spread and transmission through the community, occurring by the small-particle aerosol, is rapid. In just 2–3 weeks, incidence of the illness reaches the peak. There is evidence that influenza contributes to hospital spread of infection. It is capable of complicating and worsening the primary illness with which the subject is hospitalized.

Influenza viruses are, as a rule, highly species-specific. This means that they usually do not spill over to cause infection in other species. This characteristic is ascribed to differences in the use of cellular receptors. Human influenza viruses bind to receptors that contain terminal 2-6-linked sialyl-galactosyl moieties. On the contrary, avian viruses bind to cell-surface glycoprotein containing sialyl-galactosyl residues linked by 2-3-linkage. For this reason, an avian virus has to acquire the ability to bind cells that display 2-6 receptors to facilitate its entry into the cell and replicate in it. Then and only then, it can transmit the illness to humans and between humans. At present, we are aware of the potential routes whereby H5N1 can mutate and acquire human specificity. What we do not understand is as to which specific mutations are warranted for rendering H5N1 virus easily and sustainably transmissible among humans.

Out of the hundreds of strains of avian influenza, only four strains (H5N1, H7N3, H7N7, and H9N2) are on record to have caused infection in humans. The human infection as a result of transmission from avian reservoir has usually caused mild illness. Principal source of human infection with H5N1 is close contact with dead or sick birds (plucking, butchering, slaughtering, preparing) or exposure to feces of chickens on playgrounds.

Though, currently, H5N1 infection in humans is rare, there is evidence that the strains are becoming more virulent and pathogenic.

Since influenza is highly infective and modern travel is quite rapid, an epidemic stands good chance of developing pandemic proportions in a matter of weeks and a few months. This assertion is borne out by almost all past pandemics as well as the novel H1N1 pandemic of 2009–2010.

Invariably, one or two strains monopolize the seasonal influenza. Over the years, influenza type A strains with H1N1 and H1N2 serotypes are cocirculating. Since either type may be predominant in a given year, it becomes difficult to make predictions about the serotype and severity of the upcoming influenza season.

Q. What are clinical manifestations?

The illness has a short incubation period of sheer 1–2 days.

Usually, onset of the illness is abrupt with typical systemic symptoms comprising high fever (often with chills and rigors), severe malaise, extreme fatigue and weakness, and bodily pains (headache, myalgia) in association with respiratory tract symptoms such as nonproductive cough, sore throat, and rhinitis. Children often have additional acute otitis media or croup. Nausea and vomiting are frequent in them. Rarely, atypical presentation with febrile seizures or sepsis may be encountered.

> **BOX 1: Typical features of symptomatology of uncomplicated influenza**
> - Abrupt onset
> - Systemic: Feverishness, headaches, myalgias (extremities, long muscles of the back; eye muscles; in children: calf muscles), malaise, prostration
> - Respiratory: Dry cough, nasal discharge may be absent in elderly people who may present with lassitude and confusion instead
> - Hoarseness, dry or sore throat often appear as systemic symptoms diminish
> - Croup (only in infants and children)

The typical features of symptomatology of seasonal influenza without complications are listed in box 1.

Severity of clinical presentation varies from afebrile respiratory symptoms resembling common cold to severe prostration without major respiratory signs and symptoms, especially in the elderly. Higher the fever, more severe are the symptoms.

Classically, fever and systemic symptoms last 3 days, occasionally up to 4–8 days and gradually diminish. The cough and malaise may persist for more than 2 weeks. Second fever spikes are rare. The physical findings are summarized in box 2. Full recovery may take 1–2 weeks. In the elderly people, it may take longer.

Box 2 summarizes the classical clinical findings in uncomplicated influenza.

The patients are infectious 24 hours before the onset of symptoms and up to around 7 days

> **BOX 2: Classical clinical findings in uncomplicated influenza**
> - Fever: Rapidly peaking temperature at 38–40°C (up to 41°C, especially in children), typically lasting 3 days (up to 4–8 days), gradually diminishing; second fever spikes are rare
> - Face: Flushed
> - Skin: Hot and moist
> - Eyes: Congested and watery
> - Nose: Rhinorrhea
> - Ear: Middle ear inflammation (acute otitis media)
> - Throat: Pharyngitis; laryngeal edema (causing croup)
> - Mucous membranes: Hyperemic
> - Cervical lymph nodes: Enlarged (especially in children)

TABLE 1: Comparison of salient features of influenza and common cold

Symptoms	Influenza	Common cold
Fever	Usually high, lasts 3–4 days	Unusual
Cough	Invariable present and significant	Unusual; slight
Headache	Usual	Unusual
Fatigue/or weakness	Significant (may last up to 2–3 weeks 0)	Only mild
Bodily pains/aches	Usual and often severe	Unusual
Stuffy nose	Sometimes	Usual
Sore throat	Sometimes	Usual
Chest discomfort	Common and sometimes severe	Uncommon; mild
Complications	Bronchitis, pneumonia, acute respiratory distress syndrome; in severe cases life-threatening in severe case	Sinusitis

Adapted from: Gupte S. *Influenza*. Gurgaon (NCR): Macmillan; 2010.

thereafter. Children are even more contagious. For instance, young children can shed virus for several days before the onset of their illness and can be infectious for more than 10 days. In case of severely immunocompromised persons, virus shedding may well be for weeks or months.

During nonepidemic periods, respiratory symptoms caused by influenza may be difficult to distinguish from symptoms caused by other respiratory pathogens (see laboratory findings). However, the sudden onset of the disease, fever, and fatigue are characteristically different from the common cold (Table 1).

Q. In which way(s) do influenza and common cold differ?

For comparison of salient features of influenza and common cold, refer table 1.

Q. What are the likely complications?

Lower respiratory tract infection in the form of acute bronchitis and pneumonia (primary, secondary, or mixed) are the most frequent complication of influenza. Influenza may exacerbate the underlying cardiopulmonary disease such as asthma, chronic bronchitis, cystic fibrosis, etc. Influenza infection may also be accompanied by neurologic complications (encephalopathy, transverse myelitis), myocarditis, pericarditis, myositis, and Reye's syndrome.

Q. What is rapid influenza diagnostic test?

Rapid influenza diagnostic test is used to detect the virus in nasal secretions and one of the most common methods used to diagnose this infection. Depending on the method, it may be completed in the doctor's office in less than 30 minutes or be sent to a laboratory, with the results available the same day. It can help differentiate influenza from other viral and bacterial infections with similar symptoms that may be serious and must be treated differently. Rapid flu tests are best used within the first 48 hours of the onset of symptoms to help diagnose influenza and determine whether or not antiviral drugs are a treatment option, sometimes rapid tests are ordered to help identify outbreaks.

Rapid tests vary in their ability to detect influenza. Some types can only detect influenza A; others can detect both A and B but not distinguish between the two. Still, others can detect and distinguish between influenza A and B. However, none of them are able to differentiate between the strains of influenza A, such as H1N1.

Rapid influenza antigen test are not without demerits. It will miss up to 30% of influenza cases, may only detect 10-70% of 2009 H1N1 influenza infections, and it will occasionally be positive when someone does not actually have the flu.

Q. What are the antiviral agents presently recommended in influenza?

At present, treatment with oseltamivir (Tamifl) or zanamivir (Relenza) is recommended for all subjects with suspected or confimed inflenza who require hospitalization (Table 2).

Q. What are salient details about the recommended seasonal influenza vaccines?

Safe influenza vaccines are the "gold standard" in prophylaxis of influenza and its severe complications in vulnerable subjects. Currently, both inactivated (killed) and live attenuated vaccines are available.

The seasonal (annual) vaccine is available for influenza A and B. It contains viral strains that are most likely to produce outbreak during the subsequent season. Therefore, the vaccine strains are updated every year.

Box 3 gives the salient features of the recommended influenza vaccines.

Q. What is the usual prognosis in influenza?

Most influenza infections settle within 1 or 2 weeks regardless whether a specific treatment has been given or not, fatigue and a cough may last a while longer.

TABLE 2: Salient features of currently recommended antiviral agents in seasonal influenza

Drug	Route	Dose	Remarks
Oseltamivir	Oral	• Prophylaxis: 75 mg once a day for 7–10 days • Treatment: 75 mg twice daily for 5 days	• Transient gastrointestinal disturbance may be reduced by taking oseltamivir after a light snack
Zanamivir	Inhalation	• 10 mg twice daily for 2 days	• Avoid in chronic lung disease, asthma in particular

Centers for Disease Control and Prevention (CDC) and other recommendatory bodies have advised against the use of M2 inhibitors until the inflenza virus strains sensitive to them re-emerge in the foreseeable future.

BOX 3: Influenza vaccines

- Trivalent influenza vaccine
  - Brand name: Vaxigrip, Fluarix
    A killed, split product vaccine containing 15 µg each of the WHO-recommended two influenza A strains (novel H1N1 strain of recent pandemic rather than the old H1N1 strain) and one influenza B strain; provides 80% efficacy; licensed for use more than 6 months of age
  - Indications: Protection against influenza virus infection, especially in subjects with underlying chronic cardiac or bronchopulmonary disease, immunocompromised state, diabetes, chronic renal insufficiency, or sickle-cell anemia
  - Available as: Single dose vial, prefilled syringe or ampoule; multidose vial
  - Dose: 6–35 months: 0.25 mL (SC, IM); second dose after 4–6 weeks in subjects who have not received the vaccine earlier
  - 3 to 8 years: 0.5 mL (SC, IM); second dose after 4–6 weeks in subjects who have not received the vaccine earlier
  - 9 years: 0.5 mL (SC, IM)
  - Adverse events: Local pain, erythema and induration at the injection site, pyrexia, malaise; rarely, anaphylaxis; very rarely Guillain-Barré syndrome (GBS).
  - Contraindication: Hypersensitivity to its components
  - Caution: Avoid in children with history of GBS and severe egg allergy
  - Storage: 2 to 8°C (35–46°F)

Continued

Continued

- Live attenuated influenza vaccine
  - Brand name: FluMist
  - Live-attenuated reassortants of the three WHO-recommended strains: Two influenza A (novel H1N1 strain rather than the earlier H1N1 strain) and 1 influenza B; licensed for use after 2 years of age; superior efficacy than inactivated vaccine.
  - Available as: Prefilled, single-use sprayer containing 0.2 mL of vaccine
  - Dose: As a nasal spray. Approximately, 0.1 mL (i.e., half of the total sprayer contents) is sprayed into the first nostril while the recipient is in the upright position. An attached dose-divider clip is removed from the sprayer to administer the second half of the dose into the other nostril
- Adverse events: Mild fever, rhinorrhea, nasal congestion, sore throat, etc. which, perhaps result from effects of intranasal vaccine administration or local viral replication
- Contraindications: Children less than 2 years of age
- Precautions: Avoid in children with history of hypersensitivity to egg and GBS
- Vaccine prepared for a previous influenza season should not be administered to provide protection for any subsequent season
- Storage: 2–8°C (35–46°F)

WHO, World Health Organization; SC, subcutaneous; IM, intramuscular.

Q. What about serious secondary infections?

Serious secondary complications such as pneumonia, sepsis, and encephalitis occur in a proportion of the patients just as influenza symptoms are fading. Children who are immunocompromised or who have preexisting lung disease are most affected. Immediate medical treatment is mandatory in these cases.

CONCLUSION

Seasonal influenza, though usually a benign disease lasting for a week or so, may cause complications such as pneumonia, sepsis, and encephalitis and even death in high-risk children. The causative virus is usually influenza A and less often influenza B with the transmission of infection via aerosol, direct contact, or indirect contact. Though rapid and other diagnostic tests are available, diagnosis is generally clinical. Antiviral drugs are most effective when given within first 48 hours of onset of illness. With the development of increasing resistance to M2 inhibitors, only neuraminidase inhibitors are available for clinical use. Nonpharmaceutical measures, antiviral drug therapy and vaccination are crucial in prophylaxis of influenza and its severe complications.

KEY LEARNING POINTS

- Seasonal influenza, though usually a mild illness, may cause complications that lead to hospitalization and even death, especially in certain situations
- The causative virus is usually influenza A and less often influenza B with the transmission of infection via aerosol, direct contact or indirect contact
- Diagnosis, as a rule, is clinical but rapid and other diagnostic tests are available if required in certain cases
- Antiviral drugs (neuroaminidase inhibitors) are most effective when given within first 48 hours of onset of illness
- Antiviral drug therapy, vaccination, and supportive measures are crucial in prophylaxis of influenza and its severe complications

SUGGESTED READINGS

1. Gupte S. *Influenza*. Gurgaon (NCR); Macmillan; 2010.
2. Gupte S, Gupte N. *Pespectives in influenza*: Gurgaon (NCR): Macmillan; 2011.
3. World Health Organization. (2010). Influenza update. [online]. Available from: www.who.int/csr/disease/influenza/2010_12_17_GIP_surveillance/en/index.html. [Accessed June 2016].

SECTION 8
Envenomation

CHAPTER
33

Scorpion Sting

TM Ananda Kesavan

INTRODUCTION

Scorpions are generally found in dry, hot environments, although some species also occur in forest and wet lands. All species are nocturnal, hiding during the day under stones, wood, or tree barks. The risk of scorpion sting is higher in children in rural areas. Children will get accidental sting while playing or catching them. Except for *Hemiscorpius lepturus*, all venomous scorpion species belong to the large family Buthidae.

CASE 1

A 5-year-old female child was admitted in a local hospital 6 hours after a scorpion sting. Her main complaints were vomiting and swelling of the right big toe. Mother also noticed profuse sweating. She was treated symptomatically with antiemetics, ranitidine and injection of chlorpheniramine maleate. Thirty minutes later, she developed tachypnea and so referred to the author's center. On her way to hospital, she developed generalized tonic-clonic seizure which lasted for 3–5 minutes.

On admission: She was disoriented and dyspneic with profuse sweating and cold extremities. Pulse rate (PR): 134 beats/min, regular, low volume; respiratory rate (RR)—68 breaths/min, intercostal activity, blood pressure (BP)—90/60 mmHg with CFT >3 seconds. General examination showed profuse sweating and swelling of the right big toe. Systemic examinations were normal except mild disorientation. She was treated with oxygen, bolus of normal saline, and other supportive measures.

After 1 hour, her general condition deteriorated. PR—210/min with low volume. Chest retraction increased with grunting, CFT—4 seconds, BP—80/54 mmHg. Respiratory system showed bilateral crepitations and liver was just palpable.

Cardiovascular examination showed soft heart sounds with S3 gallop. Electrocardiogram (ECG) showed prolonged QT with ST changes. X-ray showed features of pulmonary edema. All other investigations were within normal limits.

She was treated with injection of furosemide, injection dobutamine, and prazosin table (0.5 mg) ½ stat, 6 hourly, 6 doses. Her BP improved (110/70 mmHg). She was also put on penicillin injection.

After 60 hours, she showed signs of recovery. Tachypnea decreased and BP improved. She made a rapid recovery and her repeated X-ray was normal. Dobutamine tapered and stopped antibiotics. She discharged on 7th day.

CASE REVIEW IN A NUTSHELL

The clinical profile of this 5-year-old girl admitted with a history of scorpion sting showed that there was evidence of systemic envenomation. She was initially treated with supportive measures. Later, she developed complications in the form of hypotension and pulmonary edema. Prompt treatment with intravenous fluids, inotropic support, and prazosin helped her to revert to normal. Once the child started to improve, further recovery was very rapid. She fully recovered without any residua of envenomation.

INTERACTIVE TOPIC REVIEW

Q. What is the pathophysiology of scorpion envenomation?

Scorpion venom may contain multiple toxins and other compounds. The venom is composed of varying concentrations of neurotoxin, cardiotoxin, nephrotoxin, hemolytic toxin, histamine, serotonin, phosphor diesterases, phospholipases, hyaluronidases, glycosaminoglycans, tryptophan, and cytokine releasers.

The primary targets of scorpion venom are voltage-dependent ion channels. Venom toxins alter these channels, leading to prolonged neuronal activity. Many end-organ effects are secondary to this excessive excitation. Autonomic excitation leads to cardiopulmonary effects observed after scorpion envenomation. Somatic and cranial nerve hyperactivity results from neuromuscular overstimulation. Additionally, serotonin may be found in scorpion venom and is thought to contribute to the pain.

The side chains of scorpion venom are positively charged. This is important in their ability to bind to specific membrane channel. The toxin opens the sodium channel at presynaptic nerve terminals and inhibits calcium-dependent potassium channels, thereby provoking "autonomic storm".

Stimulation of α-receptors by the toxin plays a major role, resulting in hypertension, tachycardia, myocardial dysfunction, pulmonary edema, and cool extremities. Raised angiotensin I levels facilitate the sympathetic outflow through conversion to angiotensin II. Excess catecholamines cause accumulation of endothelins and vasoconstriction.

Unopposed effects of α-receptors stimulation lead to suppression of insulin secretion, hyperglycemia, hyperkalemia, free fatty acids, and free radicals accumulation injurious to myocardium. Cardiac sarcolemmal defects, depletion of glycogen content of heart, liver, and skeletal muscles were observed in experimental animals with acute myocarditis produced by Indian red scorpion venom.

Direct effect of toxins on neurons could contribute to seizures and encephalopathy. Hemiplegia and other neurological lesions have been attributed to fibrin deposition resulting from disseminated intravascular coagulation (DIC). Acute rise in blood pressure due to sympathetic stimulation, rupture of unprotected perforating arteries, intracerebral hemorrhage, and cerebral infarction due to DIC are possibly related to central nervous system manifestations. Increased levels of interleukin (IL)-6, IL-1a and interferon-γ were seen in all patients.

Q. What are the clinical features of scorpion envenomation?

Manifestations depend upon the potency of the venom which varies with the species of scorpion. Some species produce mild flu-like illness; others cause death within an hour. Local pain, paresthesia, vomiting, salivation, sweating, and cold extremities are seen in potentially dangerous envenomation. Signs include tachycardia, hypertension, myocardial dysfunction, arrhythmias, pulmonary edema, and shock. Neurological features include convulsion, encephalopathy, aphasia, hemiplegia, DIC, and respiratory failure. Priapism, varying degrees of atrioventricular block, cardiac failure, and dilated cardiomyopathy are rare.

The toxicity and duration of the symptoms depends on the following factors:
- Scorpion species
- Scorpion age, size, and nutritional status
- Number of stings and quantity of venom injected
- Composition of the venom
- Site of envenomation: Closer proximity of the sting to the head and torso results in quicker venom absorption into the central circulation and a quicker onset of symptoms
- Age, health, and weight of the victim

- Presence of comorbidities
- Treatment effectiveness.

Q. Is there a grading system of scorpion manifestations?

On basis of clinical manifestations at the time of arrival to hospital and according to severity, they are graded in four grades.

Grade 1: Severe excruciating local pain at the sting site radiating along with corresponding dermatomes, mild local edema with seating at the sting site, without systemic involvement.

Grade 2: Signs and symptoms of autonomic storm characterized by acetyl choline excess or parasympathetic stimulation and sympathetic stimulation.

Grade 3: Cold extremities, tachycardia, hypotension, or hypertension with pulmonary edema.

Grade 4: Tachycardia, hypotension with or without pulmonary edema with warm extremities (warm shock).

Q. What precisely are the clinical features?

Clinical features are broadly classified into three groups: local, neurological, and non-neurological.

Local Signs

Screaming within seconds to minutes due to pain after the sting. Due to pain there is transient bradycardia, rise in blood pressure, mild sweating but extremities are warm. Sudden tap at and around the site of sting induces severe pain and withdrawal, is diagnostic sign of sting called "TAP sign". Severe pain without systemic involvement suggestive of benign or dry sting by venomous species. Serotonin found in scorpion venom is thought to contribute to pain associated with scorpion sting. Reappearance of severe pain accompanied by improved peripheral circulation by vasodilation suggest recovery.

Neurological Signs

Most of the symptoms are due to either the release of catecholamines from the adrenal glands and sympathetic nerves or due to the release of acetylcholine from postganglionic parasympathetic neurons.

Adrenergic signs occur at a low venom dose, while cholinergic signs occur at high venom dose concentrations, i.e., >40 µg/100 g. However, dual manifestations of the adrenergic and cholinergic signs are possible because of varying organ system sensitivities to these neurotransmitters.

Neurological signs are broadly classified as per box 1.

Non-neurological Systemic Signs

Cardiovascular signs: Usually follow a pattern of a hyperdynamic phase followed by a hypodynamic phase.

Hypertension is secondary to catecholamine and renin stimulation. It is observed as early as

---

BOX 1: Neurological signs of scorpion sting envenomation

- Central nervous system signs: Thalamus-induced systemic paresthesia occurs in all limbs, venom-induced cerebral thrombosis strokes and ataxia
- Sympathetic signs: Fever, tachypnea, tachycardia, hypertension, arrhythmias, hyperkinetic pulmonary edema, hyperglycemia, diaphoresis, piloerection, restlessness, apprehension, hyperexcitability, and seizures
- Parasympathetic signs: Bronchospasm, bradycardia, hypotension, salivation, lacrimation, urination, diarrhea, and gastric emesis (SLUDGE), rhinorrhea and bronchorrhea, loss of bowel and bladder control, priapism, dysphagia, miosis, and generalized weakness
- Somatic signs: Rigidity of muscles of the limbs and torso, involuntary muscle spasm, twitching, clonus, and contractures, opisthotonos, brisk tendon reflexes, especially prolongation of the relaxation phase, and piloerection
- Cranial nerve signs: Rotary eye movement, ptosis, nystagmus, blurred vision, mydriasis, tongue fasciculations, dysphagia, dysarthria, excessive salivation, and stridor.

within 4 minutes after the sting and lasts a few hours. Hypertension is high enough to produce hypertensive encephalopathy. Tachycardia is seen within 4 hours persist for 24–72 hours.

Cardiovascular collapse occurs secondary to biventricular dysfunction and profuse loss of fluids from sweating, vomiting, diarrhea and hypersalivation observed in 7–38% of cardiovascular cases. Transient apical pansystolic murmur is consistent with papillary muscle damage. Cardiac dysfunctions attributed to catecholamine-induced increases in myocardial metabolism, oxygen demand and to the direct effects of the toxin. Cardiological manifestation depends on degree of envenomation:
- Mild envenomation: Vascular effect with vasoconstriction hypertension
- Moderate envenomation: Left ventricular failure hypotension with and without an elevated pulmonary artery wedge pressure, depending on loss of fluid
- Severe envenomation: Biventricular cardiogenic shock.

Respiratory signs: Tachypnea is seen in almost all children. Pulmonary edema is secondary to a direct toxin-induced increased pulmonary vessel permeability effect and is also secondary to catecholamine-induced effects of hypoxia and intracellular calcium accumulation, which leads to a decrease in left ventricular compliance with resultant ventricular dilation and diastolic dysfunction. Respiratory failure may occur secondary to diaphragm paralysis, alveolar hypoventilation and bronchorrhea.

Gastrointestinal signs: Excessive salivation, dysphagia, nausea, vomiting, gastric hyperdistention (secondary to vagal stimulation), and gastric ulcers. Acute pancreatitis reported following sting by certain species, but rare in children.

Genitourinary signs: Toxin-induced acute tubular necrosis and rhabdomyolysis may lead to renal failure. Priapism may occur secondary to cholinergic stimulation.

Hematological signs: Platelet aggregation may occur because of catecholamine stimulation. Disseminated intravascular coagulation with massive hemorrhage may result from venom-induced defibrination.

Metabolic signs: Hyperglycemia may occur from catecholamine-induced hepatic glycogenolysis, pancreatitis and insulin inhibition. Increased lactic acidosis may occur from hypoxia and venom induced increased lactase dehydrogenase activity. Patients may have an electrolyte imbalance and dehydration from hypersalivation, vomiting, diaphoresis, and diarrhea.

Q. What is the role of investigations in a case of scorpion sting?

Investigations are useful to find out the extent of organ damage and need for further treatment.

Blood and urine tests: Complete blood count (CBC, leukocytosis), electrolyte imbalance (due to salivation, vomiting, and diarrhea), abnormal coagulation profile, and glucose (hyperglycemia from liver and pancreas dysfunction). Urine may show hematuria. Abnormal renal function test (RFT), liver function test (LFT), high amylase, lipase, and cholesterol level are also seen according to organ involved.

Rise in cardiac enzyme, cytokines, platelet activating factors, renin, angiotensin II, urine and serum catecholamine, serum amylase, and reduction in insulin level are also noted.

Chest X-ray: Suggestive of pulmonary edema are seen even within 3 hours of sting. These children need not be tachypneic. Unilateral pulmonary edema may be seen on chest X-ray films because of the venom effect on pulmonary vascular permeability.

Electrocardiogram: Changes are observed in 63% of children who have been envenomated. Rhythm disturbances are not dose-dependent but are related to the venom composition. Changes include sinus tachycardia, QTc prolongation, ST changes, T-wave inversion, ventricular repolarization abnormalities, bundle-branch block, and first-degree block. Electrocardiograph changes persist for 10–12 days before normalizing.

Echocardiography: Reveals left ventricular systolic dysfunction. Left ventricular dilatation with regional wall motion abnormalities is also seen. Echocardiography is more sensitive than electrocardiography for assessing myocardial compromise. Findings show a diffuse global biventricular hypokinesis with a decreased left and right ventricular ejection fraction. This dysfunction can appear just a few hours after the sting and usually normalizes within 4–8 days.

Q. How should one treat a case of scorpion sting?

Supportive care is the backbone of treatment. Stabilize the vitals followed by administration of antivenin, institution of symptomatic, and local treatment.

Systemic treatment is instituted by directing supportive care toward the organ specifically affected by the venom. Establish airway, breathing and circulation. Monitor vital signs if needed in pediatric intensive care unit (PICU). Administer intravenous fluids to prevent hypovolemia from vomiting, diarrhea, sweating, hypersalivation, and insensible water loss from a tropical environment. Institute mechanical ventilation for patients in respiratory distress.

For hyperdynamic cardiovascular changes, administration of sympathetic α-blockers is most effective in reversing this venom-induced effect. Also, nitrates can be used for hypertension and myocardial ischemia.

For hypodynamic cardiac changes, a titrated monitored fluid infusion with afterload reduction helps to reduce mortality. A diuretic may be used for pulmonary edema in the absence of hypovolemia. However, an afterload reducer such as prazosin should be the preferred choice.

Prazosin: A competitive postsynaptic α1, adrenoreceptor antagonist, it should be the first line of management, since α-receptors stimulation plays a major role in the evolution of clinical spectrum. Prazosin is a simple scientific pharmacological and physiological antidote to scorpion venom actions, it is easily available even in rural areas.

Prazosin acts by suppressing the sympathetic outflow and activating venom-inhibited potassium channels. It decreases the preload, afterload, and blood pressure without increasing the heart rate.

The agent counters vasoconstriction induced by endothelins through accumulation of cyclic guanosine monophosphate (cGMP). Prazosin by inhibiting phosphodiesterase enzyme and by inhibiting the formation of inositol triphosphate makes this possible. Cyclic GMP, a second messenger of nitric oxide in vascular endothelium and myocardium prevents further myocardial injury. The metabolic and hormonal effects of α-receptors stimulation are reversed by prazosin. Thus, prazosin is a cellular and pharmacologic antidote to the actions of scorpion venom. It is also cardioprotective.

It is available as scored 1 mg tablet. Sustained release tablets should be avoided. The dose recommended is 30 μg/kg/dose. This is given as an immediate measure in all with evidence of autonomic storm. In case of vomiting, it can be administered through nasogastric tube. After giving prazosin, lifting of the child needs to be avoided to prevent the effects of "first dose phenomenon".

The drug can be given regardless of blood pressure. There should be no hypovolemia. Blood pressure, pulse rate, and respiration must be monitored every 30 minutes for 3 hours, every hour for next 6 hours, and later every 4 hours till improvement. Prazosin should be repeated in the same dose at the end of 3 hours according to clinical response and later every 6 hours till extremities are warm.

Inotropic medications, such as digitalis, have little effect, while dopamine aggravates the myocardial damage through catecholamine like actions. Dobutamine seems to be a better choice for the inotropic effect. Gupta et al. compared dobutamine versus prazosin in children and found mortality in both groups to be equal, but the prazosin group had a quicker resolution in their pulmonary edema. Norepinephrine can be used as a last resort to correct hypotension refractory to fluid therapy. Administer atropine to counter venom-induced parasympathomimetic effects.

Diazepam is often useful to quieten a child after scorpion sting. Benzodiazepines in concert with γ-aminobutyric acid, open chloride ion channel. This effect of diazepam antagonizes the scorpion toxins' ability to stimulate specific ion channel.

Pain relief is useful since it allays anxiety and avoids myocardial stress. However, many children have only mild and tolerable pain; when severe, nonsteroidal anti-inflammatory drugs provide prolonged relief. Local ice packs and xylocaine are useful

Oral fluids, whenever feasible, should be encouraged in the presence of tachypnea and altered sensorium, carefully-balanced parenteral fluids therapy is preferred. Central venous pressure monitoring is essential when pulmonary edema is suspected.

In children with pulmonary edema with or without hypertension, management should be directed toward relieving afterload without compromising preload. The use of diuretics to minimize or reduce fluid overload seems a reasonable measure.

However, dobutamine support (5-15 mg/kg/min) with vasodilatation through sodium nitroprusside (0.3-5 mg/kg/min) or nitroglycerine (5 mg/min) infusate is strongly recommended.

Prazosin is best given 1 hour before termination of sodium nitroprusside drip or isosorbide dinitrate 10 mg every 10 minutes sublingually as an emergency measure.

Morphine, a recommended therapy in pulmonary edema, needs to be avoided in scorpion sting. Narcotics are known to worsen dysrhythmias in this situation.

Administer tetanus prophylaxis and systemic antibiotics, if signs of secondary infection occur.

Q. What is the role of scorpion antivenom?

Scorpion antivenom must be administered as early as possible through venous route and is the treatment of choice after supportive care is established. The quantity to be used is determined by the clinical severity of patients and by their evolution over time.

The antivenin significantly decreases the level of circulating unbound venom within an hour. The persistence of symptoms after the administration of antivenin is due to the inability of the antivenin to neutralize scorpion toxins already bound to their target receptors.

Perform a skin test prior to administering the antivenin. First, dilute 0.1 mL of antivenin in a 1:10 ratio with isotonic sodium chloride solution. Second, administer 0.2 mL intradermally. A positive test result is if a wheal develops within 10 minutes. The skin test has a sensitivity of 96% and a specificity of 68%.

Dose: Grade I and II—none; grade III and IV—1 vial (5 mL) in 50 mL saline IV over 30 min; if severe symptoms still persist after 1 hour, repeat one more vial.

Time guidelines for the disappearance of symptoms after antivenin administration are as follows:
- In the first hour, local pain abates
- In 6-12 hours, agitation, sweating, and hyperglycemia abate
- In 6-24 hours, cardiorespiratory symptoms abate.

Watch for anaphylaxis reaction to the antivenin, but the child is at lower risk for anaphylaxis than with other antivenins for other poisonous envenomations because of the huge release of catecholamines induced by the scorpion venom.

The best result occurs when antivenin is administered as early as possible (preferably within the first 2 hours after the sting) and with adequate quantities to neutralize the venom. A decrease in curative effects occurs with delay in serotherapy and administration of insufficient amounts.

Local treatment: Immobilize the affected part. Apply a topical or local anesthetic agent to decrease paresthesia. Administer local wound care and topical antibiotic to the wound.

Q. What kinds of treatments are contraindicated?

Lytic cocktail (pethidine + promethazine + chlorpromazine), morphine, steroids, atropine, nifedipine and angiotensin-converting enzyme inhibitors are contraindicated.

Excessive administration of fluids and atropine increase the severity of pulmonary edema. Steroids increase the necrotizing effects of circulating catecholamines and oxygen demand of myocardium. Digitalis enhances already increased myocardial contraction and oxygen requirement. Antihistamines and venom both act synergically by inhibiting Ca^+ dependent potassium activating channels lead to QTc prolongation may cause sudden death.

Q. What are the factors predicting outcome in a case of scorpion sting?

Children and elderly persons are at the greatest risk for morbidity and mortality. A smaller child, a lower body weight, and a larger ratio of venom to body weight lead to a more severe reaction.

In terms of venom lethality, the venom of *Androctonus australis* and *Leiurus quinquestriatus* are the most toxic. *Centruroides sculpturatus* venom is low in toxicity compared with most scorpions of medical importance.

Patients in rural areas tend to fare worse than patients in urban areas because of the delay in getting medical help. A worse prognosis can be expected with the presence of systemic symptoms such as cardiovascular collapse, respiratory failure, seizures, and coma.

Q. Finally, what is the cause of death in scorpion sting?

Most deaths occur during the first 24 hours after the sting and are secondary to respiratory or cardiovascular failure.

The mode of death is usually via respiratory failure secondary to anaphylaxis, bronchoconstriction, bronchorrhea, pharyngeal secretions, and/or diaphragmatic paralysis, even though venom-induced multiorgan failure.

Death within 30 minute of sting can occur due to lethal ventricular arrhythmia. Actual transport of severe scorpion sting cases to nearest big hospital delays the treatment and adds to their deaths.

Following the use of prazosin in 1980s, the mortality in the scorpion sting with pulmonary edema has reduced to <1% from 25 to 30% in the preprazasin era. As such, case fatality rate in children due to scorpion sting has declined from 13 to 3%.

CONCLUSION

Scorpion sting, a life-threatening emergency in children, may cause serious complications include anaphylaxis, cardiac arrhythmia, hyper/hypotension, and pulmonary edema. Prazosin, a competitive postsynaptic α1, adrenoreceptor antagonist, should be the first line of management, and should be given without delay. Prompt treatment of pulmonary edema is life-saving. Scorpion antivenom is now available and found to be effective, if used immediately after the sting. All health personnel, especially in rural settings, should be trained regarding the combined treatment protocols for scorpion sting.

KEY LEARNING POINTS

- Clinical features of scorpion sting can be divided into three groups, i.e., local, neurological, and other systemic features
- Degree of envenomation depends on the age of the child, species of the scorpion, site of the sting, associated comorbid condition and effective treatment
- Echocardiogram is a very useful tool to detect the extent of myocardial damage
- Serious complications include anaphylaxis, cardiac arrhythmia, hyper/hypotension, and pulmonary edema
- Treatment revolves around supportive measures, scorpion antivenom and local treatment
- Prazosin a competitive postsynaptic α1, adrenoreceptor antagonist, should be given without delay
- Scorpion antivenom is effective provided that it is administered within 30 minutes of sting
- Training of all health personnel regarding the combined treatment protocols should be extended to all rural areas of our country.

SUGGESTED READINGS

1. Abdel-Haleem AA, Meki AMA, Noaman HA, Mohamed ZT. Serum levels of IL-6 and its soluble receptor, TNF-α and chemokine RANTES in scorpion envenomed children: their relation to scorpion envenomation outcome. *Toxicon.* 2006;47:437-444.
2. Bawaskar HS, Bawakar PH. Efficacy and safety of scorpion antivenom plus prazosin compared with prazosin alone for venomous scorpion sting: randomized open label clinical trial. *BMJ.* 2011;342:c7136.
3. Bawaskar HS. Diagnostic cardiac premonitory signs and symptoms of red scorpion sting. *Lancet.* 1982;2:552-555.
4. Chippaux JP, Goyffon M. Epidemiology of scorpionism: a global appraisal. *Acta Trop.* 2008;107:71-79.
5. Gupta BD, Parakh M, Purohit A. Management of scorpion sting: prazosin or dobutamine. *J Trop Pediatr.* 2010;56: 115-118.
6. Gupte S, Raghava Rao KV, Kaushal RK. Envenomation. In: Gupte S (Ed). *The Short Textbook of Pediatrics*, 12th edn. New Delhi: Jaypee Brothers Medical Publishers; 2016:734-738.
7. Prasad R, Mishra OP, Pandey N, Singh TB. Scorpion sting envenomation in children:factors affecting the outcome. *Indian J Pediatr.* 2011;78:544-548.
8. Sarakar S, Bhattacharya P, Paswan A. Cerebrovascular manifestations and alteration of coagulation profile in scorpion sting; a case series. *Indian J Crit Care Med.* 2008;12: 15-17.

Snakebite

CHAPTER 34

BP Karunakara, K Prarthana Karumbaiah

INTRODUCTION

As per World Health Organization (WHO) statistics, India is estimated to have about 50,000 deaths per annum, the highest mortality worldwide due to snakebite. The morbidity due to snakebites is much higher than the mortality and an accurate number of those are not recorded. Hence, snakebite was included in the WHO list of notifiable neglected diseases list in 2009.

CASE 1

A 10-year-old girl while playing with her friends in a playground stepped on a snake in the bush while collecting the ball. She ran home to inform her parents that the snake had bitten her right foot. She was rushed to a hospital 10 km away. On reaching the emergency department, she was examined by the doctor. She complained of severe tingling sensation in the right foot and pain at the right inguinal region. Local examination of the area showed fang marks at the bite site. There was continuous oozing of the blood from the bite site. There was discoloration of the limb till the knee. Also, there was bilateral inguinal lymphadenopathy.

Blood tests revealed lymphocytosis, thrombocytopenia, and altered coagulation profile. She was administered 5 vials of the anti-snake venom (ASV) and injection tetanus toxoid. After 30 minutes, 10 mL of the blood was collected in a test tube and allowed to stand for 20 minutes. It was tilted to a side. Blood flowed on to the sides. Based on the 20-minute whole blood clot test (20WBCT), she was administered another 5 vials of the ASV and at 12 hours, 5 more vials of the ASV were administered. Repeating the test showed that the blood had clotted. She was treated in the hospital for the next 3 days and discharged home.

CASE 2

A 9-year-old child presented to the emergency department of a hospital in the early hours of morning, with history of a bite by a cobra when he had gone out to the fields. He was immediately rushed to the hospital where he was attended by a doctor. On examination, he had tachycardia and severe pain at the site of bite. The doctor noticed fang marks on the right foot. Local examination showed significant swelling till the thigh with bilateral inguinal lymphadenopathy. The doctor also noticed that he was not able to open his eyes completely. He was immediately started on 10 vials of ASV. When reassessed after half an hour, ptosis was still present. He was administered 5 vials of ASV and reassessed. Ptosis had disappeared. However, he required fasciotomy to relieve the swelling. After a week, he walked back home feeling better.

CASE REVIEW IN A NUTSHELL

The clinical presentation of the above cases was different. However, both the cases showed fang marks at the site of bite. Viperine bite showed continuous oozing of blood at the site of bite while Elapidae bite showed ptosis as a manifestation. The fact that in both the cases, there was bilateral painful lymphadenopathy and the swelling of the limb had crossed more than one joint show the rapidity of envenomation. The 20WBCT is the diagnostic test which gives a clue about additional requirement of the ASV.

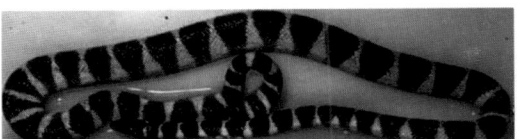

Figure 1: Sea snake *(For color version, see Plate 2)*

INTERACTIVE TOPIC REVIEW

Q. How to identify a snakebite in a given patient? What are the common symptoms associated with snakebite?

When a patient is brought to the hospital, take history of the site of bite, circumstance of the snakebite, type of the snake, and how the patient feels.

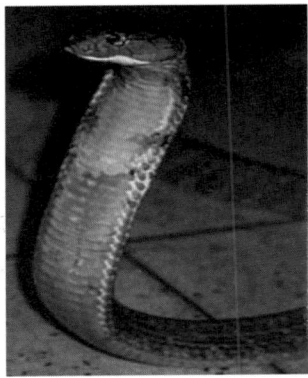

Figure 2: *Ophiophagus hannah* (king cobra) *(For color version, see Plate 2)*

Identify the site of bite. Usually, there are two puncture marks at the site of bite, though the distance and depth of bite between the marks may vary. Watch the patient for the following signs of impending dangers of snakebite envenomation:
- Nausea, vomiting, malaise, abdominal pain, weakness, drowsiness, prostration
- Prolonged bleeding from the bite site
- Ptosis
- Stiffness and tenderness of muscles
- Passage of dark brown or dark urine.

Q. Name the common poisonous snakes in India? How to identify a poisonous from a nonpoisonous snake?

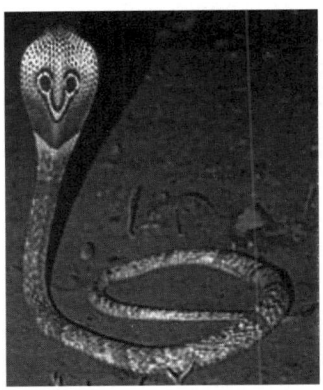

Figure 3: *Naja naja* (common cobra) *(For color version, see Plate 2)*

Of all the 15 families of snakes in the world, three major families are poisonous. They are:
1. Elapidae: Cobras, coral snakes, krait
2. Viperidae: Russell's viper, pit viper, saw-scaled viper
3. Hydrophiidae: Sea snakes (Fig. 1).

Of the 50 poisonous snakes in India, mortality is high due to the following five species—king cobra (*Ophiophagus hannah*, Fig. 2), common cobra (*Naja naja* Fig. 3), Russell's viper (*Daboia russelii*, Fig. 4), krait (*Bungarus caeruleus*, Fig. 5), saw-scaled viper (*Echis carinatus*, Fig. 6).

If a snake is brought for the identification, the following features help in the identification of the poisonous from nonpoisonous snakes:
- Most poisonous snakes have triangular heads
- May be brightly colored, e.g., coral snakes

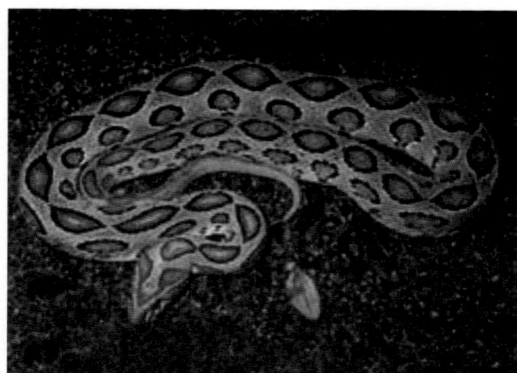

Figure 4: *Daboia russelii* (Russell's viper) *(For color version, see Plate 2)*

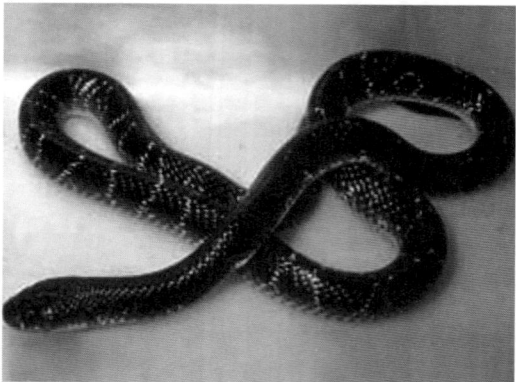

Figure 5: *Bungarus caeruleus* (Krait) *(For color version, see Plate 2)*

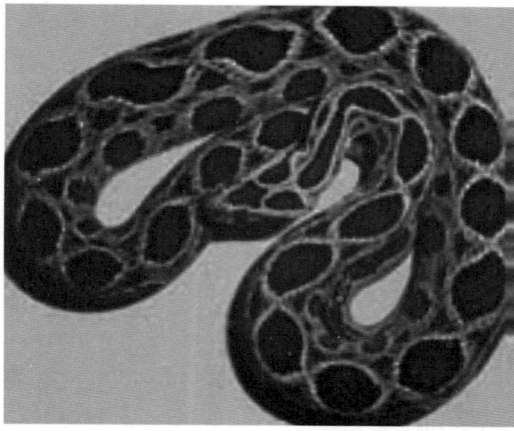

Figure 6: *Echis carinatus* (saw-scaled viper) *(For color version, see Plate 2)*

- Most poisonous snakes have vertical eye slits compared to round eye slits in nonpoisonous snakes
- Poisonous snakes have heat sensitive pits in between the their eyes and nostrils
- Rattlesnakes have a rattle on its tail and are poisonous
- Most poisonous snakes have one row of scales on their underside on the tip of the tail while nonpoisonous snakes have two rows of scales
- Poisonous snakebites have two close set of puncture marks.

Q. What are the signs of envenomation?

Local symptoms and signs in the bitten part:

Fang marks (Fig. 7), local pain, local bleeding (Fig. 8), bruising, blistering (Fig. 9), local infection, abscess formation, necrosis, lymphangitis (Fig. 10), regional lymph node enlargement, and inflammation.

Bleeding and clotting disorders (usually with Viperidae bite): Prolonged bleeding from the bite site (bleeding from recent wounds including venipunctures), spontaneous systemic bleeding (petechiae, purpura, epistaxis, gum bleeding, hemoptysis, hematemesis, melena, hematuria, vaginal bleeding, intracranial hemorrhage) (Fig. 11).

Neurological (usually Elapidae): Drowsiness, paraesthesia, ptosis (Fig. 12), external ophthalmo-

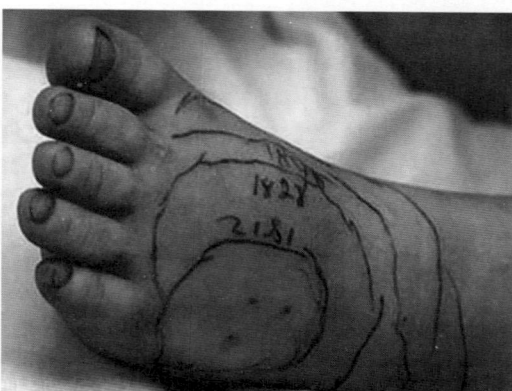

Figure 7: Fang marks *(For color version, see Plate 3)*

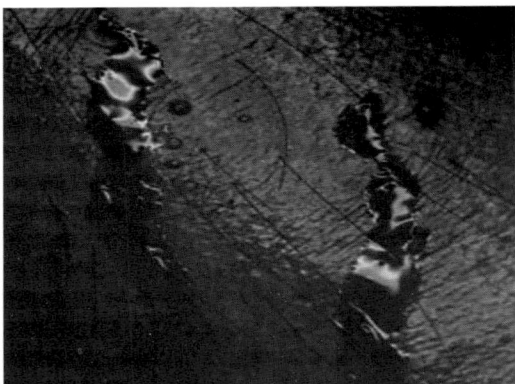

Figure 8: Local bleeding *(For color version, see Plate 3)*

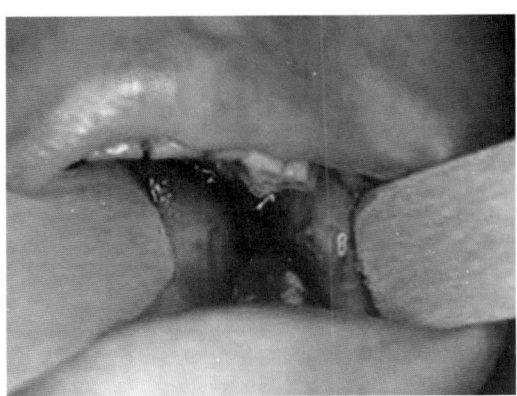

Figure 11: Bleeding from gingival sulci *(For color version, see Plate 3)*

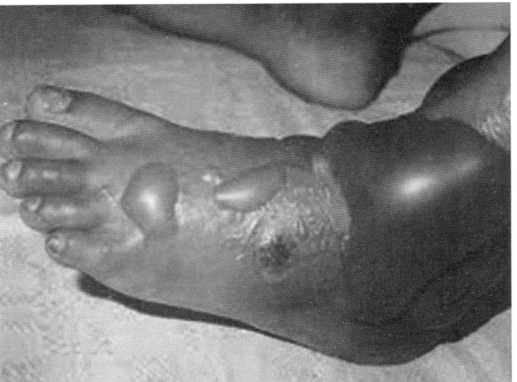

Figure 9: Bruising and blistering *(For color version, see Plate 3)*

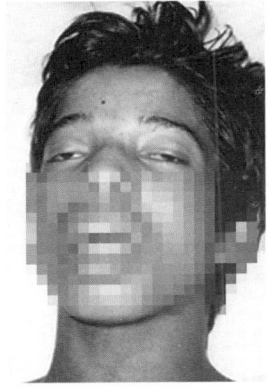

Figure 12: Ptosis *(For color version, see Plate 3)*

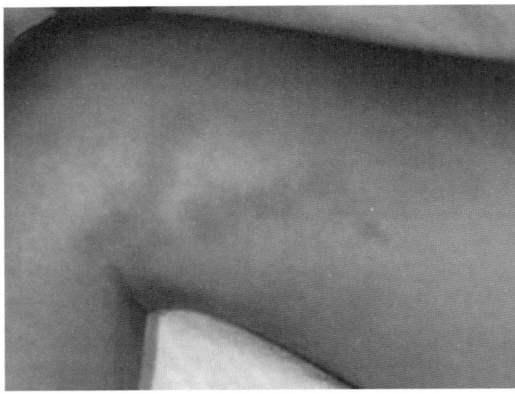

Figure 10: Lymphangitis *(For color version, see Plate 3)*

plegia, paralysis of facial muscles, difficulty in swallowing secretions, respiratory and generalized flaccid paralysis.

Cardiovascular (Viperidae): Visual disturbances, dizziness, faintness, collapse, shock, hypotension, cardiac arrhythmias, pulmonary edema, conjunctival edema.

Skeletal muscle breakdown (sea snakes, some kraits): Generalized pain, stiffness and tenderness of muscles, "broken neck sign (Fig. 13)", trismus, myoglobinuria, hyperkalemia, cardiac arrest, acute renal failure.

Endocrine: Shock, hypoglycemia.

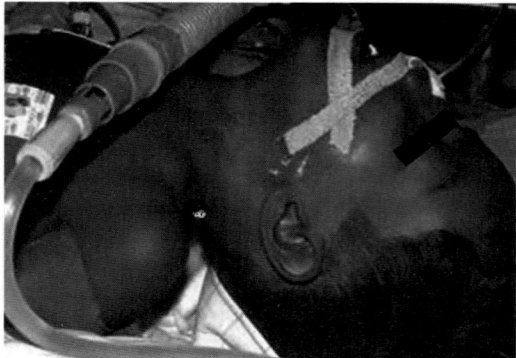

Figure 13: Broken neck sign in a child envenomed by krait (*For color version, see Plate 4*)

Q. What is the first aid for snakebite?

The first aid recommended is based around the mnemonic:

"Do it RIGHT"

It consists of:

R = Reassurance of the patient.
The patient succumbs due to the fear of being bitten by a snake rather than the envenomation.

I = Immobilize the limb.
Use bandages or cloth to hold the splints, not to block the blood supply or apply pressure. Do not apply any compression in the form of tight ligatures.

GH = Get to hospital immediately.

T = Tell the doctor of any systemic symptoms, such as ptosis, that manifest on the way to hospital.

Practices which should be discouraged are:
- Tying the tourniquet at the site of bite since it is invariably done in a wrong way
- Sucking out blood from the site of bite
- Cutting out an inch cube of skin around the bite site
- Incision, suction electric shocks, cryotherapy, and washing the wound are contraindicated.

Q. How to assess the degree of envenomation?

Table 1 describes the assessment of degree of envenomation.

TABLE 1: Degree of envenomation

No envenomation	Absence of local or systemic reactions; fang marks (±)
Mild envenomation	Fang marks + moderate pain, minimal local edema (0–15 cm), erythema + ecchymosis ± no systemic reaction
Moderate envenomation	Fang marks + severe pain, moderate local edema (15–30 cm), erythema + ecchymosis + systemic weakness, sweating, syncope, nausea, vomiting, anemia, or thrombocytopenia
Severe envenomation	Fang marks + severe pain, severe local edema (>30 cm), erythema + ecchymosis + hypotension, paraesthesia, coma, pulmonary edema, respiratory failure

Q. How to manage a case of snakebite at the emergency room?

- Reassure the patient as soon as the child is brought to the hospital
- Immobilize the limb. Use bandages or cloth to hold the splints, not to block the blood supply or apply pressure
- Check for the airway, breathing, and circulation
- Check heart rate (tachycardia may be the earliest sign of shock)
    - Respiratory rate
    - Blood pressure (hypotension may be an eminent sign)
    - Cold, clammy extremities with feeble peripheral pulses
- Check for oxygen saturation using pulse oximetry
- Start on oxygen through hood or nasal cannula
- Intravenous ringer lactate or 0.9% saline should be started to maintain circulation. Bolus may be given at 20 mL/kg (maximum 60 mL/kg) if there is shock. If there is generalized increase in capillary permeability, a selective vasoconstrictor, such as dopamine, may be given by intravenous infusion, preferably into a central vein (starting dose 2.5–5 µg/kg/min)
- If there is hypoglycemia, administer dextrose

- Anti-snake venom therapy administered at the earliest as soon as envenomation is established with an initial dose of 8–10 vials. After 6 hours, 20WBCT is done and reassessed for further doses of ASV. If the test is positive, additional dose of ASV is given and the test repeated again after 6 hours
- Tetanus toxoid should be administered
- Appropriate intravenous antibiotics are administered
- Surgical intervention (fasciotomy), if evidence of compartment syndrome.

Q. What are the indications for envenomation?

If one or more of the following are present, ASV has to be given:

Local envenomation

Local swelling involving more than half of the bitten limb (in the absence of a tourniquet) within 48 hours of the bite. Swelling after bites on the digits (toes and especially fingers).

Rapid extension of swelling (for example, beyond the wrist or ankle within a few hours of bite on the hands or feet).

Development of an enlarged tender lymph node draining the bitten limb.

Systemic envenomation

- Spontaneous systemic bleeding (clinical) or coagulopathy (20WBCT or other laboratory tests such as prothrombin time) or thrombocytopenia (<100 × 10^9/L or 100,000/mm^3) (laboratory)
- Ptosis, external ophthalmoplegia, paralysis, etc. (clinical)
- Cardiovascular abnormalities: Hypotension, shock, cardiac arrhythmia (clinical), abnormal electrocardiogram
- Acute kidney injury (renal failure): Oliguria/anuria (clinical), rising blood creatinine/urea (laboratory)
- Hemoglobin-/myoglobinuria: Dark brown urine (clinical), urine dipsticks, other evidence of intravascular hemolysis or
- Generalized rhabdomyolysis (muscle aches and pains, hyperkalemia) (clinical, laboratory)
- Supporting laboratory evidence of systemic envenoming (see above).

Q. What are the laboratory tests of importance?

Routine laboratory investigations are of little help to diagnose snakebite. Hemolysis is evident by the presence of anemia, leukocytosis, and thrombocytopenia. Prolonged clotting times and decreased fibrinogen may be present. Enzyme linked immunosorbent assay test is available to identify the species involved, based on venom antigens. Urinalysis may reveal hematuria, proteinuria, and hemoglobinuria. Electrocardiographic changes are usually nonspecific and may include rhythm disturbances, mainly bradycardia. Atrioventricular block with segment elevation (ST) segment elevation or depression. Hypokalemia and respiratory acidosis, if neuroparalysis occurs.

Q. What is the diagnostic test to determine envenomation?

Determination of hematotoxic snakebite (Viperidae): 20-minute whole blood clotting test.

In a small, new or heat cleaned, dry, glass test tube, 2 mL of freshly sampled venous blood is collected. Leave undisturbed for 20 minutes at ambient temperature. Tip the vessel once. If the blood is still liquid (unclotted) and runs out, the patient has hypofibrinogenemia ("incoagulable blood") as a result of venom induced consumption coagulopathy (WHO protocol).

Determination of neurotoxic snakebite (Elapidae)

Intravenous injection of atropine sulphate (0.6 mg for adults; 50 µg/kg for children) followed by neostigmine bromide 0.02 mg/kg for adults, 0.04 mg/kg for children is given intramuscularly.

Short-acting edrophonium chloride is ideal for this test, if available. It is given by slow intravenous injection in an adult dose of 10 mg, or 0.25 mg/kg in children.

Watch the patient for signs of improvement in neuromuscular transmission (like ptosis or ventilator capacity) over the next 30–60 minutes for neostigmine or 10–20 minutes for edrophonium.

Patients who respond convincingly can be maintained on neostigmine methylsulphate, 0.5–2.5 mg every 1–3 hours up to 10 mg/24 hours maximum for adults or 0.01–0.04 mg/kg every 2–4 hours for children by intramuscular, intravenous, or subcutaneous injection together with atropine to block muscarinic side effects.

Patients able to swallow tablets may be maintained on atropine 0.6 mg twice each day, neostigmine 15 mg four times each day, or pyridostigmine 60 mg four times each day.

Q. What is the dose of anti-snake venom to be given?

Russell's viper injects on average 63 mg (SD 7 mg) of venom in the first bite to both adults and children. As each vial of polyvalent ASV neutralizes 6 mg of Russell's viper venom, the initial dose is 8–10 vials for both adults and children. The range of venom injected was shown to be 5–147 mg. This would imply a maximum ASV dose of around 25 vials. Hence, the recommended initial dose of ASV (liquid or lyophilized ASV) is 8–10 vials administered intravenously over 1 hour.

Repeat doses for hemotoxic species is based on the 6-hour rule.

Repeat doses for neurotoxic is based on the 1–2 hour rule.

The maximum recommended dose for hemotoxic bites in 30 vials of ASV.

The maximum recommended dose for neurotoxic bites is 20 vials of ASV.

Q. How to reconstitute the anti-snake venom?

Freeze-dried (lyophilized) antivenoms are reconstituted, usually with 10 mL of sterile water for injection per ampoule.

Two methods of administration are recommended:
1. Intravenous "push" injection: Reconstituted freeze-dried antivenom or neat liquid antivenom is given by slow intravenous injection (not more than 2 mL/min)
2. Intravenous infusion: Reconstituted freeze-dried or neat liquid antivenom is diluted in approximately 5–10 mL of isotonic fluid per kg body weight (i.e., 250–500 mL of isotonic saline or 5% dextrose in the case of an adult patient) and is infused at a constant rate over a period of about 1 hour.

- No ASV test doses are to be administered. They are not predictive and carry their own risks
- Prophylactic regimens of steroids and antihistamines or adrenaline are optional
- Observation of the patient for an hour after starting intravenous ASV is very important as early anaphylactic reactions can be detected.

Q. When to stop anti-snake venom treatment?

The following response is seen if the treatment with ASV is adequate:
- Spontaneous systemic bleeding usually stops within 15–30 minutes
- Blood coagulability (as measured by 20WBCT) which is usually restored in 3–9 hours
- In shocked patients, blood pressure may increase within the first 30–60 minutes and arrhythmias, such as sinus bradycardia, may resolve
- Neurotoxic envenoming of the postsynaptic type (cobra bites) may begin to improve as early as 30 minutes after antivenom, but usually takes several hours.

Q. What are the adverse effects of anti-snake venom? How to treat them?

Early anaphylactic reactions

At the first sign of an adverse reaction, even if it is itching or a few spots of urticarial, tachycardia, or restlessness, the ASV is stopped. Epinephrine (adrenaline 0.1% solution, 1 in 1,000, 1 mg/mL) is given intramuscularly (into upper lateral thigh) in an initial dose of 0.5 mg for adults and 0.01 mg/kg body weight for children. The dose can be repeated every 5–10 minutes for a total of three doses if the patient's condition is deteriorating.

After epinephrine (adrenaline), an antihistamine anti-H1 blocker, such as chlorphenamine maleate (adults 10 mg, children 0.2 mg/kg by intravenous injection over a few minutes), should be given followed by intravenous hydrocortisone (adults 100 mg, children 2 mg/kg body weight) to prevent recurrent anaphylaxis.

In pyrogenic reactions, the patient must be given tepid sponging and antipyretics.

Intravenous fluids should be given to correct hypovolemia.

Late (Serum Sickness) Reactions

Late (serum sickness) reactions may respond to a 5-day course of oral antihistamine. Patients who fail to respond in 24–48 hours should be given a 5-day course of prednisolone.

Doses: Chlorphenamine—adults 2 mg 6 hourly, children 0.25 mg/kg/day in divided doses.

Prednisolone: Adults 5 mg 6 hourly, children 0.7 mg/kg/day in divided doses for 5–7 days.

Once the patient has recovered, the ASV can be restarted slowly for 10–15 minutes, keeping the patient under close observation. Then, the normal drip rate should be resumed.

Q. What are the complications of snakebite?

Snakebite can cause:
- Oliguria and acute kidney injury
- Severe acidosis
- Hyperkalemia
- Shock
- Septicemia
- Compartment syndrome.

Q. What are the long-term effects of snakebite?

After an initial response to ASV, there could be recurrence of symptoms over the next 24–48 hours. Months to years after the bite, there may be "endocrine problems" related to pituitary/adrenal insufficiency from infarction of the anterior pituitary which manifests as weakness, loss of secondary sexual hair, loss of libido, amenorrhea, testicular atrophy, hypothyroidism, etc.

CONCLUSION

Snakebite, a neglected tropical disease causing significant morbidity and mortality, can cause different manifestations from neurotoxins, cardiotoxins, and the phospholipases. Signs of rapid envenomation, either local or systemic, are an indication to administer ASV. The 20WBCT is a good indicator for repeating doses of ASV. Complications include oliguria and acute kidney injury, severe acidosis, hyperkalemia, shock, septicemia, and compartment syndrome.

KEY LEARNING POINTS

- Snakebite is a neglected tropical disease causing significant morbidity and mortality
- Snakebites can cause different presentations because of neurotoxins, cardiotoxins, and the phospholipases
- Signs of rapid envenomation, either local or systemic, are indications to administer anti-snake venom (ASV)
- 20-minute whole blood clotting test is a good indicator for repeating doses of ASV.

SUGGESTED READINGS

1. Ahmed SM, Ahmed M, Nadeem A, Mahajan J, Choudhary A, Pal J. Emergency treatment of a snake bite: pearls from literature. J Emerg Trauma Shock. 2008;1:97-105.
2. Kasturiratne A, Wickremasinghe AR, de Silva N, Gunawardena NK, Pathmeswaran A, Premaratna R, et al. The global burden of snakebite: a literature analysis and modelling based on regional estimates of envenoming and deaths. PLoS Medi. 2008;5:e218.
3. Mohapatra B, Warrell DA, Suraweera W, Bhatia P, Dhingra N, Jotkar RM, et al. Snakebite mortality in India: a nationally representative mortality survey. PLoS Negl Trop Dis. 2011; 5:e1018.
4. Simpson ID. The pediatric management of snakebite: the national protocol. Indian Pediatr. 2007;44:173-176.
5. World Health Organization. Influenza. [online] Available at: http://www.who.int/neglected diseases/diseases/%20 snakebites/en/index.html. Accessed on: 23 June, 2016.

SECTION 9
Gastroenterology

CHAPTER

Acute Gastroenteritis

35

BP Karunakara, V Nancy Jeniffer

INTRODUCTION

Diarrheal diseases are one of the leading causes of death in children in the developing countries and claim around 1.5–2.5 million lives per year worldwide. They are an important cause of morbidity in children in the developed world too, and incur substantial healthcare costs. During the past three decades, factors such as the widespread distribution and use of oral rehydration solutions (ORS), improved rates of breastfeeding, improved nutrition, better sanitation and hygiene, and increased coverage of measles immunization have contributed to a consistent decline in the mortality rate in developing countries from around 5/million to 1.6/million deaths of children per year due to diarrheal diseases as per World Health Organization (WHO) estimates.

CASE 1

A 3-year-old boy was brought to the casualty with history of watery moderate quantity stools, around 9–10 episodes per day for the past 2 days not associated with blood and mucus. There was history of vomiting, 2–3 episodes, nonblood/bile tinged, with history of decreased urine output, lethargy, and poor feeding. No history of fever with rash (measles)/cough/other significant problems (convulsions). No history of any comorbidities like cardiac or renal disease/diabetes/human immunodeficiency virus.

Examination: Afebrile, pulse rate of 120 beats/min, good volume, respiratory rate of 36 breaths/min, weight 12 kg, height 90 cm.

Sunken eyes, dry mucosa, lethargy, and delayed skin turgor reduced eagerness to drink.

Investigation:

Glucose random blood sugar: 114 mg/dL.

Diagnosis: Acute gastroenteritis with severe dehydration.

Treatment: Plan-C dehydration correction was started. Ringer's lactate (RL), 30 mL/kg, was given over half an hour and 70 mL/kg over the next $2\frac{1}{2}$ hours. Following dehydration correction, the child's lethargy improved and he started taking orally by next 4 hours. He was given around 100 mL ORS for any further loose stool.

Syrup zinc 20 mg/day was also started.

Course: Loose stools subsided in 3 days. He was discharged on day 3 with advice to continue zinc for a total of 14 days.

Normal diet and advice on hand hygiene and other preventive measures were also advised.

CASE REVIEW IN A NUTSHELL

This 3-year-old child was diagnosed to have acute gastroenteritis with severe dehydration (based on history and clinical examination) which amounted to 8–10% water loss from body. Hence, 10% dehydration correction (100 mL/kg) was given. Since he was more than 1 year old, intravenous (IV) fluid was given at a faster rate over a period of 3 hours. The ideal fluid for this purpose is RL which is isotonic to plasma. Zinc was given since it is known to decrease frequency, improve the consistency of stool and also prevent further episodes of gastroenteritis. There was no need of antibiotics as it was not a case of dysentery or severe malnutrition. Neither was there any focus of infection.

INTERACTIVE TOPIC REVIEW

Define Diarrhea

Diarrhea is defined as the passage of loose or watery stools. Case definition of acute diarrhea is more than three loose or watery stools per day. The volume of fluid lost through stools can vary from 5 mL/kg body weight per day (approximately normal) to more than 200 mL/kg body weight per day.

Q. What are the common complications of acute diarrhea?

These include:
- Dehydration with electrolyte imbalance/acidosis
- Hypoglycemia
- Sepsis
- Cardiovascular collapse and death.

Q. What are the causes of acute diarrhea?

Viruses are responsible for approximately 70% of episodes of acute gastroenteritis in children; *Rotavirus* is one of the best studied of these viruses (Table 1).

Q. How do you grade dehydration?

Grading of diarrheal dehydration has been described in table 2.

Q. What should be the treatment plan of dehydration?

Treatment is based on degree of dehydration (Table 3).

TABLE 1: Etiology of acute diarrhea

Pathogens	Agents
Viruses 70–80%	• Rotavirus • Enteric adenovirus • Norwalk virus • Calicivirus • Astrovirus • Parvovirus
Bacteria 10–20%	• Salmonella • Shigella • Campylobacter jejuni • Yersinia enterocolitica • Enterohemorrhagic E. coli (includes O157:H7) • Other diarrhea-genic E. coli (Cohen, 2005 [C]) • Clostridium difficile
Parasites 0–10%	• Giardia lamblia • Cryptosporidium

Q. What are the principles of treatment?

Principles of treatment are as follows:
- The treatment of a child with diarrhea is directed primarily by the degree of dehydration present
- In the vast majority of cases, rehydration should be carried out using oral rehydration therapy (ORT). Rehydration should normally be completed over a 3–4-hour period.

An ORS containing sodium 60 mmol/L, glucose 90 mmol/L, potassium 20 mmol/L, and citrate 10 mmol/L with a low osmolality of 240 mmol/L is safe and effective for the prevention and treatment of dehydration.
- No dehydration
  ○ Oral rehydration therapy: ORT is employed to replace ongoing stool losses in children with mild diarrhea and no dehydration by giving 10 mL/kg for each stool
  ○ Feeding: Continued age-appropriate feeding and increased fluid intake may be the only therapy required if hydration is normal
- Mild dehydration (3–5%)
  ○ Oral rehydration therapy: Dehydration should be corrected by giving 50 mL/kg ORT plus replacement of continuing losses during a 4-hour period. Replacement of

TABLE 2: **Grading of diarrheal dehydration**

Symptoms	Minimal or no dehydration (<3% loss of body weight)	Mild-to-moderate dehydration (3–9% loss of body weight)	Severe dehydration (>9% loss of body weight)
Mental status	Well; alert	Normal, fatigued or restless, irritable	Apathetic, lethargic, unconscious
Thirst	Drinks normally; might refuse liquids	Thirsty; eager to drink	Drinks poorly; unable to drink
Heart rate	Normal	Normal to increased	Tachycardia, with bradycardia in most severe cases
Quality of pulses	Normal	Normal to decreased	Weak, thready, or impalpable
Breathing	Normal	Normal; fast	Deep
Eyes	Normal	Slightly sunken	Deeply sunken
Tears	Present	Decreased	Absent
Mouth and tongue	Moist	Dry	Parched
Skin fold	Instant recoil	Recoil in <2 s	Recoil in >2 s
Capillary refill	Normal	Prolonged	Prolonged; minimal
Extremities	Warm	Cool	Cold; mottled; cyanotic
Urine output	Normal to decreased	Decreased	Minimal

TABLE 3: **Recommended therapy based on degree of dehydration**

Degree of dehydration	Rehydration therapy	Replacement of losses	Nutrition
Minimal or no dehydration	Not applicable	<10 kg body weight: 60–120 mL ORS for each diarrheal stool or vomiting episode; >10 kg body weight: 120–240 mL ORS for each diarrheal stool or vomiting episode	Continue breast-feeding, or resume age-appropriate normal diet after initial hydration, including adequate caloric intake for maintenance
Mild-to-moderate dehydration	ORS, 50–100 mL/kg body weight over 3–4 h	Same	Same
Severe dehydration	Lactated Ringer solution or normal saline in 20 mL/kg body weight intravenous amounts until perfusion and mental status improve; then administer 100 mL/kg body weight ORS over 4 h or 5% dextrose ½ normal saline intravenously at twice maintenance fluid rates	Same; if unable to drink, administer through nasogastric tube or administer 5% dextrose ¼ normal saline with 20 mEq/L potassium chloride intravenously	

ORS, oral rehydration solution.

continuing losses from stool and emesis is accomplished by giving 10 mL/kg for each stool; also, emesis volume is estimated and replaced. Reevaluation of hydration and replacement of losses should occur at least every 2 hours.
o Feeding: With correction of dehydration, appropriate feeding should begin

CHAPTER 35: Acute Gastroenteritis

- Moderate dehydration (6–9%)
  - Oral rehydration therapy: Dehydration is connected by giving 100 mL/kg ORT plus replacement of continuing losses during a 4-hour period. Rapid restoration of the circulating volume helps correct acidosis and improves tissue perfusion, which aids the early refeeding process. At the end of each hour of rehydration, hydration should be assessed and continuing stool and emesis losses should be calculated with the total added to the amount remaining to be given. This task may be accomplished best in a supervised setting, such as an emergency department, urgent care facility on physician's office
  - Feeding: When rehydration is complete, feeding should be resumed
- Severe dehydration (≥10%)

  Severe dehydration causes shock or a near-shock-like condition.

  A bolus IV therapy with a solution such as normal saline or Ringer's lactate is the cornerstone of its therapy.

  As per conventional recommendation, IV fluid, 20 mL/kg of body weight should be given during a 1-hour period. However, in practice, larger quantities and much shorter periods of administration may be required.

  Electrolyte levels must be determined in children with severe dehydration. Frequent clinical re-evaluation is critical. If the patient does not respond to rapid bolus rehydration, the clinician should consider the possibility of an underlying disorder, including, but not limited to, septic shock, toxic shock syndrome, myocarditis, and myocardiopathy on pericarditis. When the patient's condition has stabilized and mental status is satisfactory, ORT may be instituted with the IV line kept in place until it is certain that IV therapy is no longer needed
- When organ perfusion is restored and the patient is able to take orally well begin oral rehydration therapy
- In hypernatremic dehydration, ORT is safer than intravenous rehydration. In hypernatremic dehydration, use "slow ORT", aiming to complete rehydration over 12 hours, and monitor serum sodium to avoid a rapid reduction
- To prevent primary dehydration or recurrence of dehydration, allow unrestricted fluids, and in high-risk cases, either (a) alternate normal drinks (for example, milk or water) with ORS, or (b) give normal drinks and 10 mL/kg ORS after each watery stool
- Early feeding of appropriate foods: Children who have diarrhea and are not dehydrated should continue to be fed age-appropriate diets. Children who require rehydration should be fed age-appropriate diets as soon as they have been rehydrated. When used with glucose-electrolyte ORT, early feeding can reduce stool output as much as cereal-based ORT can. If lactose intolerant, administer milk-free diet
- Drugs are generally not necessary: Antibiotic therapy is not needed in most cases of acute gastroenteritis and may induce a carrier status in case of *Salmonella* infection. Antibiotic treatment is effective mainly in shigellosis and in the early stage of *Campylobacter* infection
- Antidiarrheal agents: In the past, antidiarrheal drugs were often employed in the treatment of acute gastroenteritis, but with little evidence of benefit. Bismuth subsalicylate has antisecretory and bactericidal properties, and it may have some effect on the clinical symptoms. There is no evidence that other agents such as cholestyramine, kaolin, pectin, loperamide, and diphenoxylate have an effect. Nowadays, none of these drugs is considered to have a role in the treatment of gastroenteritis in children. On the contrary, their use may have adverse consequences.

Q. What is oral rehydration salt?

In 1975, WHO and the United Nations Children's Fund (UNICEF) agreed to promote a single ORS (WHO-ORS) containing (in mmol/L) sodium 90, potassium 20, chloride 80, base 30, and glucose 111 (2%) for use among diverse populations. This composition was selected to allow a single solution to be used for treatment of diarrhea caused by different infectious agents and associated with varying degrees of electrolyte loss. For example, *Rotavirus* diarrhea is associated with stool sodium losses of approximately 30–40 mEq/L; enterotoxigenic *E. coli* (ETEC) infection with losses of 50–60 mEq/L; and cholera infection with losses of more than 90–120 mEq/L.

Q. What is lower osmolarity oral rehydration salts?

Oral rehydration salts with proportionally reduced concentrations of sodium and glucose with 75 mEq/L sodium, 75 mmol/L glucose, and total osmolality of 245 mOsm/L is low osmolality ORS.

A reduced osmolarity ORS has been associated with less vomiting, less stool output, and a reduced need for unscheduled intravenous infusions when compared with standard ORS among infants and children with non-cholera diarrhea. In cholera infection, no clinical difference existed between subjects treated with the lower osmolarity solution and those treated with the standard solution, apart from certain increased incidence of asymptomatic hyponatremia.

Table 4 presents composition of different ORS.

Q. What is the role of antibiotics in diarrhea?

In the event of a known causative pathogen, community-acquired secretory diarrhea and for traveler's diarrhea, antimicrobials are the drugs of choice.
- Consider antimicrobial treatment for:
    - *Persistent Shigella, Salmonella, Campylobacter,* or parasitic infections
    - Infections in the aged, immunocompromised patients, and patients with impaired resistance, sepsis, or with prostheses
    - Moderate/severe traveller's diarrhea or diarrhea with fever and/or with bloody stools
    - Quinolones (cotrimoxazole second choice)
- Nitazoxanide is an antiprotozoal and may be appropriate for *Cryptosporidium* and other infections, including some bacteria
- Rifaximin is a broad-spectrum, nonabsorbed antimicrobial agent that may be useful

An antimicrobial is recommended for patients older than 2 years with suspected cholera and severe dehydration.
- Alternative antimicrobials for treating cholera in children are cotrimoxazole (5 mg/kg trimethoprim + 25 mg/kg sulfamethoxazole, bid for 3 days), furazolidone (1.25 mg/kg, qid for 3 days), and norfloxacin.

The actual selection of an antimicrobial depends on the known resistance/sensitivity pattern of *V. cholerae* in the region, which requires the availability of a well-established and consistent surveillance system.

Q. What are the steps necessary to prevent acute gastroenteritis?

Water, sanitation, and hygiene
- Safe water
- Sanitation: Houseflies can transfer bacterial pathogens
- Hygiene: Hand washing

Safe Food
- Cooking eliminates most pathogens from foods
- Exclusive breastfeeding for infants
- Weaning foods are vehicles of enteric infection

TABLE 4: Composition of different oral rehydration solutions

Oral rehydration solutions	Glucose (g/L)	Sodium (mmol/L)	Potassium (mmol/L)	Chloride (mmol/L)	Base (mmol/L)	Osmolality
WHO ORS 2002 (reduced osmolality)	13.5	75	20	65	30	245
WHO 1975	20	90	20	80	30	311

WHO, World Health Organization; ORS, oral rehydration salts.

Micronutrient supplementation: The effectiveness of this depends on the child's overall immunologic and nutritional state; further research is needed.

Vaccines

- *Salmonella typhi:* Two typhoid vaccines currently are approved for clinical use
- *Shigella* organisms: Three vaccines have been shown to be immunogenic and protective in field trials. Parenteral vaccines may be useful for travellers and the military, but are impractical for use in developing countries. More promising is a single-dose live-attenuated vaccine currently under development in several laboratories
- *V. cholerae*: Oral cholera vaccines are recommended only in complex emergencies such as epidemics. Their use in endemic areas remains controversial. In traveller's diarrhea, oral cholera vaccine is only recommended for those working in refugee or relief camps, since the risk of cholera for the usual traveller is very low
- Enterotoxigenic *E. coli* vaccines: The most advanced ETEC vaccine candidate consists of a killed whole cell formulation plus recombinant cholera toxin B subunit. No vaccines are currently available for protection against Shiga toxin–producing *E. coli* infection
- *Rotavirus*: Currently, two vaccines have been approved—a live oral vaccine (RotaTeq™) made by Merck for use in children and GSK's Rotarix™
- Measles immunization can substantially reduce the incidence and severity of diarrheal diseases. Every infant should be immunized against measles at the recommended age.

Q. What is the role of probiotics and prebiotics in diarrhea?

Probiotics have been defined as live microorganisms in fermented foods that promote optimal health by establishing an improved balance in intestinal microflora. These products have included various species of lactobacilli or bifidobacteria or the nonpathogenic yeast *Saccharomyces boulardii*. The mechanism of action might include competition with pathogenic bacteria for receptor sites or intraluminal nutrients, production of antibiotic substances, and enhancement of host immune defenses. Limited studies have been done with sample seize in this area. Following meta-analysis suggests a positive role of their use in antibiotic-associated diarrhea.

- Prebiotics are complex carbohydrates rather than organisms used to preferentially stimulate the growth of health-promoting intestinal flora
- Oligosaccharides contained in human milk have been called the prototypic prebiotic because they foster growth of lactobacilli and bifidobacteria in the colon of breastfed neonates
- Breast milk oligosaccharides are associated with a lowered incidence of acute diarrhea. Specific recommendations regarding their use need further well-controlled human trials.

Q. What should be the dos and don'ts in the therapy of acute diarrhea?

Dos and Don'ts in the therapy of acute diarrhea have been described in box 1.

Q. Finally, what is the recommended algorithmic approach to management of diarrheal dehydration and feeding in acute diarrhea/gastroenteritis?

Flowcharts 1 and 2 provide the requisite algorithmic approaches.

CONCLUSION

Acute gastroenteritis, an extremely common problem in childhood, particularly in the first 3 years of life, is associated with a substantial number of hospitalizations and high costs. *Rotavirus* is responsible for the most severe cases. Dehydration is the main clinical feature of acute gastroenteritis. Generally, it reflects disease severity. Weight loss, prolonged capillary refill time, skin turgor, and abnormal respiratory pattern are the best individual

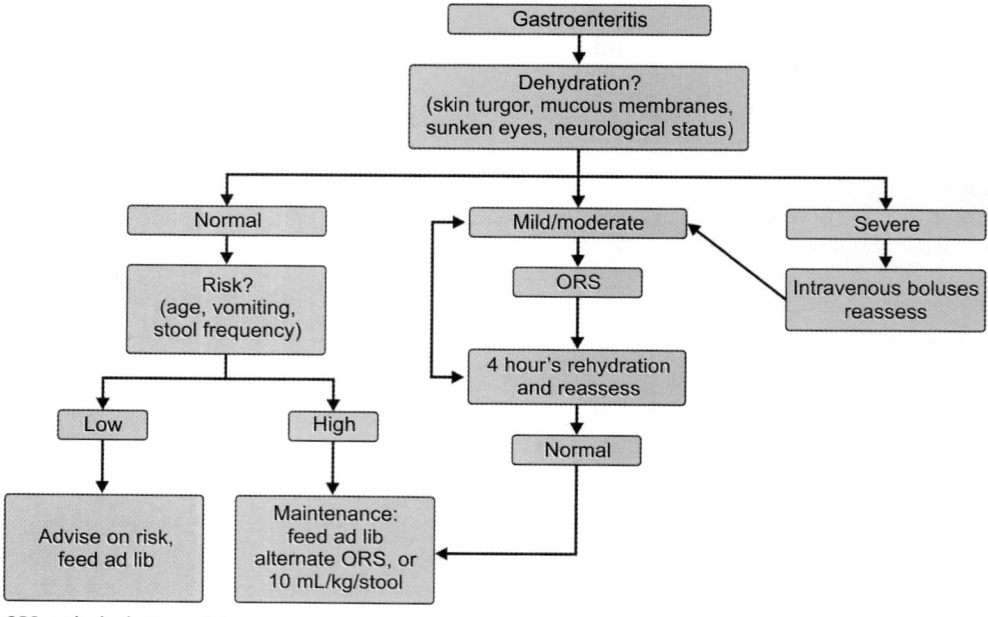

ORS, oral rehydration solution.
Flowchart 1: Algorithmic approach to management of dehydration in gastroenteritis

BOX 1: Dos and don'ts in the therapy of acute diarrhea
- Repeated cardiopulmonary cerebral assessment should be carried out after each fluid order
- Child should be shifted to oral rehydration as soon as they are able to drink
- Do not withhold fluids in children with shock in view of elevated urea/creatinine
- Contraindications to oral rehydration are if there are any signs of shock, ileus or intestinal obstruction, comatose/unconscious patients, and patients with persistent vomiting
- Evidence of warm shock such widening of pulse pressure, tachycardia and tachypnea fulfilling systemic inflammatory response syndrome (SIRS) criteria is suggestive gastrointestinal (GI) sepsis and warrants antibiotic therapy
- Diarrhea can be among the initial signs of nongastrointestinal tract illnesses, including meningitis, bacterial sepsis, and pneumonia, otitis media and urinary tract infection. Vomiting alone can be the first symptom of metabolic disorders, congestive heart failure, toxic agent ingestion, or trauma. To rule out other serious illnesses, a detailed history and physical examination should be performed as part of the evaluation of all children with acute gastroenteritis.

clinical signs of dehydration. Microbiological investigations are generally not needed. Rehydration is the key treatment and should be applied as soon as possible. Reduced osmolality oral rehydration solution should be used,

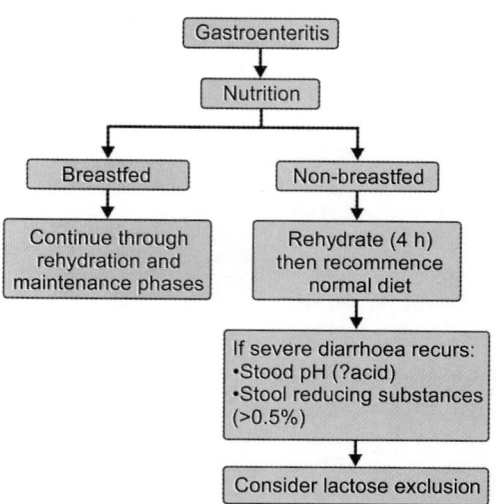

Flowchart 2: Algorithmic approach to management of feeding in gastroenteritis

and it should be offered ad libitum. Regular feeding should not be interrupted and should be carried on following initial rehydration. As a rule, in most cases, regular milk (lactose-containing) formulas are appropriate.

> **KEY LEARNING POINTS**
>
> ☞ Gastroenteritis in children is usually of viral etiology
> ☞ Most children with acute gastroenteritis develop varying grades of dehydration which, if left untreated or inappropriately treated, is responsible for morbidity and mortality
> ☞ Appropriate treatment of acute gastroenteritis include the following:
>   – Use of oral rehydration for dehydration
>   – Hypotonic oral rehydration solution (ORS)
>   – Fast oral rehydration over 3–4 hours
>   – Rapid realimentation with normal feeding
>   – Use of special formula is unjustified
>   – Use of diluted formula is unjustified
>   – Continuation of breastfeeding at all time
>   – Supplement with ORS for ongoing losses

SUGGESTED READINGS

1. Atherly-John YC, Cunningham SJ, Crain EF. A randomized trial of oral vs intravenous rehydration in a pediatric emergency department. *Arch Pediatr Adolesc Med.* 2002;156:1240-1243.
2. Awasthi S, INCLEN Childnet Zinc Effectiveness for Diarrhea (IC-ZED) Group. Zinc supplementation in acute diarrhea is acceptable, does not interfere with oral rehydration, and reduces the use of other medications: a randomized trial in five countries. *J Pediatr Gastroenterol Nutr.* 2006;42:300-305.
3. Centers for Disease Control and Prevention (CDC). Managing acute gastroenteritis among children: Oral rehydration, maintenance, and nutritional therapy. *MMWR.* 2003;52:1-16.
4. CHOICE study group. Multicenter, randomized, double-blind clinical trial to evaluate the efficacy and safety of a reduced osmolarity oral rehydration salts solution in children with acute watery diarrhea. *Pediatrics.* 2001;107:613-618.
5. Meyers A. Fluid and electrolyte therapy for children. *Curr Opin Pediatr.* 1994;6:303-309.
6. Patwari A, Gupte S, Anderson RA. Pediatric gastroenterology. In: Gupte S (Ed). *The Short Textbook of Pediatrics*, 12th edn. New Delhi: Jaypee Brothers Medical Publishers; 2016:549-583.

Acute Dysentery

CHAPTER 36

BP Karunakara, SN Vishwas

INTRODUCTION

Dysentery is an infectious gastrointestinal disorder, characterized by inflammation of the intestines, mainly colon, associated with fever, dehydration, mucopurulent and bloody diarrhea, and tenesmus. The World Health Organization defines dysentery as an episode of diarrhea in which there is blood in loose and watery stool. Dysentery spreads mainly through fecal-oral route of transmission (through contaminated food and water and poor sanitation). It is a major cause of childhood morbidity and mortality, especially in developing countries in Africa, Asia, Central and Latin America. Shigellosis is an important cause of diarrheal deaths. Shigellosis, also known as acute bacillary dysentery, is characterized by passage of loose stools mixed with blood and mucus, accompanied by fever, tenesmus, and abdominal pain. It has been reported that not less than 140 million cases of shigellosis occur worldwide with 600,000 deaths annually. About 60% of deaths are seen in children under 5 years of age.

CASE 1

A previously healthy 10-year-old boy was brought to the pediatric outpatient department with history of fever for 2 days with loose stools since 1 day (10–12 episodes). Last 2 episodes of loose stools were bloody. He had vomiting thrice. Oral intake had considerably reduced. Preceding history of eating food (and drinking water) in roadside shop was present.

On examination, temperature 101°F, pulse rate 120 beats/min, respiratory rate 24 breaths/min, and blood pressure (BP) 80/60 mmHg. Peripheries were cold. Clot formation time was prolonged. Lips and tongue (mucus membranes) were dry. Per abdomen—diffuse tenderness was present. No mass palpable.

Investigations: Neutrophilic leukocytosis. Stool routine showing leukocytes (pus cells) with guaiac test positive (for blood).

Stool culture: *Shigella* is sensitive to ceftriaxone.

Diagnosis: Dysentery with severe dehydration.

Treatment: Child was administered intravenous fluid bolus, 20 mL/kg. Following 2 boluses, BP was 96/60 mmHg, and child was started on severe dehydration correction. Ceftriaxone was also started.

Pending stool culture report, ceftriaxone was started. Child was better by 6 hours of admission, was changed to maintenance intravenous fluids. By day 2 of admission, child was better with decrease in loose stools, was off intravenous fluids, and was taking orally well. Stool culture was positive for *Shigella* and was sensitive to ceftriaxone; antibiotics were given for 7 days, and then the child was discharged.

CASE REVIEW IN A NUTSHELL

The clinical profile of this 10-year-old boy was in keeping with the diagnosis of acute dysentery. The culture report showing *Shigella* lent support to the clinical impression. Correction of severe dehydration along with ceftriaxone proved effective in controlling dysentery and accompanying dehydration.

INTERACTIVE TOPIC REVIEW

Q. What is dysentery?

Dysentery is manifested by passing of loose stools mixed with blood and mucus, accompanied by fever, abdominal cramps, and tenesmus (a symptom characterized by incomplete sense of evacuation with rectal pain). Most common causative organism is *Shigella*, so commonly known as acute bacillary dysentery.

Q. What are the causative organisms?

An acute bacillary dysentery is most commonly caused by *Shigella* species, enteroinvasive *Escherichia coli*, *Campylobacter*, *Salmonella* (bacteria), and *Entamoeba histolytica*; rarely, giardiasis, balantidiasis, and cryptosporidiosis in immunocompromised children.

Q. How does *Shigella* cause dysentery?

Shigella is divided into four serotypes: (i) *S. sonnei*, (ii) *S. boydii*, (iii) *S. dysenteriae*, and (iv) *S. flexneri*. *S. dysenteriae* type I and *S. flexneri* are common in developing countries. *Shigella* is facultative, nonmotile, Gram-negative bacilli. They invade intestinal epithelial cells. Virulence factors are smooth polysaccharide cell wall antigen and a toxin (shiga toxin) which is both cytotoxic and neurotoxic that causes watery diarrhea. *Shigella* invades and multiplies within the colonic epithelial cells causing cell death and mucosal ulcer but rarely invades bloodstream. Histological findings include cellular infiltration with mixed round cells, neutrophilic in majority, and disorganization of crypts with branching and dilatation. The inflammatory process extends to muscularis mucosa and submucosa with resultant edema.

Q. What are the clinical features of dysentery?

Children may present with fever, loose stools (with blood), severe abdominal pain, dehydration, and rectal pain. Some children can present with fever, headache, vomiting, and convulsions suggestive of *Shigella* encephalopathy.

Q. What are the complications of dysentery?

Shigella may be associated with large number of life-threatening complications (particularly caused due to *S. dysenteriae* type 1). Children can have rectal prolapse (Fig. 1), arthritis, conjunctivitis, arthralgia, intestinal perforation, hemorrhage, toxic megacolon, irritable bowel syndrome, and protein losing enteropathy. Hemolytic uremic syndrome and Guillain-Barré syndrome may be some of the fatal complications. Protein energy malnutrition can be one of the long-term complications.

Q. How is it diagnosed and what is the role of investigations?

Diagnosis is made clinically by typical features of bacillary dysentery with blood and mucus in stool although some cases may present with mild-to-moderate diarrhea. Dehydration is not a conspicuous feature. History is suggestive of eating food or drinking water outside.

Complete blood picture may show leukocytosis. Fecal smear stained in iodine may show leukocytes (>10 per high power field). Confirmation is made by stool culture. Fresh stool samples before initiation of therapy are

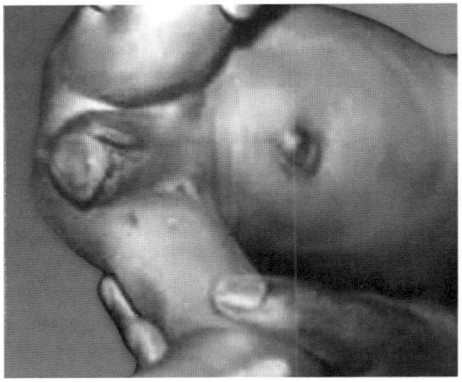

Figure 1: Rectal prolapse in a child with dysentery *(For color version, see Plate 4)*

preferred because the chances of recovering the organisms are high. Samples that cannot be cultured immediately should be kept in buffered glycerol saline transport medium.

Polymerase chain reaction (PCR) is used to detect bacteria, especially an immunocapture PCR, which employs amplification to detect bacteria captured by specific antibodies coupled either beads or polystyrene plates is the method of choice.

Direct stool PCR is preferred to deoxyribonucleic acid probe hybridization technique in which strains should be cultured several times.

Q. How do you manage a child with dysentery?

Appropriate rehydration (oral or intravenous) therapy is an integral component of the therapy and antibiotic therapy. Fluid management based on dehydration status (oral rehydration solution supplementation can be done). The decision to start antimicrobial therapy should always be taken after adequate hydration and individual evaluation of various factors, including the likelihood of extraintestinal dissemination of the infection and its severity. The empirical choice of the antimicrobial agent must be made individually for each case, considering the safety and the cost of drugs, the pathogens most likely to be infecting the patient and up-to-date knowledge of the susceptibility pattern of locally circulating strains. Empirically, patient can be started on ceftriaxone (100 mg/kg/day), cefixime (10 mg/kg/day), or ciprofloxacin (10–20 mg/kg/day). Laboratory confirmation is necessary, especially for antimicrobial sensitivity pattern. Zinc supplementation is helpful in reducing diarrheal episodes (duration of 14 days). Use of appropriate antibiotic hastens recovery, shortens duration of stay, and excretion of pathogen in stool and possibly prevents complications. Antibiotics are usually given for 5–7 days.

Q. How do you prevent acute dysentery?

Main route of transmission is through water, food, and person-to-person contact. The prevention and control strategy is essentially provision of safe water supply, adequate sanitation facilities, maintenance of good personal hygiene, and food safety. Handwashing with plenty of soap and water is the single effective preventive strategy against dysentery.

CONCLUSION

Acute dysentery is an important public health problem with high morbidity and mortality mainly among children in developing countries where overcrowding and poor personal hygiene are rampant. *S. dysenteriae* species are notorious for producing not only large scale epidemics, but also pandemics with several serious complications including hemolytic uremic syndrome. Mainstay of treatment is appropriate use of antibiotics. Preventive long time measures, like improved sanitation and personal hygiene, should be emphasized and reached to masses through health education.

KEY LEARNING POINTS

- Acute dysentery is caused most commonly by bacteria (*Shigella*) and protozoa
- It spreads through food and water associated with poor sanitation
- *S. dysenteriae* species are notorious for producing not only large scale epidemics, but also pandemics with several serious complications including hemolytic uremic syndrome
- Diagnosis is essentially clinical
- Mainstay of treatment is appropriate use of antibiotics
- Preventive long time measures, like improved sanitation and personal hygiene, should be emphasized and reached to masses through health education.

SUGGESTED READINGS

1. Sur D, Ramamurthy T, Deen J, Bhattacharya SK. Shigellosis: challenges and management issues. *Indian J Med Res*. 2004;120:454-462.
2. Kweon MN. Shigellosis: the current status of vaccine development. *Curr Opin Infect Dis*. 2008;21:313-318.
3. Sangeetha AV, Parija SC, Mandal I, Krishnamurthy S. Clinical and microbiological profiles of shigellosis in children. *J Health Popul Nutr*. 2014;32:580-586.

CHAPTER 37

Variceal Bleed

Rajeev Khanna

INTRODUCTION

Variceal hemorrhage secondary to portal hypertension (PHT) is an important cause of gastrointestinal bleeding (GIB) in children. Prevalence rate varies due to geographical locale, socioeconomic status, and referral center. Around one-third of cases of GIB in children from the developed world and 45–90% from the developing world are due to variceal hemorrhage. The difference in prevalence rates are largely due to the fact that extrahepatic venous obstruction is largely a disease of poor socioeconomic status and predominantly presents with GIB. On the other hand, variceal bleed in a child with cirrhosis is usually a late event.

In order to understand various causes of PHT, one should remember the anatomy of hepatic vasculature. Portal vein is formed by the union of superior mesenteric and splenic veins, and provides 80% of the vascular supply of the liver. Remaining 20% is supplied by the hepatic artery. The smallest branches of portal venules, hepatic arterioles, and bile ductules are located in the portal tracts (triads) of hepatic acini. Blood flows from the portal tracts towards central vein (smallest tributary of hepatic venules) via sinusoids which are lined by endothelial cells and are spaced in between adjoining hepatocytes. Numerous hepatic venules join together to form three hepatic veins which open into inferior vena cava (Fig. 1).

Portal hypertension is theoretically defined as a pressure difference of more than 5 mmHg between portal vein and inferior vena cava. The various causes of PHT can be classified on the basis of anatomical level of obstruction—prehepatic, hepatic, and posthepatic, the hepatic causes are further classified into presinusoidal, sinusoidal, and postsinusoidal. An objective measurement of PHT can be done by measuring hepatic venous pressure gradient (HVPG), which is the difference between wedge hepatic venous pressure and free hepatic venous pressure. However, in prehepatic as well as presinusoidal causes, the HVPG is normal despite PHT being very prominent clinically. In fact, the spleen size and severity of PHT decreases if we move from portal vein towards hepatic veins (Fig. 2).

CASE 1

A 5-year-old boy presented with 1 day history of passage of black liquid sticky stools associated with abdominal distention and irritability. He had a background of biliary atresia and was operated with Kasai portoenterostomy at 56 days of life following which he cleared his jaundice with passage of pigmented stools. He subsequently had three episodes of cholangitis which were treated with intravenous antibiotics. On examination, he was tachycardic, tachypneic, and irritable. He had a low volume pulse with cold clammy extremities. He was pale, mildly icteric with palmar erythema, and grade three clubbing. He had firm, irregular, and enlarged liver with splenomegaly and moderate ascites. Central nervous system examination revealed evidence of grade 2 encephalopathy.

CASE 2

An 8-year-old boy presented with 2 bouts of massive hematemesis followed by passage of black liquid tarry stools for 2 days. He had previous history of two such episodes in the past when he was managed with intravenous fluids and blood transfusion, and was found to have splenomegaly. He was born premature and had a history of necrotizing enterocolitis and umbilical vein catheterization. There was no history of jaundice, abdominal distention, itching, altered sensorium, or irritability. On examination, he was tachycardic with evidence of postural hypotension. He had pallor with moderate splenomegaly (6 cm below costal margin). There were no other stigmata of chronic liver disease. His growth parameters revealed short stature (height <2 standard deviations).

CASE REVIEW IN A NUTSHELL

Case 1 apparently is a known cirrhotic with features of chronic liver disease and PHT. Acute variceal bleed has precipitated an episode of decompensation in this child in the form of ascites and hepatic encephalopathy. On the other hand, Case 2 is a child who apparently is a noncirrhotic and presented with a third episode of well-tolerated bleed.

INTERACTIVE TOPIC REVIEW

Q. When should we suspect variceal hemorrhage in a child presenting with gastrointestinal bleeding?

Massive hematemesis followed by melena in a child with splenomegaly with or without stigmata of chronic liver disease indicate bleeding from esophageal or gastric varices. Gastric variceal bleed is rare in children, but if present, is usually torrential and life-threatening. Laboratory pointers of varices as a cause of GIB are evidence of hypersplenism (presence of any 2 out of 3: hemoglobin <10 g/dL, white blood cells <4,000/mm^3, platelets <100,000/mm^3) and aspartate amino-transferase to platelet ratio index (<0.5) calculated as aspartate aminotransferase (in IU/L) divided by platelets (10^9/L).

Q. What are the important differentials we should consider in a child?

Nonvariceal causes of massive GIB in children include vascular malformation of gastrointestinal tract and ulcer perforating into an artery. Nasal and oropharyngeal causes should be excluded by proper history and examination. Classically, GIB is classified as upper or lower on the basis of location of the bleeding, either proximal or distal to the ligament of Treitz. It has now been reclassified into three categories: (i) upper, (ii) mid, and (iii) lower GIBs, defined as bleeding above the ampulla of Vater, from the ampulla of Vater to the terminal ileum, and distal to terminal ileum, respectively; the important causes in childhood have been summarized in table 1.

Q. How can we differentiate noncirrhotic from cirrhotic causes of portal hypertension and why is it important?

Table 2 lists important causes of PHT in children. One has to take proper history and look for stigmata of chronic liver disease in every child with suspected PHT (Box 1). It is important to differentiate cirrhotic versus noncirrhotic causes of PHT in order to determine prognosis and future management. Variceal bleeding in a cirrhotic child is usually an ominous sign, indicates decompensation, and thus guides in listing for liver transplantation. Variceal bleed initiates numerous alterations in cirrhotics—increased protein load to intestine, hyperammonemia, hepatic encephalopathy, bacterial translocation, spontaneous bacterial peritonitis, sepsis, hemodynamic instability, acute kidney injury, hepatorenal syndrome,

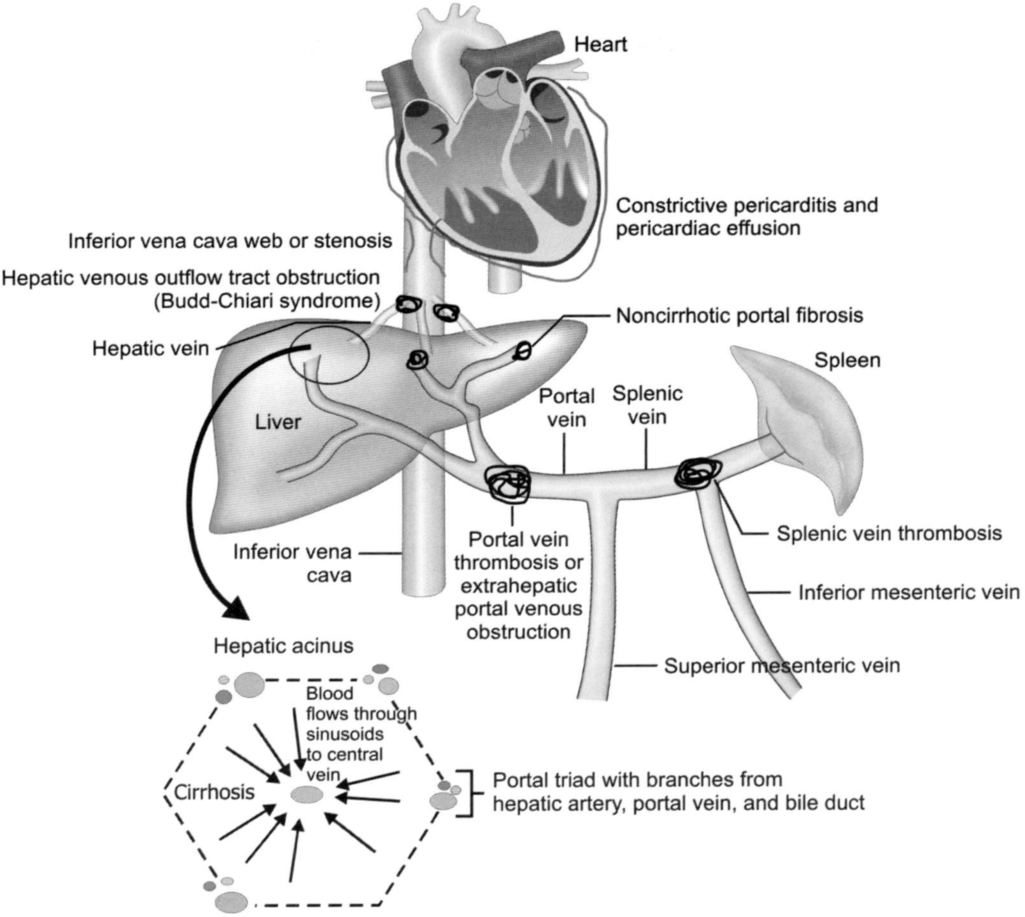

CHAPTER 37: Variceal Bleed | 253

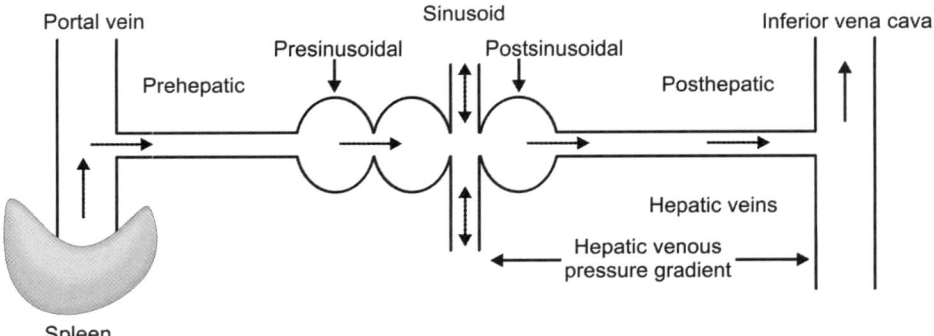

Figure 1: Anatomy of portal circulation and sites of blockage in various causes of portal hypertension marked with alphabets in blue

Figure 2: Diagramtic representation of portal vein circulation into the liver. Hepatic venous pressure gradient is indicated by the difference in the pressure gradient between the hepatic sinusoids and inferior vena cava

TABLE 1: Common causes of gastrointestinal bleeding in children depending on the location

	Site of bleed	Causes	Approach
Upper gastrointestinal bleeding	Proximal to ampulla of Vater	• Stress gastritis • Peptic ulcer • Variceal hemorrhage • Vascular malformation • Mallory-Weiss tear • Caustic injury	• Upper gastrointestinal endoscopy
Mid gastrointestinal bleeding	From ampulla of Vater to ileocecal junction	• Meckel's diverticulum • Vascular malformation • Crohn's disease • Nonsteroidal anti-inflammatory drugs induced ulcers • Small intestinal duplication • Small intestinal tumors • Hemobilia	• Meckel's scan • Small bowel enteroscopy • Capsule endoscopy • Computed tomography or magnetic resonance enterography • Angiography
Lower gastrointestinal bleeding	Distal to ileocecal junction	• Rectal polyp • Anal fissure • Colitis—infectious, inflammatory bowel disease • Milk protein allergy (allergic proctocolitis) • Hemorrhoids and rectal varices • Rectal prolapse • Solitary rectal ulcer	• Colonoscopy • Sigmoidoscopy

TABLE 2: Causes of portal hypertension in children on the basis of site of anatomic block

Prehepatic	Presinusoidal	Sinusoidal	Postsinusoidal	Posthepatic
• Portal vein thrombosis (extrahepatic portal venous obstruction) • Splenic vein thrombosis • Splanchnic arteriovenous fistula • Storage disorders (Gaucher's disease)	• Noncirrhotic portal fibrosis • Congenital hepatic fibrosis • Nodular regenerative hyperplasia • Schistosomiasis • Sarcoidosis	• Cirrhosis • Biliary atresia • Progressive familial intrahepatic cholestasis • Wilson's disease • Autoimmune hepatitis • Sclerosing cholangitis	• Veno-occlusive disease (Irradiation, drugs, toxins)	• Budd-Chiari syndrome • Congestive heart failure • Constrictive pericarditis • Tricuspid regurgitation

and disseminated intravascular coagulation. These changes are, however, not seen in noncirrhotics. As we can see, case 1 suffered some of these complications in view of cirrhotic background, whereas case 2 apparently had extrahepatic portal venous obstruction (EHPVO) and remained relatively well, except for hemodynamic instability.

Q. What should be our approach in managing a child with acute variceal bleed?

An approach to management of a child with acute variceal bleed is mentioned in flowchart 1. Child should be immediately assessed for hemodynamic and oxygenation status. Fluid

BOX 1: Clinical, laboratory, and imaging pointers towards etiology in a child with portal hypertension

- History
  - Decompensation-hepatic encephalopathy or ascites (cirrhosis)
  - History of umbilical vein catheterization, umbilical sepsis, necrotizing enterocolitis, recurrent diarrhea in infancy (EHPVO)
  - Family history of prothrombotic events (Budd-Chiari syndrome or EHPVO)
  - Ongoing liver disease (Biliary atresia or PFIC)
  - Recurrent jaundice (autoimmune hepatitis)
  - Cola-colored urine (Wilson's disease)
  - Itching (cholestatic liver disease—sclerosing cholangitis, PFIC)
  - Recurrent cholangitis (congenital hepatic fibrosis, sclerosing cholangitis)
- Examination
  - Firm, sharp, enlarged (cholestatic) or shrunken (cirrhotic) liver
  - Massive splenomegaly (>8 cm below costal margin) (EHPVO, NCPF)
  - Peripheral stigmata-palmar erythema, spider nevi, paper-dollar sign, facial telangiectasia, scratch marks, clubbing, testicular atrophy, gynecomastia, skin bleeds (severe cholestasis or advance cirrhosis)
  - Eye signs: Cataract (galactosemia), Kayser-Fleischer ring (Wilson's disease), posterior embryotoxon (Alagille's syndrome), vertical gaze palsy (Niemann-Pick disease type C)
  - Abdominal veins and caput medusa (excludes prehepatic portal hypertension)
  - Back veins (Budd-Chiari syndrome with inferior vena cava block)
  - Ascites—puddle sign, shifting dullness, fluid thrill (cirrhosis)
  - Ascites disproportionate to liver dysfunction (Budd-Chiari syndrome)
  - Hepatic encephalopathy—behavioral abnormalities, personality changes, alteration of sleep rhythm, flapping tremors (asterixis), extensor plantars (cirrhosis)
  - Specific syndromic features (CHF)*
- Laboratory
  - Normal or near normal liver functions (EHPVO, NCPF)
  - Hypoalbuminemia, deranged international normalized ratio (cirrhosis)
  - Evidence of hemolysis (Coombs' test positive—autoimmune, Coombs' test negative—Wilson's disease)
- Imaging
  - Portal vein replaced by bunch of collaterals or cavernoma, perisplenic collaterals (EHPVO)
  - Evidence of portal biliopathy (gall-bladder or pericholedochal varices) (EHPVO, NCPF)
  - Dilated thickened portal vein with pruning of peripheral branches (withered tree appearance) (NCPF)
  - Hypoechoic or isoechoic nodules with echogenic rim on ultrasound; hyperintense on T1 on magnetic resonance imaging (nodular regenerative hyperplasia)
  - Cystic dilatations of the intrahepatic bile ducts with renal cysts (CHF with autosomal recessive polycystic kidney disease/autosomal dominant polycystic kidney disease)
  - Dilatation, beaded appearance and strictures of biliary system (sclerosing cholangitis)

CHF, congenital hepatic fibrosis; EHPVO, extrahepatic portal venous obstruction; NCPF, noncirrhotic portal fibrosis.

Note: *Certain features point towards specific syndromes associated with congenital hepatic fibrosis: Joubert syndrome (dysgenesis of cerebellar vermis, Dandy-Walker malformation), Meckel-Gruber syndrome (central nervous system and cardiac malformations, polydactyly), Bardet-Biedl syndrome (obesity, retinitis pigmentosa, hypogonadism), Jeune syndrome (asphyxiating thoracic skeletal dystrophy), congenital glycosylation disorder type 1b (protein losing enteropathy).

resuscitation should be initiated with crystalloids while waiting for packed red cell transfusion. Preferably, two large bore cannulas should be inserted to facilitate large volume infusions. Packed red cells should be transfused to maintain hemoglobin between 7 and 8 g/dL with a goal to maintain tissue perfusion. Particular attention should be given to persistent tachycardia as

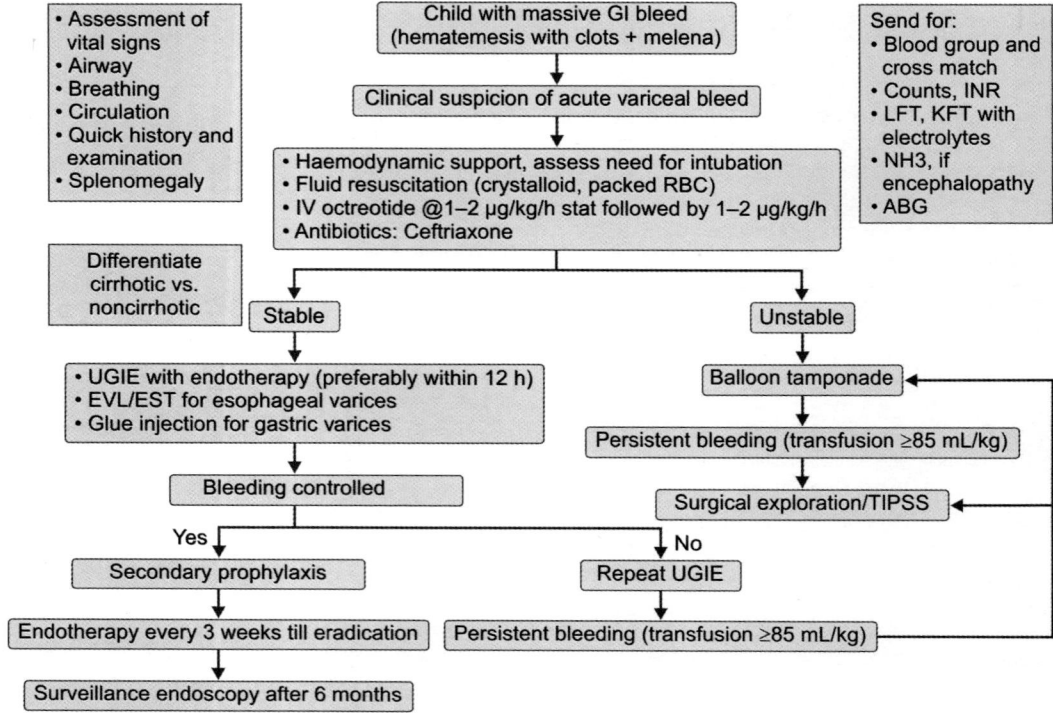

CLD, chronic liver disease; GI, gastrointestinal; RBC, red blood cells; EVL, endoscopic variceal ligation; EST, endoscopic sclerotherapy; UGIE, upper gastrointestinal endoscopy; TIPSS, transjugular intrahepatic portosystemic shunt; INR, international normalized ratio; LFT, liver function test; KFT, kidney function test; ABG, arterial blood gas.

Flowchart 1: Management approach to a child with acute variceal bleed

an indicator of compensated shock. Central venous oxygen saturation and venous lactate serve as useful markers of adequate tissue perfusion. Transfusion of fresh frozen plasma or cryoprecipitate may be guided on the basis of deranged coagulation and decision should be individualized. Overtransfusion with blood products can be hazardous and can lead to volume overload, brain edema, and chances of rebleed, although transfusion policy should take into consideration other factors like patient's age, ongoing bleeding, presence of lung disease, or cyanotic congenital heart disease. Splanchnic vasoconstrictors in the form of octreotide should be started—a stat dose of 1–2 µg/kg intravenously followed by maintenance infusion of 1–2 µg/kg/h to be continued for 3–5 days. Broad spectrum antibiotics, preferably third-generation cephalosporin, should be started in all cirrhotics. Child should be monitored continuously for hemodynamic status and once stabilized, he should be taken immediately for endoscopy, preferably within 12 hours of admission. If the child remains hemodynamically unstable with persistent bleeding, balloon tamponade should be attempted with a triple lumen Sengstaken-Blakemore tube or a four-lumen Minnesota tube. Gastric balloon should be inflated up to a volume (50, 150, and 250 mL) that depends upon the size of the tube and patient. Esophageal balloon needs to be inflated only in case of torrential bleed, and should be under manometric guidance (up to a maximum pressure of 30–45 mmHg). The tube is then fixed with a gentle traction around the patient's nose to compress the gastroesophageal junction, thus reducing blood flow to varices. Gastric (and esophageal) channel should be continuously aspirated. Balloons need to be deflated every 12 hours in order to prevent gastroesophageal

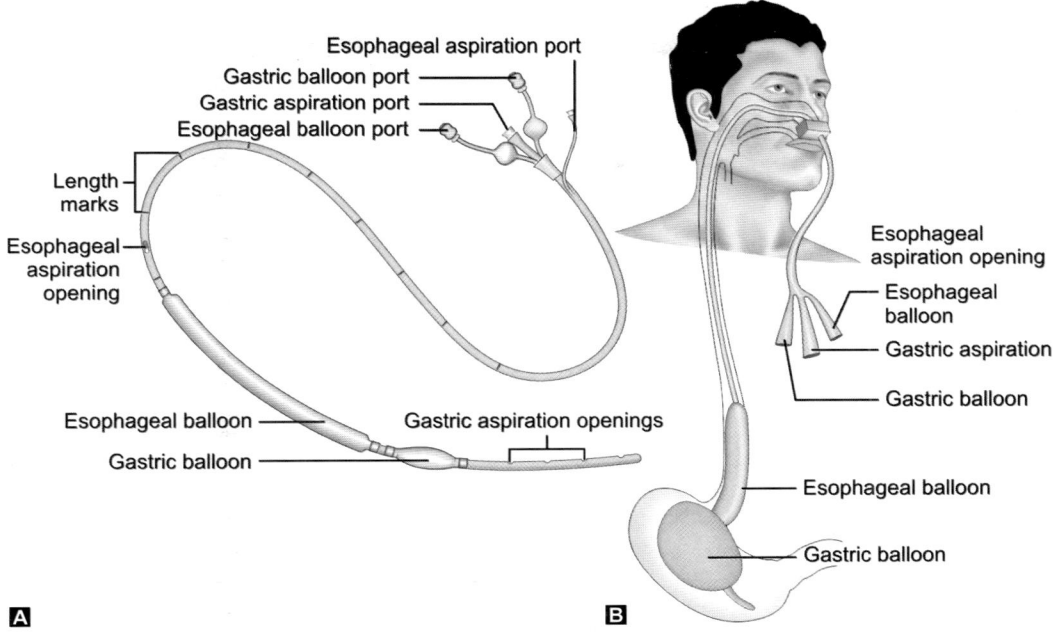

Figure 3: **A,** Four-lumen Minnesota tube (Sengstaken-Blakemore tube is a triple lumen tube and does not have esophageal aspiration channel). **B,** Sengstaken-Blakemore tube after insertion and inflation of gastric and esophageal balloons

necrosis or perforation (Fig. 3). Endoscopy should be attempted as soon as bleeding seems controlled.

Q. What are the endoscopic techniques used to control variceal bleeding?

Either endoscopic sclerotherapy (EST) or endoscopic variceal ligation (EVL) is used for control of bleeding due to ruptured esophageal varices. The goal of endoscopic management is to find the cause, localize the site of bleeding, and control acute variceal bleeding. There are numerous systems for grading of esophageal and gastric varices. For statistical comparison and to maintain uniformity in reporting, varices have now been reclassified as small (<5 mm in diameter) and large (>5 mm in diameter). Apart from size, presence of red color signs over the varices should be looked carefully (Box 2). In an adult with cirrhosis, presence of large esophageal varices (>5 mm), isolated gastric varix, red color signs, tense ascites, child status C (score ≥10), and HVPG more than 12 mmHg predict variceal bleed.

In EST, a sclerosant is injected either intravariceally or paravariceally through the endoscope beginning 2–3 cm above gastroesophageal junction. This causes thrombosis, fibrosis and obliteration of superficial varices as well as perforators. Various sclerosing agents used are absolute alcohol (99.5%), ethoxysclerol or polidocanol (1%, 3%), sodium tetradecyl sulfate (1%, 3%), sodium morrhuate (5%), and ethanolamine oleate (5%). In EVL, a multiband applicator is used and varices are sucked into the plastic cap followed by application of bands. Varices are banded sequentially in a spiral fashion starting just above the gastroesophageal junction. For gastric variceal obliteration, tissue adhesive or glue is used—N-butyl 2-cyanoacrylate or isobutyl 2-cyanoacrylate. As the glue hardens within 20 seconds of coming in contact with blood, the technique needs endoscopic expertise. Table 3 gives a comparison of EVL versus EST.

BOX 2: Endoscopic grading of varices
- Conn's classification for grading of esophageal varices:
    - Grade I: Small varices which disappear on air insufflation
    - Grade II: Nonconfluent varices which persist on air insufflation occupying <25% of esophageal lumen
    - Grade III: Large confluent varices occupying 25–50% of esophageal lumen
    - Grade IV: Very large varices occupying >50% of esophageal lumen
- Red color signs:
    - Red wale marks: Dilated venules arranged longitudinally on the varices
    - Cherry red spots: Small red spots about 2 mm in diameter on the surface of the varices
    - Hemocystic spots: Round dark red blood blisters about 4 mm of large in diameter
    - Diffuse redness: A diffuse red discoloration of the variceal surface
- Sarin's classification for gastric varices:
    - Gastroesophageal varices (GOV) (in continuity with esophageal varices)
        - GOV-1: Varices extending along the lesser curvature
        - GOV-2: Varices extending along greater curvature
    - Isolated gastric varices (IGV) (not in continuity with esophageal varices)
        - IGV-1: Isolated varices in fundus
        - IGV-2: Isolated varices other than in fundus

Q. What is the role of secondary prophylaxis for acute variceal bleed?

Secondary prophylaxis to prevent further episodes of variceal bleed is used in the form of endoscopic therapy (EVL or EST) or nonselective β-blockers (NSBB). Endotherapy is repeated at 3 weekly intervals till variceal eradication, and after that every 6 months and then yearly. Nonselective β-blockers, like propranolol or carvedilol, can also be used either alone or in combination with endotherapy to prevent further bleed. The NSBBs cause both β-1 and β-2 blockage, thus decreasing cardiac output and splanchnic vasodilatation, leading to decrease in PHT and incidence of variceal bleed. Propranolol is used in a dose of 0.5–2 mg/kg/day (maximum 8 mg/kg/day). Therapeutic efficacy is assessed by reduction in heart rate by 25% from baseline, thus theoretically bringing HVPG down to less than 12 mmHg. Major side effects are hypotension and exacerbation of asthma.

Q. What is the role of radiological interventions in control of acute variceal bleed?

In case of refractory variceal bleed uncontrollable by balloon tamponade and/or second endoscopy within 24 hours, consideration

TABLE 3: Comparison of endoscopic variceal ligation versus endoscopic sclerotherapy for endoscopic management of varices

	Endoscopic variceal ligation	Endoscopic sclerotherapy
Cost	Moderate*	High
Indications	Large varix, children >3 years	Any size of varices till eradication, feasible in small children
Complications	Less (4%)	High (25%)—ulcer, stricture
Rebleeding	Less (4%)	High (25%)
Variceal eradication	96%	92%
Sessions needed	3.9	6.1
Recurrence	More (17%)	Less (10%)
Effect on gastric varix	Increase	Increase isolated gastric varices-1, decrease gastro-esophageal varices-1
Effect on gastropathy	Increase	Increase

*One time cost of endoscopic variceal ligation is almost 2–3 times than endoscopic sclerotherapy, but considering the number of sessions needed to eradicate varices, the cost is less.

should be given to insertion of transjugular intrahepatic portosystemic shunt (TIPSS) which is an artificial nonsurgical portosystemic shunt. A catheter is introduced through the internal jugular vein into one of the hepatic veins and a needle tract is created through the hepatic parenchyma between the portal and hepatic veins. Stent is deployed over the guide wire after dilatation of tract. Reduction of portal pressures is demonstrated. In a cirrhotic patient, TIPSS serves as a bridge to liver transplantation, taking care of portal hypertensive complications. However, synthetic functions and encephalopathy may worsen. Another radiologic technique is balloon-occluded retrograde transvenous obliteration where a bleeding gastric varix is embolized through transjugular or transfemoral route via a naturally available gastrorenal shunt.

Q. Is there any role of surgery in control of acute variceal bleed?

With advent of expertise in endoscopic and radiological techniques, emergency surgery to control variceal bleed has become word of the past. Esophageal transection with devascularization and splenectomy surgeries were done in old days. Assessment of shunt surgery should be done after control of acute variceal bleed with computerized tomography or magnetic resonance imaging to identify shuntable veins. Indications for shunt surgery in the setting of EHPVO include complications related to PHT (recurrent bleeds, bleeding from gastric varices, severe portal hypertensive gastropathy or colopathy, hepatopulmonary syndrome, portal biliopathy), massive splenomegaly, symptomatic hypersplenism (recurrent infections or bleeds due to leukopenia or thrombocytopenia, respectively), poor growth, and poor quality of life. Cirrhotic children should be listed for liver transplantation on a priority basis.

CONCLUSION

Acute variceal bleed from PHT is an important cause of GIB in pediatric practice. Careful hemodynamic assessment, usage of crystalloids and packed red blood cells, splanchnic vasoconstrictors, timely endoscopy, and antibiotics form the core of therapy. Assessment to determine the underlying cause of PHT (cirrhotic ve. noncirrhotic) in order to determine prognosis, management, and future plan is crucial.

KEY LEARNING POINTS

- Massive gastrointestinal bleed in a child with splenomegaly point toward variceal hemorrhage
- Judicial packed red cells transfusion, splanchnic vasoconstrictors, and timely endotherapy are cornerstones of management
- Endoscopic sclerotherapy and band ligation are equally effective in controlling variceal bleeding with some differences in adverse effect profile
- Radiological interventions, like transjugular intrahepatic portosystemic shunt, is indicated in refractory bleeds
- Surgery in the form of shunts should be considered in noncirrhotic children with complications related to portal hypertension.

SUGGESTED READINGS

1. Yachha SK. Portal hypertension in children: an Indian perspective. *J Gastroenterol Hepatol.* 2002;17:S228-S231.
2. Khanna R, Sarin SK. Noncirrhotic portal hypertension-diagnosis and management. *J Hepatol.* 2014;60:421-441.
3. Krishna YR, Yachha SK, Srivastava A, Negi D, Lal R, Poddar U. Quality of life in children managed for extrahepatic portal venous obstruction. *J Pediatr Gastroenterol Nutr.* 2010;50:531-536.
4. Ling SC. Advances in the evaluation and management of children with portal hypertension. *Semin Liver Dis.* 2012;32: 288-297.
5. Morris JM, Oien KA, McMahon M, Forrest EH, Morris J, Stanley AJ, et al. Nodular regenerative hyperplasia of the liver: survival and associated features in a UK case series. *Eur J Gastroenterol Hepatol.* 2010;22:1001-1005.
6. Poddar U, Bhatnagar S, Yachha SK. Endoscopic band ligation followed by sclerotherapy: is it superior to sclerotherapy in children with extrahepatic portal venous obstruction? *J Gastroenterol Hepatol.* 2011;26:255-259.
7. Srinath A, Shneider BL. Congenital hepatic fibrosis and autosomal recessive polycystic kidney disease. *J Pediatr Gastrotenterol Nutr.* 2012;54:580-587.
8. Shneider BL, Bosch J, de Franchis R, Emre SH, Groszmann RJ, Ling SC, et al. Portal hypertension in children: expert pediatric opinion on the report of the Baveno v Consensus Workshop on Methodology of Diagnosis and Therapy in Portal Hypertension. *Pediatr Transplant.* 2012;16:426-437.

CHAPTER

38

Acute Hepatitis

Rajeev Khanna

INTRODUCTION

According to the Pediatric Acute Liver Failure Study Group, acute hepatitis, having a multifactorial etiology with preponderance of viral infections and drug induced injury, is characterized by acute onset of liver dysfunction secondary to an inflammatory process lasting for less than 6 months. It usually presents with a combination of features comprising jaundice, nausea, vomiting, and pain over right upper quadrant. In a large majority of children with acute febrile illness, the syndrome is diagnosed incidentally on routine blood tests. When it is complicated by coagulopathy or encephalopathy, the term "acute liver failure" is applied. It should be clinically differentiated from acute cholestasis, which may be caused by biliary obstruction or cholangitis, and presents with a typical triad of fever, pain abdomen, and jaundice (Charcot's triad), and is associated with predominant elevation of alkaline phosphatase (ALP) and γ-glutamyl transpeptidase (GGT).

Notwithstanding advances in understanding of pathophysiology and molecular biology of acute hepatitis in the recent decades, therapy remains symptomatic and supportive.

CASE 1

An 8-year-old girl presented to outpatient department with complains of anorexia and lethargy for 10 days, vomiting for 5 days, and yellowish discoloration of eyes and urine with pain right upper quadrant for 3 days. There was no history of fever, reduced urine output, pallor, cola-colored urine, irritability, or altered sensorium. On examination, she was icteric with tender hepatomegaly.

CASE 2

A 12-month-old boy presented to emergency with complains of high grade fever for 3 days, irritability and poor feeding for 1 day, and skin and mucosal bleeds for 1 day. There was no history of jaundice, reduced urine output, or pallor. He was the second child born to consanguineous parents and the older sibling was healthy. Family had a recent visit to countryside. On examination, he was pale, edematous, tachycardic, tachypneic with cervical lymphadenopathy, and numerous petechiae over skin. He had right-sided pleural effusion with massive hepatosplenomegaly and mild ascites. He was irritable and inconsolable with a Glasgow Coma Scale of 11.

CASE 3

A 12-year-old boy presented to emergency with high grade fever associated with chills and rigors for 4 days, yellowish discoloration of eyes for 1 day, and passage of cola-colored urine associated with pallor for 1 day. There was no history of reduced urine output, irritability, altered sensorium, seizures, etc. On examination, he was icteric and pale with tender hepatomegaly and mild splenomegaly.

CASE 4

An 11-year-old girl from a rural background presented with a 3-week history of low grade fever, anorexia and weight loss (10%), and 1-week history of central pain abdomen and vomiting. There was no history of jaundice, altered sensorium, irritability, skin or mucosal bleeds, reduced urine output, or chronic drug intake. Examination revealed mild pallor, mild hepatomegaly, splenomegaly, and generalized tenderness over abdomen. Blood tests revealed leukopenia with relative lymphocytosis, elevated transaminases (two times upper limit of normal), normal bilirubin and prothrombin time.

CASE REVIEW IN A NUTSHELL

Case 1 presented with a typical prodrome of anorexia, lethargy, and vomiting, followed by jaundice suggesting a diagnosis of acute viral hepatitis. The illness in young children below 5 years of age is mostly anicteric with nonspecific features and may go undiagnosed. Older children mostly present with jaundice. Subsidence of fever with appearance of jaundice is helpful to differentiate acute viral hepatitis from typhoid hepatitis. Most of the cases are afebrile. Biochemical tests reveal marked elevation of transaminases (in 1,000s) with high bilirubin. In the tropics, the most common cause of acute hepatitis in children is hepatitis A followed by E. In view of common feco-oral route of transmission, hepatitis A and E can sometimes be seen together or with typhoid fever. Acute liver failure develops in 0.05% of cases with hepatitis A and E. Diagnosis is confirmed by the demonstration of immunoglobulin (Ig) M antibodies against hepatitis A or E virus. A proportion of children with hepatitis A (<5%) develop a prolonged cholestatic pattern with rising bilirubin and ALP and normalization of transaminases. Hepatitis B also sometimes causes acute hepatitis in children, particularly in the setting of horizontal transmission (injections with contaminated syringes, blood transfusion, and close household contacts) in areas with moderate and high endemicity with a prevalence of 4–8% and more than 8%, respectively. Immunoglobulin M antibody against hepatitis B core antigen (IgM Anti-HBc) establishes the diagnosis, which is usually associated with presence of surface antigen (HBsAg), early antigen (HBeAg), and low viral load (hepatitis B virus-deoxyribonucleic acid). One should be vigilant to look for signs of acute liver failure in all such children (Box 1). Following exclusion of hepatotropic viruses as a cause of acute hepatitis, one should always look for nonhepatotropic viruses, particularly Epstein-Barr virus, *Cytomegalovirus* (CMV), herpes simplex virus, and parvovirus B19.

Case 2 is a young infant with fever, hepatosplenomegaly, lymphadenopathy, bleeds, and altered sensorium. Although, the illness in this case seems acute, but in view of massive hepatosplenomegaly, one should not miss chronic liver disease from early infancy. History of consanguinity is important to look for metabolic disorders and familial hemophagocytosis syndromes. Recent visit to countryside or endemic zones is important for various zoonotic infections. The illness in this boy fits into the definition of dengue hemorrhagic fever as per World Health Organization (WHO)

BOX 1: Parameters for early identification of acute liver failure in a child with acute hepatitis

Clinical features indicating acute liver failure
- Liver span: Shrinking liver size
- Pupil size: Dilatation or inequality of pupils
- Vital signs: Hypertension, bradycardia (Cushing's reflex) indicating raised intracranial pressure
- Sensorium and behavior: Irritability, combative behavior, alteration of sleep rhythm
- Reflexes: Exaggerated deep tendon reflexes, extensor plantars

1997 classification, and into severe dengue as per modified WHO 2009 classification. Liver involvement in dengue ranges from asymptomatic elevation of transaminases to acute liver failure. Hepatomegaly and elevated transaminases are present in up to 80 and 90% of children with dengue fever, respectively, whereas liver failure is rare. Transaminases are mostly in 100s but in up to 10% of cases, they may go more than 1,000 (severe dengue) indicating a component of ischemic hepatitis. Aspartate transaminase (AST) is more prolonged than alanine transaminase (ALT) in dengue because of ischemia or shock, and also by release from muscles (break-bone fever). Aspartate transaminase/alanine transaminase ratio of more than 1 helps in differentiating from acute viral hepatitis where ALT is more prolonged due to predominant hepatic insult. Dengue infection is also commonly associated with secondary hemophagocytosis which is likely in this case in view of hepatosplenomegaly, effusion, lymphadenopathy, and possible organ failure. Primary hemophagocytic lymphohistiocytosis (HLH) presents in infants and young children with a clear familial inheritance and with defects in lymphocyte granule mediated cytotoxic pathway. The immune abnormality in these children is often triggered by infections or vaccination. Secondary HLH generally develops in older children or adults secondary to specific infections, malignancies, or rheumatological disorders, the later one is termed as macrophage activation syndrome. Both primary and secondary HLH are associated with profound cytokine storm and have similar pathogenesis, diagnostic criteria, and treatment protocols.

Case 3 presented with an acute febrile illness associated with jaundice, pallor, and cola-colored urine. Persistent fever, pallor, splenomegaly, and cola-colored urine point toward diagnosis of complicated malaria (Black water fever). Malaria should always be considered in areas with high endemicity when a child presents with high grade fever and jaundice. Jaundice (bilirubin >3 mg/dL) is one of the biochemical characteristics classifying severe malaria and warrants prompt antiprotozoal therapy. Cola-colored urine indicates intravascular hemolysis and can also be seen in fulminant Wilson's disease and glucose-6-phosphate dehydrogenase (G6PD) deficiency. Exposure to oxidant drugs precipitating G6PD deficiency like primaquine, sulfonamides, methylene blue, naphthalene, and vitamin K should be looked up.

Case 4 presented with afebrile illness with systemic features with mildly deranged transaminases. Her clinical and laboratory findings fit into a systemic infection, liver being a bystander in this process. Differentials include typhoid fever, tuberculosis, leptospirosis, brucellosis, leishmaniasis, acquired immune deficiency syndrome (AIDS), and Gram-negative sepsis. Typhoid hepatitis presents in third week of untreated illness with hepatomegaly and pain abdomen—other complications like perforated ulcer, encephalopathy, myocarditis, and cholecystitis may be present. Ratio of ALT/lactate dehydrogenase is significantly low (<4.0) in typhoid fever and this helps in differentiating from acute viral hepatitis, where it is high (>5.0). Tuberculosis is another differential and should be considered in the setting of poor socioeconomic status or rural background. Liver involvement in tuberculosis can be due to miliary, granulomatous, or localized hepatic tuberculosis. Clinical features include fever, abdominal pain, and hepatomegaly. Elevated ALP and aminotransferases are seen in 83 and 42% of such patients, respectively. Hepatic tuberculosis can occur in the absence of pulmonary tuberculosis. Diagnosed can be achieved by liver biopsy which may show caseating granulomas with demonstration of acid-fast bacilli on smear or polymerase chain reaction. Jaundice is uncommon in both typhoid and tubercular hepatitis. Leptospirosis presents with a biphasic illness—anicteric illness, followed 2–3 weeks later by jaundice, hemorrhagic manifestations, and renal failure. Liver enzymes elevate 2–3 times of upper limit of normal. Brucellosis and leishmaniasis have a more protracted course with prolonged fever, hepatosplenomegaly, and lymphadenopathy, and should be considered depending on endemicity and following

CHAPTER 38: Acute Hepatitis

> **BOX 2: Causes of liver involvement in sepsis**
> **Increased bilirubin load**
> - Red blood cells lysed by bacterial products (e.g., exotoxin) or immunological mechanisms
>
> **Hepatic dysfunction**
> - Hepatocellular injury (hepatitis and/or necrosis)
> - Hepatic ischemia
> - Decreased bilirubin uptake; dysfunction of basolateral transport proteins like sodium taurocholate cotransporting polypeptide
> - Decreased transport of conjugated bilirubin; dysfunction of canalicular transport proteins (bile salt export pump and multidrug resistance associated protein-2)
>
> **Decreased bile flow**

exclusion of other common etiologies. Liver dysfunction may develop in the setting of human immunodeficiency virus infection and may present acutely. Various causes include concomitant infection with hepatitis B or C, AIDS cholangiopathy (caused by *Cryptosporidium*, CMV, Microsporidium, *Mycobacterium*), AIDS related acalculous cholecystitis (caused by CMV or cryptosporidium), opportunistic infections directly infecting liver (*Mycobacterium, Cryptococcus, Histoplasma, Coccidioides*), and antiretroviral drugs induced liver injury especially nevirapine, efavirenz, ritonavir, stavudine, zidovudine, and didanosine. Lastly, Gram-negative sepsis can cause liver dysfunction, various causes of which have been enumerated in box 2. Jaundice in the range of 2–10 mg/dL is often seen in children with sepsis. Cholestatic enzymes, ALP and GGT, are elevated 1–3 times, whereas transaminases are just modestly elevated. In event of septic shock, transaminases may jump up to thousands in the setting of ischemic hepatitis (shock liver).

INTERACTIVE TOPIC REVIEW

Q. What are the various causes of acute hepatitis?

There are various causes of acute hepatitis in the pediatric age group. Also, one should note that certain liver conditions, particularly metabolic or transport defects, may be present right from birth and may come into picture when such infants are specifically tested for their liver functions. Acute hepatitis should be clinically differentiated from acute cholestasis, which may be caused by biliary obstruction or cholangitis, and presents with a typical triad of fever, pain abdomen, and jaundice (Charcot's triad), and is associated with predominant elevation of ALP and GGT.

Q. What are the parameters for diagnosing acute liver failure?

The parameters for diagnosing acute liver failure have been described in box 3.

Q. What is the etiology of liver involvement in sepsis?

Etiology of liver involvement in sepsis has been described in box 2.

Q. When should we suspect Wilson's disease in the setting of acute hepatitis?

Wilson's disease is a disorder of copper metabolism associated with ATP7B mutation leading to disordered handling of intracellular copper within the hepatocytes, thus causing impaired incorporation of copper into ceruloplasmin and poor excretion through the bile canaliculi. Biochemically, the disease is characterized by low serum levels of ceruloplasmin (>20 mg/dL), elevated urinary

> **BOX 3: Definition of pediatric acute liver failure as defined by Pediatric Acute Liver Failure Study Group**
> **Children from 0 to 18 years of age with:**
> - No known evidence of chronic liver disease
> - Biochemical evidence of acute liver injury
> - Hepatic based coagulopathy defined as a prothrombin time (PT) more than 15 s or international normalized ratio (INR) more than 1.5 not corrected by vitamin K in the presence of clinical hepatic encephalopathy, or a PT more than 20 s or INR more than 2.0 regardless of the presence or absence of clinical hepatic encephalopathy

excretion of copper (24-h levels >40 µg), and high liver tissue copper (>250 µg/g of liver tissue). In the age group 5-10 years, over 80% affected children present with hepatic involvement and rest with neuropsychiatric symptoms; in the second decade, 50% present with hepatic and neuropsychiatric symptoms; and in adulthood, 25% present with hepatic whereas 75% with neuropsychiatric symptoms. Fulminant Wilson's disease presents acutely with coagulopathy, high transaminases (AST/ALT ratio >4 due to hemolysis), low ALP (due to high copper and low zinc, thus interfering with ALP activity), high bilirubin, and intravascular hemolysis. Mortality is high without liver transplantation.

Q. How does autoimmune hepatitis present and how can it be diagnosed?

Autoimmune hepatitis (AIH) is a chronic liver disease associated with presence of autoantibodies against liver antigens. Acute presentation is seen in 40% of cases, sometimes with ALF. It commonly presents in adolescent girls but the disorder may be seen in young children including infants. There may be family history of other autoimmune conditions. History of fever and features of autoimmune disorders (skin rashes, arthralgia/arthritis, thyroiditis, autoimmune anemia, inflammatory bowel disease, vitiligo, insulin dependent diabetes, and nephrotic syndrome) would indicate etiologic possibility of AIH. History of diarrhea with or without blood could point to an association with inflammatory bowel disease or celiac disease, respectively. Commonest presentation of AIH is episodes of relapsing jaundice (without typical prodrome), with progressive fatigue, anorexia, and weight loss over a period of months to years. Autoimmune hepatitis can be diagnosed by demonstration of hypergammaglobulinemia; elevated IgG; and presence of anti-nuclear or anti-smooth muscle antibodies (type 1) or anti-liver kidney microsomal antibodies (type 2). Almost two-thirds of cases belong to type 1 category. Type 2 AIH is more common in young children and has a more severe and relapsing course.

Q. What are the types of drug induced liver injury presenting as acute hepatitis?

The diagnosis of drug induced liver injury depends on a careful history taking and temporal association with intake of drug with derangement of liver functions. In the setting of acute hepatitis, two distinct patterns have been defined on the basis of R value (ALT times upper limit of normal/ALP times upper limit of normal). An R value of more than 5, 2-5, less than 2 suggests hepatocellular, mixed, and cholestatic, respectively—hepatocellular having worst prognosis. Two basic types of drug reactions have been defined. First is immunoallergic type shown by phenytoin, sulfonamides, and nitrofurantoin, where there is absence of a dose-effect relationship. The injury manifests anytime from 2 to 10 weeks after starting the drug. The illness is usually associated with fever and extrahepatic manifestations like rash and lymphadenopathy. Eosinophilia and autoantibodies may be demonstrable. The disease subsides rapidly on withdrawal of offending drug and reappears rapidly in a few days of reintroduction. Another type is mediated through metabolic idiosyncrasies, e.g., isoniazid and pyrazinamide, where the onset of liver injury ranges from 2 weeks to 6 months with absence of dose relation to the injury. Coadministered drugs may affect metabolic pathways and augment liver injury. Unlike in the previous type, fever and extrahepatic manifestations are not seen. Recovery may not be dramatic with drug withdrawal and children may continue to worsen or recover slowly. Rechallenge after recovery may result in recurrence of manifestations but some may show phenomenon of tolerance.

Q. What is Reye's syndrome and what are its clinical and laboratory features?

Reye's syndrome is a severe systemic disorder of children and adolescents associated with a high mortality. It has a biphasic behavior in typical cases—viral respiratory infection, apparent remission with a brief interval of 3-5 days before onset of the severe syndrome, which is characterized by persistent vomiting followed by cognitive confusion, seizures, and then coma. A progressive gradual evolution of the syndrome is also described. There is a strong association with influenza A and B and Varicella zoster infection followed by salicylate usage. Biochemically, it is characterized by profound hypoglycemia, moderately elevated transaminases, and hyperammonemia. Salicylate use interferes with β-oxidation activity at the 3-hydroxyacyl-coenzyme A mitochondrial dehydrogenase stage. Metabolic disorders like primary and secondary β-oxidation defects, gluconeogenetic defects, and urea cycle disorders may present with a Reye's-like syndrome.

Q. Should we consider liver abscess in the differential of acute hepatitis?

Liver abscess presents with a triad of fever, pain abdomen, and hepatomegaly, and does not present with acute hepatitis. Very rarely, jaundice or deranged liver enzymes may develop in the setting of biliary compression secondary to a huge abscess or as a part of sepsis.

CONCLUSION

Acute hepatitis should be suspected when a child presents with a combination of features comprising jaundice, nausea, vomiting, and pain over right upper quadrant. In a large majority of children with acute febrile illness, the condition becomes apparent just incidentally on routine blood tests. Though etiology is multifactorial, it should be clinically differentiated from acute cholestasis. The term "acute liver failure" should be reserved for cases in whom acute hepatitis is accompanied by coagulopathy or encephalopathy. Despite advances in molecular biology and pathophysiology, therapy continues to be supportive.

KEY LEARNING POINTS

- Acute hepatitis, a clinical syndrome characterized by acute onset of liver dysfunction (usually over a period 4 weeks), indicated by elevation of transaminases with variable synthetic dysfunction
- In a large majority of children with acute febrile illness, the syndrome comes into light just incidentally on routine blood tests
- Etiology is multifactorial
- It should be clinically differentiated from acute cholestasis, which may be caused by biliary obstruction or cholangitis and presents with a typical triad of fever, pain abdomen, and jaundice (Charcot's triad)
- When accompanied by coagulopathy or encephalopathy, it is termed "acute liver failure", which has been described variously by different workers
- Therapy is by and large supportive.

SUGGESTED READINGS

1. Davidson A, Acute hepatitis. In: Kelly DA (Ed). *Diseases of the Liver and Biliary System in Children*. London: Blackwell; 1999:65-76.
2. Gupte S. Acute hepatitis. In: Gupte S, Horvath K (Eds): *Pediatric Gastroenterology, Hepatology and Nutrition*. New Delhi: Jaypee Brothers Medical Publishers; 2008:602-613.
3. Matthai J, Paul S. Acute hepatitis. In: Bavdekar A, Matthai J, Sathiyasakeran M, Yachha Sk (Eds). *IAP Speciality Series on Pediatric Gastroenterology*. New Delhi: Jaypee Brothers Medical Publishers; 2008:145-160.

CHAPTER

39

Acute Pancreatitis

Utpal Kant Singh, Suraj Gupte, Sarah Sege

INTRODUCTION

The term acute pancreatitis denotes an acute inflammation of pancreas with variable involvement of surrounding tissues and organs as well as distant organs in the body. Manifestations include abdominal pain, nausea, and vomiting. Often, the patient presents with one or more complications that have a huge impact on morbidity and mortality.

Severe acute pancreatitis means acute pancreatitis with other organ system failure or local complications in the form of necrosis, abscess, or pseudocyst. Around 20–25% cases of acute pancreatitis belong to this class.

The condition is infrequent in children. However, when it occurs, emergency and intensive handling become mandatory for an acceptable prognosis. Despite treatment, mortality in severe cases is high with a variation between 20 and 60% in different documentations.

CASE 1

A 12-year-old boy presented with severe upper abdominal pain radiating to back, nausea, and vomiting of 12 hours duration. He was recovering from mumps.

Examination: Sick-looking boy with moderate dehydration. Temperature 38°C, respiratory rate 26 breaths/min, pulse rate 110 beats/min, blood pressure (BP) 105/60 mmHg. Abdominal distention ++ epigastric tenderness ++.

Investigations:
- Hemoglobin 10.5 g/dL, normocytic normochromic picture
- Total leukocyte count 18,000/cmm
- Differential leukocyte count polys 75%, lymphocytes 20%, monocytes 2%, eosinophils 3%
- C-reactive protein (CRP) 35 mg/dL
- Serum amylase 1,150 units/L, lipase 675 units/L
- Blood sugar 140 mg/dL
- Calcium 7.2 mg/dL
- Transaminases slight rise
- Serum bilirubin 2.3 mg/dL.

Abdominal ultrasonography: Hypoechogenicity indicating enlarged pancreas.

Treatment: The boy was treated on supportive lines, including fluid resuscitation, oxygen, analgesia, correction of hyperglycemia, and hypocalcemia. Nasogastric feeding was started after stabilization.

Course: Since fever recurred on the 5th day and lingered on despite antipyretic therapy with rise in leukocytosis contrast-enhanced computed tomography (CECT) scan was done after 7 days of hospitalization. It showed enlarged, poorly enhancing, and inflamed pancreas with a single peripancreatic fluid collection; dilated loops of colon. At this stage, ceftriaxone was started. He showed good response and was discharged after 2 weeks hospital stay.

CASE REVIEW IN A NUTSHELL

The clinical presentation of this 12-year-old boy with severe epigastric pain and tenderness, abdominal distention nausea, vomiting, and fever while he was convalescing from mumps is typical of acute pancreatitis. The investigations lent support to the clinical suspicion. He was rightly managed on conservative supportive lines with good response. The recurrence of fever on the 5th day raised the suspicion of a complication. As per standard protocol, at this stage a computed tomography (CT) scan showed evidence of single pancreatic fluid collection which meant a CT score of 3 indicating a moderate necrosis which could be the result of a superadded infection. Addition of an antibiotic (imipenem) to arrest the infection and further necrosis proved useful. In subsequent week or so he showed good recovery. Whether addition of antibiotic earlier as a prophylactic measure is of advantage, remains debatable. Currently, opinion does not favor use of prophylactic antibiotics.

INTERACTIVE TOPIC REVIEW

Q. What are the causes of acute pancreatic in pediatric practice?

Common causes of acute pancreatitis in children include:
- Infections: Usually viral infections
- Abdominal injury
- Systemic diseases
- Drugs: Sodium valproate
- Congenital defects: Choledochal cyst
- Metabolic: Hypertriglyceridemia
- Idiopathic.

Q. Are all cases severe enough to report as emergency?

No. Only 20–25% cases are with severe acute pancreatitis. Rest has mild illness.

Mild cases have only pancreatic interstitial edema and no complications unlike severe cases who suffer from pancreatic necrosis and complications.

Q. What is the precise definition of severe acute pancreatitis?

The term severe acute pancreatitis is reserved for cases in whom there is organ system failure, local complications, such as necrosis, abscess or pseudocysts, or both.

Q. What kind of complications can occur in the disease?

Both local and remote complications can occur in acute pancreatitis (Box 1).

Q. What is its pathophysiology?

Inflammatory involvement of pancreas triggers activation of trypsinogen to active trypsin. Trypsin activates proenzymes and precursors of elastase, carboxypeptidase, and phospholipase A. This leads to complications, both local and systemic.

Without treatment, sepsis and multiorgan failure syndrome may follow with serious outcome.

BOX 1: Complications of acute pancreatitis

- Local complications:
  - Necrosis
  - Pseudocyst
  - Abscess
- Systemic complications:
  - Gastrointestinal bleed
  - Intestinal obstruction
  - Intestinal perforation
  - Vascular aneurysms
  - Splenic infarct
  - Acute respiratory distress syndrome
  - Pleural effusion
  - Pericardial effusion
  - Myocardial depression
  - Shock
  - Disseminated intravascular coagulation
  - Hyperglycemias
  - Hypocalcemia
  - Acute tubular necrosis
  - Fat necrosis

Q. What is the diagnostic approach?

Clinical presentation with acute abdominal pain and nausea, vomiting, and abdominal distention must arouse suspicion.

In the absence of bowel sounds, tachycardia, low BP, and cutaneous bleeds, disease is likely to be severe. However, the following investigative support is required:
- Serum amylase and/or serum lipase levels more than 3 times upper range of normal
- Plain X-ray of chest and abdomen for pleural effusion, ileus (local or generalized) and colon cutoff sign
- Ultrasonography for:
  - Diffuse enlargement of pancreas and decrease in pancreatic echocardiography texture compared to the left lobe of the liver
  - Structural pancreatic: Biliary abnormalities, e.g., choledochal cyst, gallstones, dilatation of pancreatic biliary tree.
- Computed tomography may be required in difficult cases.

Q. What is the computed tomography severity index?

The CT severity index is given in table 1.

Q. Is there any relationship with overweight and obesity?

Yes, obsess adolescent stand enhanced risk of more severe disease.

Q. Which is the investigation of choice for detection of complications?

Contrast-enhanced CT is excellent for detecting parenchymal necrosis.

Q. How about magnetic resonance imaging?

This too can be employed. Though somewhat less sensitive than CECT, its advantage lies in avoiding radiation.

Q. Are there any hematological and serum markers for predicting severity?

First, CRP more than 150 mg/dL at 48 hours.
Secondly, high hematocrit (>40%) is predictive of a severe attack.

Q. Any other markers for predicting severity of disease?

Other markers for predicting severity of disease include:
- Tumor necrosis factor
- Interleukin-1 (IL-1), IL-6 and IL-8
- Procalcitonin
- High polymorpholeukocyte elastase.

Q. What is the standard approach to management of severe pancreatitis?

This is on the following lines:
- Resuscitation and rehydration
- Oxygen

TABLE 1: The computed tomography severity index

Grade	Findings	Points	Necrosis (%)	Additional points	Severity index
A	Normal pancreas	0	0	0	0
B	Enlarged pancreas	1	0	0	1
C	Pancreatic inflammation and/or peripancreatic fat	2	<30	2	4
D	Peripancreatic fluid collection (single)	3	30–50	4	7
E	Perpancreatic fluid collection (2 or more)	4	>50	6	10

Note: Computed tomography grade points are added to the points assigned for percentage of necrosis.

- Nasogastric tube placement
- Analgesics
- Nutrition
- Antibiotics.

Q. Regarding relief of pain by administering analgesics, will nonsteroidal anti-inflammatory drugs be sufficient?

No. Prompt relief of pain is important in pancreatitis. Hence, powerful analgesics such as morphine meperidine or fentanyl need to be used.

Q. When is pancreatic stenting needed?

Pancreatic stenting is needed in traumatic pancreatitis and pancreatitis with pseudocyst.

Q. When is endotherapy needed?

Endotherapy is needed in acute gallstone pancreatitis.

Q. Is there any indication for surgery?

Yes, surgical intervention is in order in:
- Choledochal cyst
- Gallstones.

Q. How frequent can recurrence be?

Recurrence occurs when the etiologic condition is left untreated. It is, therefore, mandatory that condition predisposing to the attack is identified and treated.

Q. Is there any role of antibiotics in prophylaxis against pancreatic infection?

Though once strongly recommended, routine use of antibiotics is no longer recommended in acute pancreatitis, except when CT severity index exceeds 8. However, strict infection control measures need to be in place.

CONCLUSION

Acute pancreatitis may infrequently in children more than 10 years of age. Severe acute pancreatitis warrants high index of suspicion, prompt diagnosis and energetic treatment in the form of fluid resuscitation and rehydration, oxygen therapy, nasogastric tube placement, strong analgesics, timely initiation of enteral feeds to maintain intestinal barrier, and blood flow and antibiotics. Specific management of complications revolves around endotherapy and stenting. Surgical intervention is indicated in subjects with choledochal cyst and gallstones. Mortality in severe acute pancreatitis, which constitutes 20–25% of all cases of acute pancreatitis, is very high in spite of treatment.

LEARNING POINTS

☞ Acute pancreatitis occurs infrequently in children, the usual age group being 10–18 years, and usually follows trauma and infections

☞ High index of suspicion in clinical presentation with high pancreatic enzyme levels and imaging studies, especially CT scan

☞ Acute pancreatic is of varying severity, the severe acute pancreatitis being responsible for high morbidity and mortality in children

☞ Early and aggressive fluid and electrolyte correction along with analgesic, oxygen therapy, organ support, and enteral nutrition constitute the hallmark of management

☞ Specific management of complications revolves around endotherapy and stenting

☞ Surgical intervention is indicated in subjects with choledochal cyst and gallstones.

SUGGESTED READINGS

1. Fischer JM, Gardner TB. The "golden hours" of management in acute pancreatitis. *Am J Gastroenterol*. 2012;107:1146-1150.
2. Gupte S, Anderson RA. Pediatric hepatology and pancreatology. In: Gupte S (Ed). *The Short Textbook of Pediatrics*, 12th edn. New Delhi: Jaypee Brothers Medical Publishers; 2016: 588-611.
3. Podar B. Severe acute pancreatitis. In: Udani S, Ugra D, Chugh K, Khilnani P (Eds). *IAP Specialty Series on Pediatric Intensive Care*. Gwalior: IAP National Publication House/Jaypee Brothers Medical Publishers; 2013:446-453.
4. Villatoro E, Mulla M, Larvin M. Antibiotic therapy for prophylaxis against infection of pancreatic necrosis in acute pancreatitis. *Cochrane Database Syst Rev*. 2010:CD002941.

SECTION 10
Nutrition

CHAPTER

40

Severe Acute Malnutrition

BP Karunakara, K Anitha

INTRODUCTION

Severe acute malnutrition (SAM) is a major public health issue in children below the age of 5 years. Children with SAM have a limited ability to respond to stress, making them vulnerable to high risk of morbidity and mortality. It should be emphasized that nearly all physiological, biochemical, and immunological systems in the body are changed in a malnourished individual. It is thus vital to treat these children proactively with short duration of highly intensive treatment regimes, aiming to rehabilitate the child in a few weeks. Severe acute malnutrition without complications can be effectively managed at the community level. Facility based in-patient care is essential when SAM has progressed to a stage where children have medical complications that are life-threatening. Successful treatment of sick children with severe malnutrition depends on appropriate medical nutrition therapy and effective management of complications in a step wise manner. The principle of "continuum of care"—from home and community to the health center and back, has to be applied to have an effective management of SAM. This chapter emphasizes on understanding case based management of SAM according to the new World Health Organization (WHO) guidelines.

> **CASE 1**
>
> **History:** A 2 years and 3 months old boy was brought to the emergency department with history of loose stools, vomiting since 2 days, and refusal of feeds since 1 day. The child had history of repeated infections in the past and had been unwell for a while. There is history of faulty feeding and irregular immunizations. Mother also feels that the child has poor interest in surroundings and failure to gain weight. The family history and birth history are noncontributory.
>
> **Examination:** The child was conscious, had a respiratory rate (RR) 48 breaths/min, no severe respiratory distress, and looks pale. The child's axillary temperature was 34°C and pulse rate (PR) 150 beats/min with low volume peripheral pulses and prolonged clot formation time (CFT). He is severely wasted, has bipedal pitting edema (grade +++). He weighted 7.6 kg, had a length of 78 cm, and a mid-upper arm circumference of 11 cm.
>
> **Salient Investigations:** Hemoglobin (Hb)—8.5 g/dL; peripheral film—microcytic hypochromic cells; blood sugar—34 mg/dL; chest X-ray—bronchopneumonia.
>
> He was diagnosed as suffering from complicated SAM with acute gastroenteritis, hypoglycemia bronchopneumonia, and anemia.
>
> His acute complicated malnutrition, including gastroenteritis, dehydration, hypoglycemia, and bronchopneumonia were treated according to the WHO guidelines. Thereafter, he was referred for community-based care for further management.

CHAPTER 40: Severe Acute Malnutrition

CASE REVIEW IN A NUTSHELL

This child has acute gastroenteritis. Examination and anthropometry show that he has SAM. The presence of bipedal pitting edema, lethargy and refusal of feeds classifies him as a case of complicated SAM, which requires hospitalization and in-patient management.

INTERACTIVE TOPIC REVIEW

Q. Define severe acute malnutrition?

In children between the ages of 6–59 months, SAM is defined as:
- Weight/height or weight/length less than –3 Z score or
- Presence of visible severe wasting or
- Presence of bipedal edema of nutritional origin or
- Mid-upper arm circumference less than 115 mm.

In children aged less than 6 months, SAM is defined as:
- Weight/length less than –3 Z score or
- Visible severe wasting or
- Bipedal edema.

Q. What are the admission criteria for a child with severe acute malnutrition?

In children 6–59 months, any of the following:
- Mid-upper arm circumference less than 115 mm with or without any grade of edema
- Weight/height less than –3 standard deviation (SD) with or without any grade of edema
- Bilateral pedal edema +/++ (children with edema +++ always need in-patient care) with any of the following complications:
  - Anorexia
  - Fever or hypothermia
  - Persistent vomiting
  - Severe dehydration
  - Apathetic, unconscious
  - Convulsions
  - Hypoglycemia
  - Severe anemia (severe palmar pallor)
  - Severe pneumonia
  - Extensive superficial infection
- Any other sign that a clinician thinks requires admission.

Infants less than 6 months: Any of the following:
- Infant is too weak or feeble to suckle effectively (independently of his/her weight-for-length)
- Weight/length less than –3 Z score (in infants >45 cm)
- Visible severe wasting (in infants <45 cm)
- Presence of bipedal edema.

Note: Out patient management is not recommended for children aged 6 months or less with severe acute malnutrition.

Q. Describe grading of nutritional edema?

Edema caused by acute malnutrition starts from both feet, extending upwards to the arms, face, and entire body. It is pitting in nature and does not change with time of the day or posture. It is elicited by applying thumb pressure gently for at least 3–5 seconds on the dorsum of each foot (Table 1).

TABLE 1: Classification of nutritional edema

Observation	Classification
No edema	(0)
Bilateral edema in both feet (below the ankles)	+/(Grade 1)
Bilateral edema in both feet and legs (below the knees)	++/(Grade 2)
Bilateral edema observed on both feet, legs, arms, face	+++/(Grade 3)

Q. What is appetite test?

Appetite test is an important criterion to differentiate a complicated case from an uncomplicated case of SAM and, therefore, decide if a patient should be sent for in-patient or out-patient management. Children with SAM who have poor appetite are at immediate risk of death and they will not take sufficient amount of the diet at home. It is usually conducted in a quiet area with ready-to-use therapeutic food (Table 2). The child should not have taken any food for the last 2 hours.

TABLE 2: Criteria for passing appetite test

Body weight (kg)	Minimum amount of RUTF to be consumed for passing the appetite test (mL or grams)
>4	15
4–6.9	25
7–9.9	35
10–14.9	50

RUTF, ready to use therapeutic food.

Q. What are the principles of management in complicated severe acute malnutrition?

- Triage: Aim is to assess if the severely malnourished child has a life threatening problem:
  - Assessment of airway and breathing: Check whether the child has severe respiratory distress or central cyanosis, proceed to next step if airway and breathing are normal as in this case
  - Assessment of circulation: This child has cold peripheries with weak, fast pulse and prolonged CFT:
    – Make sure the child is warm
    – Now, check whether the severely malnourished child is lethargic or unconscious
    – If yes, he requires intravenous glucose and rehydration.
   Since this child is not unconscious or lethargic, he requires oral rehydration solution (ORS) and oral glucose
  - Check whether child has coma or is convulsing:
    – If yes, position the child, manage airway, check and correct hypoglycemia and hypocalcemia and assess need for anticonvulsants if convulsions continue
    – This child is not comatose or convulsing; hence proceed to the next step
  - Check for signs of severe dehydration:
    – Since this child has SAM, proceed to further assessment before starting intravenous fluids.

- The principles of further management of this case are based on the following three phases:
  1. Stabilization: In this phase, child is stabilized and started on F-75 diet. This phase lasts 1–2 days
  2. Transition: This phase lasts 2–3 days. There is transition from starter to catch up diet
  3. Rehabilitation: Child enters this phase when he has good appetite and finishes 90% of the feed, major reduction of edema and no other medical problems.

INTERACTIVE TOPIC REVIEW

The 10 steps of management are described below:

Step 1: Treat or prevent hypoglycemia

- The general random blood sugar (GRBS) of this child at admission is found to be 36 mg/dL (hypoglycemia <54 mg/dL)
- Immediately treat the hypoglycemia by administering 50 mL of 10/dL glucose through a nasogastric tube (NGT). Then start F-75 feeds every 30 minutes for 2 hours (giving one fourth volume of the total recommended) to prevent further episodes of hypoglycemia. But if the child is found lethargic, unconscious or convulsing, administer 5 mL/kg of 10% glucose through intravenous route, followed by 50 mL of 10% glucose by NGT
- Repeat the GRBS after 2 hours or early if warranted by the clinical condition. If the GRBS cannot be checked, assume all severely malnourished children as hypoglycemic and treat accordingly since hypoglycemia may also occur if the malnourished child has not been fed for 4–6 hours
- Administer antibiotics as hypoglycemia may be a feature of underlying infection (described in step 5)

Step 2: Treat or prevent hypothermia

- This child has hypothermia since he feels cold to touch and the measured axillary temperature is found to be 34ºC (hypothermia-axillary temperature <36.0ºC or 96.8ºF)

- Immediately rewarm the child: Either cloth the child (including head), cover with a warmed blanket and increase the ambient temperature with available but safe heat source or put the child on the mother's bare chest (skin to skin) and cover them, remove wet linen or clothing
- Hypoglycemia and hypothermia usually occur together, hence the child has to be rewarmed as early as possible while correcting for hypoglycemia. Administer the first dose of antibiotics if not given in step 1
- Take temperature every 2 hours and every 30 minutes if heater is used. Stop rewarming when it rises above 36.5°C
- Severe hypothermia is when the temperature is less than 32°C, in addition to the above give warm humidified oxygen, 5 mL/kg of 10% dextrose intravenous or 50 mL/kg of 10% dextrose by NGT and warm using overhead warmer and give warmed intravenous fluids.

Step 3: Treat or prevent dehydration

- It is difficult to estimate dehydration status in this child using clinical signs alone as he is severely malnourished. This is because the clinical signs of dehydration may already be present in SAM (e.g., slow skin pinch, sunken eyes). Dehydration may be overestimated in a wasted child and underestimated in an edematous child as dehydration can coexist with edema. Therefore, assume that all children with SAM, presenting with watery diarrhea and cold peripheries may have dehydration and treat accordingly. Rehydrate cautiously, use oral route or NGT whenever possible.

Oral rehydration

The procedure for oral rehydration solution therapy is given in table 3.

TABLE 3: Oral rehydration solution

How often to give ORS (ReSoMal)	Amount to give
Every 30 min for first 2 h	5 mL/kg weight
Alternate hours for up to 10 h	5–10 mL/kg

ORS, oral rehydration solution; ReSoMal, oral rehydration salts or ORS for severely malnourished children.

- Starter diet is given in alternate hours (e.g., 2, 4, 6) with reduced osmolarity ORS (e.g., 3, 5, 7) until the child is rehydrated
- Monitor the vital signs every half hour for the first 2 hours, then hourly
- Signs of improved hydration status: Child is less lethargic, slowing of respiratory and pulse rates from previous high rate, skin pinch is less slow
- Signs of over hydration: Increase of pulse rate by 15 beats/min and RR by 5 breaths/min, engorged jugular veins, puffiness of eyes, tender hepatomegaly. Stop ORS if any of the above mentioned signs appear
- If diarrhea continues after rehydration, give ORS after each loose stool to replace on going losses as follows
  - For children less than 2 years, give approximately 50 mL after each loose stool
  - For children 2 years and older, give 100 mL after each loose stool
- Continue breastfeeding with increased frequency if the child is breastfed.

Intravenous rehydration

If this child is found to be unconscious, he requires intravenous rehydration as follows:
- Intravenous fluid of choice: Half saline and 5% glucose or Ringer lactate and 5% glucose
- Rate: At 15 mL/kg over the first hour
- Assess vital signs at the start and every 5–10 minutes. In case of an improvement in the hydration status, repeat the Intravenous fluids over the next 1 hour and switch to oral or nasogastric rehydration with ORS, 10 mL/kg/h up to 10 hours. Subsequently, initiate feeding with starter formula
- If the child fails to improve or deteriorates during the intravenous rehydration (i.e., increase in pulse rate by 15 beats/min or RR by 5/min), assume that the child has septic shock.

Treatment of septic shock

In this case, if the child does not show an improvement after corrective steps for hypothermia and dehydration, one must assume septic shock and begin treatment as follows:

- Give maintenance intravenous fluid (4 mL/kg/h)
- Review antibiotic treatment
- Start dopamine
- Initiate refeeding as soon as possible.

Step 4: Correct electrolyte imbalance

- Potassium: Give supplemental potassium at 3–4 mEq/kg/day for at least 2 weeks
- Magnesium: On day 1, give 50% magnesium sulphate intramuscular once (0.3 mL/kg) up to a maximum of 2 mL. Thereafter, give extra magnesium (0.4–0.6 mmol/kg/day) orally for 2 weeks.
- Sodium: When rehydrating, give low sodium containing rehydration fluid [(e.g., oral rehydration salts or ORS for severely malnourished children (ReSoMal)] give food without added salt to avoid sodium overload.

Step 5: Treatment of infections

In view of complications like hypoglycemia and hypothermia which may be the signs of underlying sepsis, this child will require antibiotics as described below:
- Injection ampicillin 50 mg/kg/dose 6 hourly
- Injection gentamicin 7.5 mg/kg once a day.

Step 6: Micronutrient supplementation

- Vitamin A: Since this child has edematous malnutrition, give a single dose of 50,000 IU (half of oral dose of 100,000 IU since the child weighs <8 kg) intramuscularly
- Folic acid 1 mg/day (give 5 mg on day 1)—for at least 2 weeks
- Zinc 2 mg/kg/day—for at least 2 weeks
- Copper 0.3 mg/kg/day
- Multivitamin supplement (without iron)
- Elemental iron 3 mg/kg/day to be started in rehabilitation phase when child starts gaining weight.

Step 7: Start feeding cautiously

The essential features of feeding during the stabilization phase are as follows:
- Type of feed—starter formula (F-75) which contains 75 kcal and 0.9 g protein per 100 mL
- Total volume of feeds required in this child with edematous malnutrition 100 mL/kg/day
- Frequency: 8–12 feeds over 24 hours
- Encourage continued breastfeeding
- Monitor: Amount of feeds offered and left over, frequency of vomiting and watery stools and daily body weight
- During this phase, the edematous child is expected to lose weight with reduction in diarrhea and a gradual return of appetite.

Step 8: Achieve catch-up growth (rehabilitation phase)

A gradual transition is recommended to avoid the risk of heart failure which can occur if children suddenly consume large amounts.
- Replace starter formula F-75 with the same amount of catch-up formula F-100 every 4 hours for 48 hours. F-100 contains 100 kcal and 2.9 g protein per 100 mL
- Increase each successive feed by 10 mL until some feed remains unconsumed, which is about 30 mL/kg/feed
- Gradually replace F-100 with modified family foods (kichuri/halwa) containing the equivalent amount of kilocalories.

Assessment of weight gain:
- Poor: Less than 5 g/kg/day
- Moderate: 5–10 g/kg/day
- Good: More than 10 g/kg/day.

Formula for calculating weight gain:

$$\text{Weight gain in g/kg/day} = \frac{(W_2 - W_1) \times 1{,}000}{W_1 \times \text{number of days from } W_1 \text{ to } W_2}$$

W_1 = initial or lowest weight in kg
W_2 = weight in kg on the day of calculation

Step 9: Provide sensory stimulation and emotional support

- Provide tender loving care (smiling, laughing, patting, touching, etc.)
- Parental or caregiver involvement when possible
- Structured play therapy 15–30 min/day
- Physical activity as soon as the child is well enough.

Step 10: Prepare for discharge and follow up after recovery

Criteria for discharge
- The child has achieved weight gain of more than 15% and has satisfactory weight gain for 3 consecutive days, i.e., more than 5 g/kg/day
- Weight/height Z score more than −2 SD
- Edema has resolved
- Child eating an adequate amount of nutritious food that the mother can prepare at home
- All infections and other medical complications have been treated
- Child is provided with micronutrients
- Immunization is updated.

Discharge after providing treatment for helminthic infections: Give a single dose of 200 mg albendazole for children aged 12–23 months, 400 mg albendazole for children aged 24 months or more.

This child is now referred to community-based care for further management. A plan is made with the parents for regular follow-up visits where they are educated regarding causes of malnutrition and avoidance of its recurrence. The child has to be followed up by health providers in the program till he reaches a weight-for-height of −1 SD.

Q. How do you treat infections in a child with severe acute malnutrition?

Adding routine antibiotic agents to nutritional therapy may increase recovery rates and decrease mortality among children with SAM.
- If the child appears to have no complications give oral amoxicillin 15 mg/kg every 8 hours for 5 days
- If child has complications, select antibiotic as shown below:
  - All admitted cases with any complications other than shock, meningitis or dysentery: Give injection ampicillin 50 mg/kg/dose 6-hourly and injection gentamicin 7.5 mg/kg once a day for 7 days. Add injection cloxacillin 100 mg/kg day 6 hourly if staphylococcal infection is suspected
  - For septic shock or worsening/no improvement in initial hours: Give 3rd generation cephalosporins like injection cefotaxime 150 mg/kg/day in 3 divided doses or ceftriaxone 100 mg/kg/day in 2 divided doses along with injection gentamicin 7.5 mg/kg in single dose
  - For meningitis: Give intravenous cefotaxime 50 mg/kg/dose 6 hourly or ceftriaxone 50 mg/kg 12 hourly plus injection amikacin 15 mg/kg/day divided in 8 hourly doses
  - For dysentery: Give ciprofloxacin 15 mg/kg in 2 divided doses per day for 3 days. If child is sick or has already received ciprofloxacin, give injection ceftriaxone 100 mg/kg once a day or divided in 2 doses for 5 days.

Duration of antibiotic therapy:
- Suspicion of clinical sepsis: At least 7 days
- Urinary tract infection: 7–10 days
- Culture positive sepsis: 10–14 days
- Meningitis: At least 14–21 days
- Deep seated infections like arthritis and osteomyelitis: At least 4 weeks.

If the condition does not improve after 5 days of antibiotic treatment, check for sites of infection and potentially resistant organisms and take appropriate measures. Revise therapy based on sensitivity report. If there is partial improvement after 5 days, complete a full 10-day course.

Q. How do you prevent development of congestive cardiac failure in a child with severe acute malnutrition?

Cardiac failure may occur due to the inability of the heart to adapt to increased fluid load, electrolyte imbalance or severe anemia and is a common cause of unexpected sudden death. It is, therefore, important to monitor for signs of cardiac failure during stabilization and transition.

Following are the steps to be followed in preventing congestive cardiac failure in a child with SAM:

- Cautious feeding, give only the prescribed amount of feeds
- Avoid blood transfusion and only transfuse if child is severely anemic (Hb <4 g/dL). Cautiously use packed cells 10 mL/kg or whole blood 15 mL/kg, give diuretic (frusemide-1 mg/kg) at start of transfusion, transfuse slowly for over 3 hours.
- Give IV rehydration only when absolutely necessary and change to oral rehydration as soon as possible.

Treating congestive cardiac failure:
- Position the child in an upright sitting position and provide oxygen
- Stop all fluids and feeds
- Administer diuretic (frusemide—1 mg/kg).

Q. How do you manage a case of severe acute malnutrition below the age of 6 months?

Stabilization phase:
- Initial steps of management i.e., hypoglycemia, hypothermia, dehydration, infection, and septic shock are same as for older children
- Wherever possible breastfeeding or expressed milk is preferred in place of starter diet
- If the production of breast milk is insufficient initially, combine expressed breast milk and noncereal starter diet initially
- For babies who are not breastfed, give noncereal based starter diet
- Give good diet and micronutrient supplements to the mother.

Rehabilitation phase:
- Provide support to mother to give frequent feeds and try to establish exclusive breast feeding
- Supplementary suckling technique can be practiced to enhance breast feeding till lactation is established. In this technique, the baby while feeding at the breast will also be simultaneously sucking at a NGT, the end of which will be put in a cup with supplemental milk. The cup is initially placed 5–10 cm below the level of the nipple to help the weak infant suck, and gradually lowered down to 30 cm
- In artificially fed infants without any prospects of breastfeeds, the infant should be given diluted catch-up diet (catch-up diet diluted by one third extra water to make volume 135 mL in place of 100 mL).
- Discharge the infant from the facility when gaining weight for 5 days and has no medical complications
- On discharge, the nonbreastfed infants should be given locally available animal milk with cup and spoon or infant formulas if the parents can afford this.

Q. When do you say that the child has "failure to respond"?

The criteria of child's failure to respond is shown in table 4:

TABLE 4: Child's failure to respond-criteria

Failure to respond-criteria	Approximate time after admission
Failure to regain appetite	Day 4
Failure to start to lose edema	Day 4
Edema still present	Day 10
Failure to gain at least 5 g/kg/day	For 3 successive days after feeding on catch-up diet

In such cases, check for lack of adherence to treatment, malabsorption syndromes, psychological causes, infections like tuberculosis, human immunodeficiency virus, and urinary tract infection.

CONCLUSION

The management of SAM is either community based or hospital based, based on the severity and the presence or absence of complications. The objectives of hospital based treatment are to manage complications and reduce the mortality. It also aims at improving the physical and psychosocial growth of children with SAM.

The present emphasis is on early identification and treatment at the community level to improve the outcome of malnutrition. Finally, prevention of SAM by improving maternal and child nutrition by good infant and young child feeding practices will go a long way in reducing the burden of this disease.

KEY LEARNING POINTS

- Severe acute malnutrition is an emergency
- Objectives of hospital based treatment are to manage complications and reduce the mortality. As well as to improve the physical and psychosocial growth
- Prevention of severe acute malnutrition by improving maternal and child nutrition by good infant and young child feeding practices will go a long way in reducing the burden of this disease.

SUGGESTED READINGS

1. Bhatnagar S, Lodha R, Choudhury P, Sachdev HP, Shah N, Narayan S, et al. IAP guidelines on hospital based management of severely malnourished children (adapted from WHO Guidelines). *Indian Pediatr.* 2007;44:443-461.
2. Government of India. 2011 Operational guidelines on facility based management of children with severe acute malnutrition, Ministry of health and family welfare. [online]. Available at: www.cmamforum.org/Pool/Resources/India-Operationalguidelines-facility-based-management-SAM-2011.pdf. Accessed on: 20 June 2016].
3. Gupte S, Gomez M. Severe acute malnutrition (SAM): state-of-the-art management. In: Gupte S (Ed). *Pediatric Nutrition*, 2nd edn. New Delhi: Jaypee Brothers Medical Publishers; 2011:233-241.
4. Sachdev HP, Kapil U, Vir S. Consensus Statement National Consensus Workshop on Management of SAM Children through Medical Nutrition Therapy. *Indian Pediatr.* 2010;47:661-665.
5. World Health Organization. WHO child growth standards and the identification of severe acute malnutrition in infants and children. A joint statement by WHO and UNICEF. [online] Available on: www.who.int/nutrition/publications/severemalnutrition/978924 Accessed on: 23 June 2016.

SECTION 11
Hemato-oncology

CHAPTER 41

Bleeding Child

V Nancy Jeniffer, BP Karunakara

INTRODUCTION

Bleeding in infancy and childhood is a common problem. However, clinical evaluation of a bleeding child, though a diagnostic challenge, in a systematic manner is mandatory for deciding about the appropriate therapy. It begins with a detailed history, with emphasis on the child's age, sex, past medical history, clinical presentation and family details. Symptoms such as bruising and epistaxis occur frequently in children without underlying bleeding disorder, and so determining which child requires further investigation can be difficult.

Type and pattern of bleeding are important indicators of possible diagnoses. Mucocutaneous bleeding such as petechiae, bruising, epistaxis, gastrointestinal bleeding and/or menorrhagia suggests disorders of platelets, von Willebrand disease (VWD), etc. There may be prolonged bleeding following surgery and/or dental extractions. In contrast, spontaneous or excessive bleeding into soft tissues, muscles and joints, or delayed surgical bleeding suggests disorders of coagulation factors.

Undoubtedly, therapy is dictated by the underlying cause of bleeding. Platelet function disorders need desmopressin, antifirinolytic agents, or transfusion of platelets.

CASE 1

A 4-year-old boy presented to the emergency department with history of profuse nasal bleed following trauma to the nose for the past half an hour. He has had history of frequent oral and skin bleeds following minor trauma. There was no history of joint bleeding or bleed into soft tissues and muscles. Similar complaints associated with excessive menstrual bleed were present in the mother.

Examination: Child was lethargic, tachycardiac with feeble pulses, and respiratory rate of 30 breaths/min. Blood pressure normal. Saturation in room air maintained. Oral and nasal cavities are full of blood. Little's area shows erosion. Multiple ecchymosis present on the skin. Systemic examination is within normal limits.

Immediate treatment: Child was given intravenous bolus of normal saline. Oral cavity suctioned. Nasal packing done. Bleeding is controlled with fresh frozen plasma (FFP) transfusion awaiting von Willebrand factor antigen (VWF Ag) assay and VWF:RCO which are later found to be low.

Investigations: Complete blood count (CBC), peripheral smear, prothrombin time (PT), international normalized ratio (INR), activated partial thromboplastin time (aPTT) sent. Platelet count normal. aPTT prolonged.

CASE 2

A 5-year-old male child, a known case of hemophilia presented to the emergency department with history of head injury 15 minutes back and loss of consciousness after he fell from a height of 6 steps at home while playing. On the way to the hospital, he had one episode of convulsion.

Examination: He was found to be unconscious. Pulse rate 120 beats/min, tachycardia, blood pressure 90/60 mmHg, SpO_2–88% with poor respiratory efforts at a rate of 30 breaths/min.

Investigations: CBC, PT, aPTT, INR and neuroimaging ordered.

Treatment and course: Intravenous (IV) midazolam was given; he was intubated and put on ventilator.

10 mL/kg IV bolus of normal saline. Tachycardia decreases.

Factor VIII is arranged and transfused immediately at major factor dose (50 IU/kg) over 20 minutes.

Neuroimaging following urgent factor replacement showed right epidural hemorrhage with cerebral edema and midline shift. IV mannitol was started and child was operated by neurosurgeons and bleed evacuated.

He regained consciousness on day 2 of surgery. He was continued on ventilation for two more days and extubated on day 4. Factor VIII was continued at major factor dose for 1 week on alternate days.

He was discharged on after 10 days of hospital stay (on antiepileptic drugs).

CASE REVIEW IN A NUTSHELL

Hemophilia and VWD are the most common inherited bleeding disorders encountered in the emergency department. In both these cases, stabilization of the airway, breathing and circulation takes priority.

Mucocutaneous bleeding (case 1) may be the result of primary hemostatic disorders such as vascular abnormalities, VWD, thrombocytopenia and platelet dysfunction. There is family history of similar complaint in the mother without history of joint or soft tissue bleeds. Most children with epistaxis have spontaneous anterior nasal bleeding without airway compromise or hemodynamic instability. Rapid assessment of general appearance, vital signs, airway stability, and mental status are still necessary to identify children who require airway intervention and/or fluid resuscitation. Airway intervention may be needed for patients who are spitting or regurgitating blood and in those with hemorrhagic shock.

Initial laboratory tests in this child include complete blood count, peripheral blood smear, mean platelet volume, VWF antigen assay, VWF ristocetin cofactor activity and factor VIII activity. Platelet function should be tested by platelet aggregation once thrombocytopenia and VWD have been excluded.

In the second case, child is a known case of hemophilia. As mentioned above stabilization of airway and circulation takes priority. Child should be taken up for surgery only after factor VIII is administered. In hemophiliac children with known history of inhibitors, factor VII can be transfused.

INTERACTIVE TOPIC REVIEW

Q. What is primary and secondary hemostasis?

Hemostasis is a complex process that leads to the formation of a blood clot at the site of vessel injury. This process is divided into three components:
1. Primary hemostasis, which starts immediately after endothelial damage and is characterized by vasoconstriction, platelet adhesion and aggregation, resulting in the formation of a platelet plug (Fig. 1).
    For a firm platelet plug, it is necessary to have healthy blood vessels, VWF and sufficient and well-functional platelets. Diseases of these three players cause primary hemostatic disorders including vascular anomalies, VWD, thrombocytopenia and platelet function disorders.
2. Secondary hemostasis is the formation of fibrin through the coagulation cascade (Fig. 2).
    Coagulation cascade has three pathways:
    I. Intrinsic
    II. Extrinsic
    III. Common.

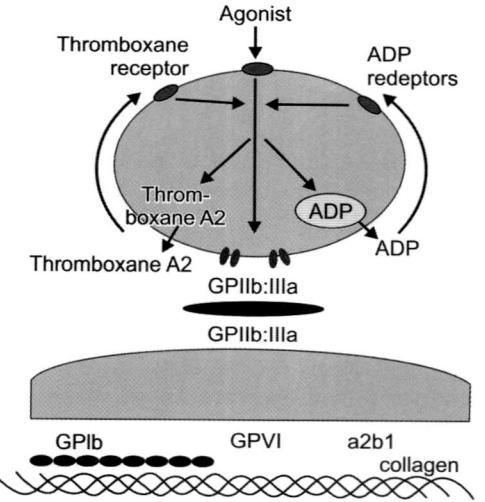

Figure 1: Primary hemostasis. von Willebrand factor binds to the exposed collagen. Platelets are tethered to the site of the injured endothelium through the binding of VWF to the glycoprotein Ib (GPIb). They attach to the collagen by participation of other receptors including GPVI and α2β1. After activation, the GPIIb:IIIa changes conformation and binds fibrinogen ( ) or VWF, initiating platelet aggregation. Adenosine 5′-diphosphate (ADP) and thromboxane A2 are released, supporting aggregation

Intrinsic pathway involves the contact activation factors [factor XII (FXII), FXI, high-molecular-weight kininogen (HMWK) and prekallikrein (PK)], FIX and FVIII. FVIII acts as a cofactor for the FIXa-mediated activation of FX.

Extrinsic pathway involves the tissue factor (TF) and FVII complex which activates FX.

Intrinsic and extrinsic pathways come together in the common pathway. Common pathway involves the FXa-mediated generation of thrombin from prothrombin and subsequent generation of fibrin from fibrinogen.

3. Fibrinolysis.

Q. How do you clinically evaluate a child with hemostatic disorders?

Children with underlying bleeding disorders usually have bruises on parts of the body that are involved in falls or trauma. Small bruises can be seen on forehead, knees, and shins in all children from the time they begin to crawl. If these bruises are larger or more than one would

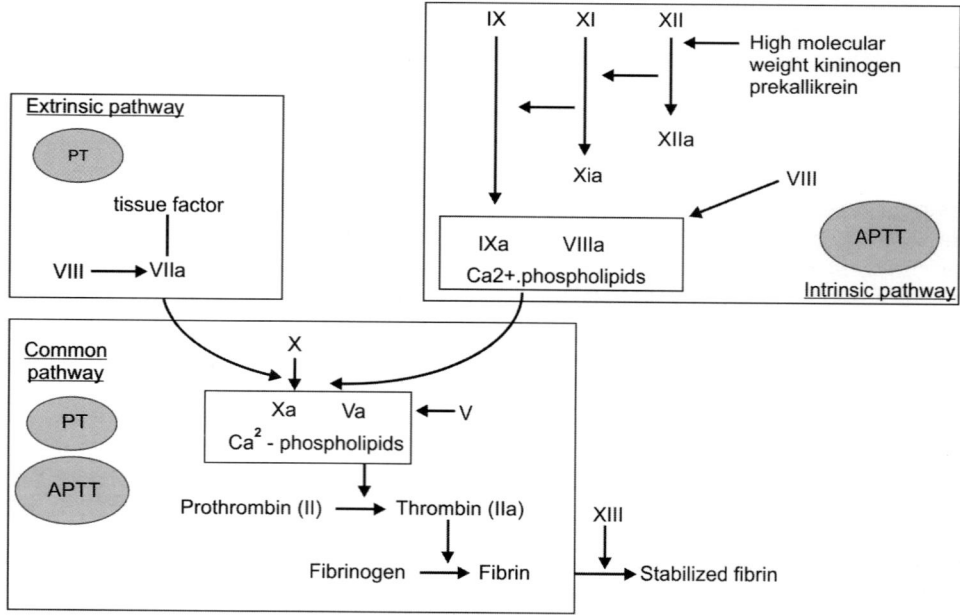

PT, prothrombin time; APTT, activated partial thromboplastin time.

Figure 2: The classical coagulation model: Two pathways, intrinsic and extrinsic, come together in the common pathway at the level of factor X

TABLE 1: Clinical abnormalities associated with inherited bleeding disorder

Coagulation defects	
FXIII deficiency	Poor wound healing, severe scar formation
Platelet function defects	
Hermansky-Pudlak syndrome	Oculocutaneous albinism
Chediak-Higashi syndrome	Oculocutaneous albinism, infections, neutrophil peroxidase-positive inclusions
Arthrogryposis-renal dysfunction-cholestasis (ARC) syndrome	Arthrogryposis, renal dysfunction, cholestasis
MYH9-related disorders	Cataracts, sensorineural hearing defect, nephritis
Leukocyte adhesion deficiency type III	Recurrent severe infections, delayed separation of the umbilical cord, neutrophilia
Thrombocytopenia	
Wiskott-Aldrich syndrome	Eczema, immunodeficiency
Thrombocytopenia with absent radii, amegakaryocytic thrombocytopenia with radioulnar synostosis	Skeletal defects
DiGeorge/velocardiofacial syndrome	Cleft palate, cardiac defects, facial anomalies, learning disabilities
Paris-Trousseau/Jacobsen syndrome	Cardiac defects, craniofacial anomalies, mental retardation
X-linked thrombocytopenia and dyserythropoiesis with or without anemia/ X-linked thrombocytopenia	Thalassemia Microcytosis of red blood cells, unbalanced hemoglobin chain synthesis resembling β-thalassemia minor

expect, a bleeding disorder must be ruled out. Before crawling, bruising is unusual and one should keep the possibility of nonaccidental trauma in mind. Uncommon sites of bruising such as the back, buttocks, arm, and abdomen should also trigger suspicion for child abuse.

Mucocutaneous bleeding points to primary hemostasis such as VWD, platelet dysfunction/deficiency or a vascular disorder.

Deep hematomas, hemarthroses, or evidence of chronic joint abnormalities in boys suggests hemophilia.

Acquired bleeding disorders present in the context of coexisting illness. Lymphadenopathy and/or organomegaly favor diagnosis of an infiltrative process like a malignancy or a storage disease.

Evidence of liver failure points to an acquired coagulation factor deficiency. Presence of additional congenital anomalies suggests a syndromic bleeding disorder as mentioned in table 1. The symptoms of acquired disorders, including ITP, usually present over days, whereas symptoms of a longer duration are suggestive of a congenital disorder such as congenital platelet disorders or VWD. The shedding of the umbilical stump, heel prick, immunizations, minor surgical interventions, including circumcision and adenotomy, and the time that their child started to crawl may be necessary history to diagnose bleeding disorders in childhood in history.

A mild bleeding disorder may manifest later in childhood or even in adulthood following more significant challenges to the hemostatic system such as surgery, dental extractions or menstruation.

Q. What are laboratory tests you would like to do in a bleeding child and how do you interpret laboratory investigation in a bleeding child?

Initial tests to screen for bleeding disorders should include a CBC, blood film, PT and aPTT. CBC (blood collected into EDTA) is performed to exclude thrombocytopenia. The CBC also provides information about additional cytopenias, and other WBC and RBC abnormalities. Peripheral blood film (blood collected into EDTA) provides additional information regarding platelet number, size, clumping and granularity. Evaluation of WBC morphology allows identification of malignant blasts, granulocyte inclusions, such as Dohle-like bodies or other WBC abnormalities. Evaluation of RBC morphology is important to exclude a microangiopathic process as evidenced by presence of fragmented red blood cells, microcytosis, macrocytosis and other RBC abnormalities.

Prothrombin time/INR (Flowchart 1) measures the extrinsic and common pathway in the coagulation cascade. A prolonged PT/high INR (with normal aPTT) suggests FVII deficiency, or use of vitamin K antagonists (VKA) such as warfarin. *aPTT (blood collected into citrate)* measures the intrinsic and common pathways of coagulation (FXII, FXI, FIX, FVIII, FX, FV, FII, fibrinogen).

The *aPTT* is less sensitive than the PT to deficiencies of the common pathway factors. An abnormally prolonged aPTT (with normal PT/INR) suggests FVIII or FIX deficiency and FXI deficiency.

Since an aPTT within the reference range does not rule out mild FVIII, FIX or FXI deficiency, factor assays need to be conducted if specific deficiencies are suspected. Though FXII deficiency also causes a prolonged aPTT, it is not associated with clinical bleeding.

A prolonged aPTT may be seen in severe VWD because of an associated FVIII deficiency.

In the presence of heparin and other inhibitors, *aPTT* is also prolonged.

Usually, heparin contamination occurs in specimens drawn from arterial or central venous catheters.

Combined prolongation of PT/INR and aPTT may result from inherited deficiencies of individual factors in the common pathway: FX, FV, FII and fibrinogen, or from the rare inherited deficiency of the vitamin K-dependent coagulation factors. However, more frequently,

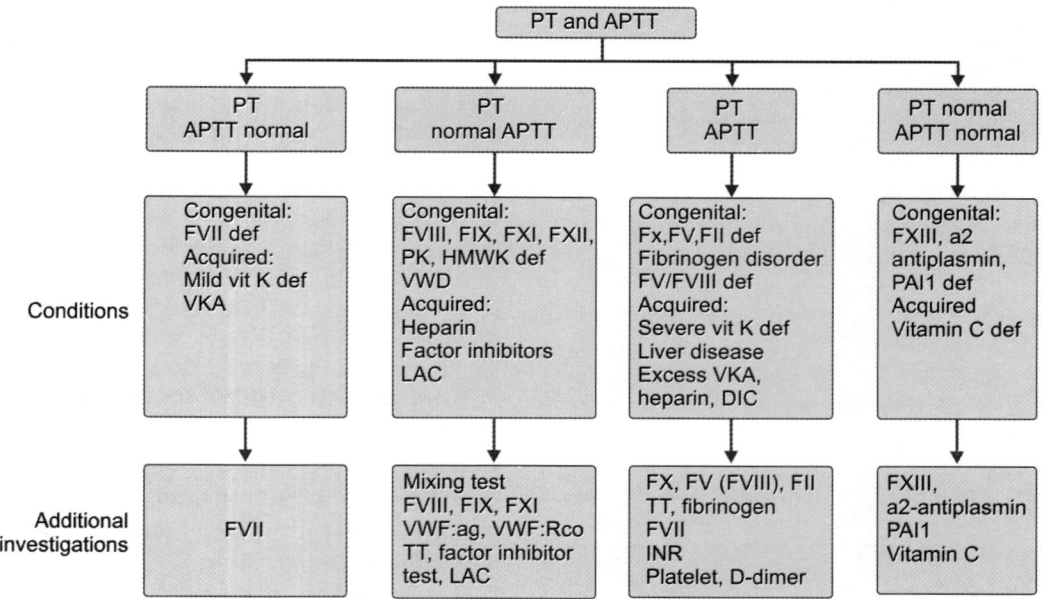

PT, prothrombin time; APTT, activated partial thromboplastin time VKA, vitamin K antagonists; VWD, von Willebrand disease; DIC, disseminated intravascular coagulation; TT, thrombin time; PAI, plasminogen activator inhibitor; LAC, lupus anticoagulant.

Flowchart 1: Extrinsic and common pathway in the coagulation cascade combined abnormalities of aPTT and PT/INR are the outcome of acquired deficiencies of multiple coagulation factors.

A *mixing study* (patient plasma 1:1 normal plasma; blood collected into citrate) should be done when an abnormal PT and/or an aPTT is identified. The patient's plasma is mixed with normal plasma in a 1:1 ratio, and the screening tests are repeated.

The mixing test differentiates between factor deficiency (mixing corrects the PT or aPTT) and the presence of an inhibitor (mixing does not correct the PT or aPTT). The most common inhibitor that results in noncorrection of the aPTT with mixing is a lupus anticoagulant. This is often an incidental finding in children and is not associated with clinical bleeding. Specialized assays will confirm its presence. Specific factor inhibitors also interfere with correction of screening tests by mixing with normal plasma. Specific inhibitor assays are warranted for confirmation.

Thrombin time (TT) and fibrinogen measurement (blood collected into citrate): TT measures the thrombin-induced conversion of fibrinogen to fibrin PT, aPTT and TT.

Urea clot lysis test (blood collected into citrate) measures the solubility of the clot with the addition of urea. An abnormal test suggests severe FXIII deficiency or hypofibrinogenemia. Clot solubility is increased only at a very low levels of FXIII levels (<3%) and therefore does not detect mild/moderate deficiencies. A quantitative assay of FXIII should be used to confirm the result of this screening test.

Platelet function analyzer, PFA-100® (blood collected into citrate) comprises an instrument in which primary, platelet-related hemostasis is simulated (building a stable platelet plug). The time required to obtain full occlusion of the aperture is reported as the closure time. Low levels of VWF and thrombocytopenia are reflected as prolonged closure time, decreased hematocrit, and some platelet function abnormalities (e.g., severe disorders such as Bernard-Soulier syndrome and Glanzmann thrombasthenia) useful especially for screening very young children for VWD or severe platelet function disorders as very little amount of blood is required as opposed to platelet aggregometry.

Testing for defects in primary hemostasis

von Willebrand factor antigen and activity (ristocetin cofactor assay) (blood collected into citrate): These tests measure the level and the activity of VWF for the diagnosis of VWD.

Platelet function testing (blood collected into citrate): The most common method of assessing platelet function is light transmission aggregometry in which the increase in light transmission through a rapidly stirred sample of citrated platelet-rich plasma is recorded as platelets aggregate.

Fibrinolysis inhibitors

Abnormalities of *fibrinolysis inhibitors (blood collected into citrate)*, such as α2-AP and plasminogen activator inhibitor (PAI)-1, can cause rare bleeding disorders because of increased fibrinolysis.

Genetic testing

The genetic mutations associated with inherited hemostatic disorders are gradually being revealed.

Q. What are the vascular anomalies causing bleeding in children?

These are various forms of structural anomalies, such as hereditary hemorrhagic telangiectasia, disorders of the connective tissue (including Ehlers–Danlos disease and osteogenesis imperfecta) and small vessel vasculitis.

Q. What is the treatment for platelet function disorders?

Treatment of platelet function disorders consists of:
- Desmopressin,
- Antifibrinolytic agents, or
- Transfusion of platelets.

Desmopressin works well in many disorders. Therapeutic efficacy of desmopressin should, therefore, be tested.

Platelet transfusions should be reserved for severe bleeding complications, which do not respond to medical therapy, and platelet defects that cannot be managed by desmopressin therapy. Alloantibodies either to human leucocyte antigens or missing GPs may easily occur.

Recombinant factor VIIa is a good alternative in patients who no longer respond to platelet transfusions.

CONCLUSION

Management of bleeding child in emergency room follows the initial same protocol of securing the ABCs of the patient with additional measures to diagnose the type of the bleeding disorder based on history, physical examination and stepwise laboratory assessment.

KEY LEARNING POINTS

- Evaluation of a bleeding child must include detailed history and physical examination before ordering investigations
- Pattern and types of bleeding (petechiae, bruising, epistaxis, gastrointestinal bleeding and/or menorrhagia; mucocutaneous bleeding; spontaneous or excessive bleeding into soft tissues, muscles and joints, or delayed surgical bleeding) are important indicators of possible diagnoses
- Stepwise laboratory evaluation is important
- Therapeutic modalities depend on the underlying cause of bleeding
- Therapy of platelet function disorders comprises desmopressin, antifibrinolytic agents or transfusion of platelets.

SUGGESTED READINGS

1. Ansell J, Hirsh J, Hylek E, Jacobson A, Crowther M, Palareti G. Pharmacology and management of the vitamin K antagonists: American College of Chest Physicians Evidence-Based Clinical Practice Guidelines. *Chest.* 2008;133:160S-198S.
2. Blanchette VS, Breakey VR, Revel-Vilk S (Eds). *Sick Kids Handbook of Pediatric Thrombosis and Hemostasis.* Basel, Switzerland: Karger; 2013:14-24.
3. Lokeshwar MR, Balasubramanam P, Kanakia S. Immune thrombocytopenic purpura. In: Gupte S, Gupte SB, Gupte M (Eds). *Recent Advances Pediatrics—24 Hot Topics.* New Delhi: Jaypee Brothers Medical Publishers; 2015:311-340.
4. Sobti P, ChandraJ, Gupte S. Pediatric haematology. In: Gupte S (Ed). *The Short Textbook of Pediatrics*, 12th edn. New Delhi: Jaypee Brothers Medical Publishers; 2016:633-664.
5. van Herrewegen F, Meijers JC, Peters M, van Ommen CH. Clinical practice: the bleeding child. Part II: disorders of secondary hemostasis and fibrinolysis. *Eur J Pediatr.* 2012;171:207-214.

CHAPTER 42

Tumor Lysis Syndrome

Sirisha Rani

INTRODUCTION

Malignancies such as acute lymphoblastic leukemia (ALL), Burkitt's lymphoma or leukemia and other malignancies with high proliferative, index or tumor burden are more prone for tumor lysis syndrome (TLS), and also highly chemosensitive tumors and increased lactate dehydrogenase levels also markers of increased TLS risk. In some cases, TLS can lead to acute renal failure and even death. The key to the prevention and management of TLS include awareness of its causes, physiologic consequences, predisposing risk factors, and identification of high-risk patients. Implementation of appropriate prophylactic measures, vigilant monitoring of electrolyte levels in patients undergoing chemotherapy, and initiation of more active treatment measures when necessary are essential.

CASE 1

A 3-year-old boy presented with fever of 4 days duration, generalized edema, and reduced urine output. On examination, he had mild pallor, significant cervical lymphadenopathy, abdominal distention, and anasarca. His blood pressure (BP) was normal.

His complete blood picture (CBP) revealed hemoglobin (Hb) of 8.9 g/dL, white blood cell (WBC)-3800 and neutrophils were 24%, platelets were 1.4 lakhs. Ultrasound abdomen showed mild hepatosplenomegaly, periportal lymph nodal enlargement, and focal hypoechoic lesions in liver and spleen. Potassium was 5.8 MEqL, sodium 132 mEqL, uric acid 13 mgdL, phosphate 8.9 mgdL, and calcium was 6.8 mgdL. Though clinically it was thought to be acute nephritis, with over all pictures after initial investigations, acute leukemia was suspected. Bone marrow examination revealed Burkitts leukemia.

He was treated with hyperhydration, diuretics and nebulization for hyperkalemia and hyperphosphatemia. He was given rasburicase for hyperuricemia and anuria. After which his urine output gradually improved over next 24 hours.

He achieved remission with induction chemotherapy, currently off treatment for 1.5 years.

CASE 2

A 4-year-old boy presented to pediatrician with history of cough for 1 week and feeling weak. He was found to have rhonchi, which was not relieved by nebulization and oral antibiotics. He received oral steroids to control wheezing. On day 2 of treatment, he started having headache, vomiting, and increasing weakness. He was investigated and found to have WBC of 63,000, Hb 9.5 g/dL, platelets were 78,000. Peripheral smear examination showed blasts. Potassium was 6.2 mEq/L, sodium 135 mEq/L, uric acid 17 mg/dL, phosphate 7.8 mg/dL, and calcium 8.1 mg/dL. His chest X-ray showed, widened mediastinum and bone marrow morphology and flow cytometry confirmed T cell ALL.

> He was treated with hyperhydration and for hyperkalemia and hyperphosphatemia. He was given rasburicase for hyperuricemia as his urine out was also low along with high tumor lysis markers.
> He was started on induction chemotherapy as per UK ALL 2003 protocol after his tumor lysis got stabilized. Currently he is 2 years off-treatment and is well.

CASE REVIEW IN A NUTSHELL

Case 1

Though clinical features like acute febrile illness, anasarca, reduced urine output pointing towards acute nephritis, BP being normal, and significant cervical lymphadenopathy makes it less likely. With ultrasound showing hypoechoic lesions in liver and spleen, one tends to think of septicemia and abscess, biochemical profile strongly point towards malignancy. Careful smear examination and critical analysis of biochemistry will help in planning further tests like bonemarrow examination or lymph node biopsy and management.

Case 2

Before giving steroids to control wheezing, critical review of our diagnosis is required as conditions like T cell ALL or T-lymphoblastic lymphoma can present like reactive airway disease. However, if there are focal signs, associated weakness or other features like superior vena cava compression symptoms like distress, edema of the face, venous engorgement, bone pain, organomegaly, lymphadenopathy, significant fever, or any atypical feature like in this case, feeling weak at presentation are warning signs and symptoms as giving steroids in those cases can result in massive TLS and its consequences.

INTERACTIVE TOPIC REVIEW

Q. What is tumor lysis syndrome?

Tumor lysis syndrome is as a result of massive and abrupt release of cellular components into bloodstream by cancer cells; characterized by hyperuricemia, hyperkalemia, hyperphosphatemia, hypocalcemia, and uremia.

Q. What are the risk factors for tumor lysis syndrome?

Due to the serious and potentially fatal consequences of TLS, there are set guidelines for the stratification of patients according to risk, optimal use of prophylactic measures and implementation of appropriate treatment (Table 1).

Q. What is the incidence of tumor lysis syndrome?

In a case review study of 102 patients with high-grade non-Hodgkin lymphoma (NHL), laboratory TLS was found in 42% of patients, however, clinically symptomatic or life threatening emergencies requiring specific therapy with TLS, occurred in only 6%.

In another study of 1,791 pediatric patients with NHL, 78 children, 4.4%, developed TLS.

Within the subgroup Burkitt's lymphoma and Burkitt's ALL (B-ALL), the rate of TLS was 8.4% and 26.4%, respectively, suggesting B-ALL patients are at the highest risk for TLS.

TABLE 1: Risk factors for tumor lysis syndrome

Risk	Low risk	Intermediate risk	High risk
Tumors	• Stage 4 neuroblastoma • Hepatoblastoma • Hodgkin's lymphoma • CML, etc.	• Standard count ALL with normal uric acid • AML • DLBCL	• Burkitt lymphoma or Burkitt leukemia • Lymphoblastic Lymphoma • High count ALL, high levels of uric acid at diagnosis

CML, chronic myelogenous leukemia; ALL, acute lymphoblastic leukemia; AML, acute myeloid leukemia; DLBCL, diffuse large B-cell lymphoma.

In another retrospective study of 788 patients (433 adults, 322 children), the overall incidence of hyperuricemia and TLS was 18.9% and 5.0%, respectively. The rates were 14.7 and 3.4% in patients with acute myeloid leukemia (AML), 21.4 and 5.2% in those with ALL, and 19.6 and 6.1% in patients with NHL, respectively. Finally, the rate of hyperuricemia was 18.9% in both the adult and pediatric populations, whereas rates of TLS were 4.8% and 5.3%, respectively.

Q. What is clinical tumor lysis syndrome, laboratory tumor lysis syndrome, and Cairo-Bishop scoring?

Cairo and Bishop developed a system for defining clinical tumor lysis syndrome (CTLS), laboratory tumor lysis syndrome (LTLS) based on modifications to the Hande-Garrow classification. As per this, LTLS is considered to be present if levels of two or more serum values of uric acid, potassium, phosphate, or calcium are more than or less than normal at presentation or if they change by 25% within 3 days before or 7 days after the initiation of treatment. Clinical tumor lysis syndrome requires the presence of LTLS in addition to one or more of the following significant clinical complications: renal insufficiency, seizures, cardiac arrhythmias, or sudden death. Initial symptoms of TLS may include nausea, vomiting, diarrhea, anorexia, lethargy, edema, fluid overload, hematuria, congestive heart failure, cardiac dysrhythmias, seizures, muscle cramps, tetany, syncope, and possible sudden death. Though symptoms can occur before initiation of chemotherapy, they are more after the initiation of it (Table 2).

With all the above information, patients are stratified into low, intermediate, and high-risk groups. Stratification is based on type of malignancy, white blood cell counts, and type of therapy and is listed in table 3. Low-risk patients are defined as those with indolent NHL or other slowly proliferating malignancies. Patients with rapidly proliferating malignancies are considered to be of intermediate risk for development of TLS. High-risk patients are defined as those having Burkitt's lymphoma, lymphoblastic lymphoma, and B-ALL. Patients with ALL and AML are stratified by WBC count.

Q. How to prevent and manage the problem?

Prompt initiation of TLS management is must because of fatal complications that can occur with it. Recognition of risk factors, close monitoring of at-risk patients, and appropriate interventions are the key to prevent or manage TLS.

TABLE 2: Cairo-Bishop scoring

	Lab tumor lysis syndrome	Clinical lab tumor lysis syndrome
Parameters	Two or more of the following changes: • At presentation, elevation of uric acid, potassium, phosphate or reduced calcium or • 25% change in values 3 days before or 7 days after treatment initiation	• Renal insufficiency • Seizures • Congestive cardiac failure • Cardiac arrhythmias or death • Other symptoms: Nausea, vomiting, diarrhea, anorexia, lethargy, edema, fluid overload, muscle cramps

TABLE 3: Risk by white blood cell count or malignancy

	High risk	Intermediate risk	Low risk
Lymphoma	• Burkitt lymphoma or leukemia • Lymphoblastic lymphoma	Diffuse large B-cell lymphoma	Indolent NHL or Hodgkins
ALL	High WBC of >100,000	Count 50,000–100,000	<50,000
AML	WBC more than 50,000	10,000–50,000	<10,000

ALL, acute lymphoblastic leukemia; AML, acute myeloid leukemia; NHL, non-Hodgkin lymphoma; WBC, white blood cell.

Hydration with fluids and alkalinization: Aggressive hydration and diuresis are essential in preventing and managing TLS. The combination of hydration and enhanced urine flow promotes the excretion of uric acid and phosphate. Diuretics may be necessary to maintain adequate urine output. Alkalinization with sodium bicarbonate has been recommended previously, as uric acid is better soluble with pH of 7.0, especially while using allopurinol. However, it is not required while using recombinant urate oxidase (rasburicase) as it does not increase the solubility of xanthine and hypoxanthine. In the absence of increased urine output, increasing urinary pH greater than 7.0 was ineffective in preventing uric acid crystallization, in fact, it may lead to metabolic alkalosis and calcium phosphate precipitation, hence, currently alkalinization is not recommended.

Allopurinol: Ever since its introduction in 1965, till now allopurinol is standard approach in preventing or managing TLS. It blocks the conversion of xanthine and hypoxanthine to uric acid (Flowchart 1).

Allopurinol when converted *in vivo* to oxypurinol, acts as a competitive inhibitor of xanthine oxidase, thereby blocking the conversion of the purine metabolites to uric acid reducing incidence of uric acid crystal obstructive uropathy. In pediatric patients, uric acid levels improved in 88% of patients and stabilized in 7% (mean time to response, 1 day in both cases).

Rasburicase: Recombinant urate oxidase (rasburicase) is recommended for the treatment of pediatric patients with hyperuricemia with LTLS or CTLS and in the initial management of patients considered to be at high risk of developing TLS as a preventive measure. In addition, for patients in the intermediate-risk group, rasburicase is recommended if hyperuricemia develops despite prophylactic treatment with allopurinol. Rasburicase is a recombinant urate oxidase that converts uric acid into allantoin (Flowchart 1). Allontoin quickly gets excreted in urine, because of its easy water solubility.

Rasburicase is contraindicated in patients with a known glucose-6-phosphate dehydrogenase (G6PD) deficiency. Screening for G6PD deficiency should include taking history of any drug induced hemolytic anemia, ethnic background, and enzyme assay. As per Food and Drug Administration (FDA), recommended dose of rasburicase is 0.15–0.2 mg/kg once daily in 50 mL of normal saline as an intravenous infusion over 30 minutes for 5 days. It is also effective at lower doses and shorter duration. Regular monitoring of uric acid levels is must and it is a good guide to adjust the usage. In certain cases, with massive tumor lysis, increase the administration schedule to twice day. The length of treatment is related to control of plasma uric acid levels, and therefore, clinical judgment should be used. Adverse reactions are rare and include anaphylaxis, rash, nausea, vomiting, headache, hemolysis, methemoglobinemia, fever, neutropenia, respiratory distress, and sepsis.

Management of hyperphosphatemia: Treating hyperphosphatemia is very important in pediatric patients even though asymptomatic. Initial treatment consists of eliminating phosphate from fluids, adequate hydration, and the administration of phosphate binders. For severe hyperphosphatemia, hemodialysis, peritoneal dialysis, or continuous venovenous hemofiltration can be used. Aluminum hydroxide 50–150 mg/kg/day is administered in divided doses orally or nasogastrically every

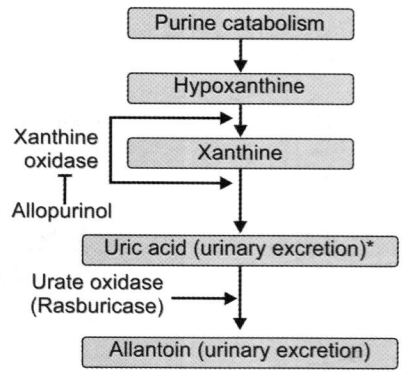

*A normal endpoint of purine metabolisms in humans.
Flowchart 1: Allopurinol in tumor lysis syndrome

6 hours for 2 days. Other phosphate binders, like calcium carbonate, sevelamer hydroxide, and lanthanum carbonate are also used and are more palatable. Calcium carbonate should not be used in patients with elevated calcium levels.

Management of hyperkalemia: First step should be giving potassium free fluids. Prompt response needed if serum potassium is greater than 7.0–7.5 mEq/L or the electrocardiogram (ECG) shows widening of QRS complex. For asymptomatic patients, the standard treatment is sodium polystyrene sulfonate 1 g/kg with 50% sorbitol administered orally. Avid giving per rectally as it can cause septicemia in neutropenic patients. For symptomatic patients, use rapid-acting insulin (0.1 U/kg administered intravenously) and glucose infusion (25% dextrose 2 mL/kg). Sodium bicarbonate (1–2 mEq/kg administered via intravenous push) can be given to induce influx of potassium into cells. Calcium gluconate (100–200 mg/kg/dose) via slow infusion with electrocardiogram (ECG) monitoring for bradycardia can be given for treatment of life threatening arrhythmias. Try to avoid giving sodium bicarbonate and calcium through the same line. Potassium should be monitored regularly along with ECG and cardiac rhythm follow-up.

Management of hyperkalemia: For asymptomatic patients, no intervention is recommended. Symptomatic patients may be treated with calcium gluconate 50–100 mg/kg intravenously, administered slowly with ECG monitoring. Avoid giving excessive calcium as its precipitation can result in obstructive uropathy.

Q. When to consider dialysis?

Dialysis usage has been significantly reduced after the introduction of rasburicase. However, 1–3% cases may still require dialysis. In view of coexisting problems like neutropenia (which can increase risk of infections with indwelling dialysis catheter) and bleeding tendency, dialysis is avoided as possible, as rasburicase can improve the situation even from established renal failure scenario. However, it requires careful monitoring of electrolytes, fluid status, and hemodynamic status.

CONCLUSION

Tumor lysis syndrome is one of the common oncological emergency which requires immediate treatment because of the severe consequence that may occur in case of any delay in recognizing and treating it. It is very important to start preventive measures in high risk patients and treat the established TLS aggressively. Awareness about the pattern of TLS, its complications, and management guidelines is essential for pediatricians to control the morbidity and mortality as they are the first contacts in these cases. It requires multidisciplinary approach with team consisting of pediatric hematologist, intensivist, and nephrologist. Regular monitoring of electrolytes in at-risk patients, and appropriate interventions are the key to preventing or managing TLS.

> **KEY LEARNING POINTS**
> - Tumor lysis syndrome, one of the common oncological emergencies, needs preventive measures in high-risk patients and aggressive therapy in established ones
> - In order to control morbidity and mortality, awareness about the pattern of TLS, its complications, and management guidelines is essential for pediatricians who are the first contacts in these cases
> - It requires multidisciplinary approach with team consisting of pediatric hematologist, intensivist, and nephrologist
> - Regular monitoring of electrolytes in at-risk patients, and appropriate interventions are the key to preventing or managing TLS.

SUGGESTED READINGS

1. Coiffier B, Altman A, Pui CH, Younes A, Cairo MS. Guidelines for the management of pediatric and adult tumor lysis syndrome: an evidence-based review. *J Clin Oncol.* 2008;26:2767-2778.
2. Howard SC, Jones DP, Pui CH. The tumor lysis syndrome. *N Engl J Med.* 2011;364:1844-1854.
3. Rheingold SR, Langen BJ. Tumor lysis syndrome: In: Pizzo PA, Poplack DG (Eds). *Principles and Practice of Pediatric Oncology*, 5th edn. Philadelphia: Lippincott Williams and Wilkins; 2006:14-37.
4. Plon SE, Malkin D. Childhood cancer and heredity. In: Pizzo PA, Poplack DG (Eds). *Principles and Practice of Pediatric Oncology*, 5th edn. Philadelphia: Lippincott Williams and Wilkins; 2006:14-37.

… SECTION 12: Homeostasis

Fluid and Electrolyte Imbalance

CHAPTER 43

PK Pruthi

INTRODUCTION

Disturbances of water and electrolyte imbalance are a frequent occurrence in pediatric clinical practice both as a primary and secondary manifestation of disease processes. Dehydration is a well accepted term used to describe situations in which invariably there are combined water and electrolyte deficits and in practice is used interchangeably with saline depletion.

Electrolytes play a vital role in maintaining homeostasis within the body. They help to regulate cardiac and neurological functions, fluid balance, oxygen delivery, and acid-base balance. The accurate evaluation of water and electrolyte deficit is necessary to achieve a successful outcome. There is a tendency to equate changes in plasma sodium with changes in total body sodium status, e.g., low plasma sodium is assumed to indicate sodium deficiency and treated with administration of saline, while in effect the low sodium could be due to excess water in the body.

Interpretation of changes in plasma sodium requires information about the presence or absence of a fluid deficit and in particular assessment of the effective intravascular volume. Careful assessment of urinary electrolytes is required, particularly in patients with obvious fluid deficit and also as confirmation of a low effective intravascular volume in patients with expansion of extracellular fluid (ECF) compartment, e.g., congestive cardiac failure, nephrotic syndrome and hepatic failure.

The evaluation of the patients with a complex fluid and electrolyte problem not only requires serial biochemical monitoring, but equally importantly serial clinical evaluation, body weight, sodium and water balance recordings. It is the combination of clinical and biochemical data which allows successful management.

The most serious disturbances involve abnormalities in levels of sodium, potassium and water content of the body.

CASE 1

A 1-year-old child, weighing 9 kg, presented with diarrhea for 3 days. The child was passing loose stools 3–4 times in a day. His preillness weight was 10 kg.

Examination: His pulse rate was 108/min, low volume, blood pressure (BP) 90/65 mmHg. The child was moderately dehydrated, skin turgor is lost and eyes are sunken. He has passed urine 1 hour ago.

Investigations: Hemoglobin (Hb)—10.5 g/dL, total leukocyte count (TLC) 9,500/cm^3, blood urea nitrogen (BUN)—20 mg/dL, serum creatinine—0.5 mg/dL, serum sodium—136 mEq/L, serum potassium—4.2 mEq/L, serum chlorine—104 mEq/L, bicarbonate (HCO$_3$)—20 mEq/L.

Diagnosis: Acute gastroenteritis with moderate dehydration.

Treatment:
- Total fluid deficit (1 kg weight loss) = 1 L
- Maintenance requirement fluid calculation—by Holliday-Segar method = 100 mL/kg/day × 9 = 900 mL
- Replacement for diarrheal fluid loss (4 episodes in 24 h) 10 mL/kg for each episode
- For 4 episodes 4 × 10 × 9 = 360 mL
- Sodium deficit from isotonic fluid deficit = 1 L × 135 mEq = 135 mEq (1 kg body weight has 1 L of fluid)
- Ongoing electrolyte loses—the patient has at present normal sodium and potassium, but estimated sodium and potassium loses are 80 mEq of sodium and 80 mEq of potassium in next 24 hours.

Procedure:
- Initial bolus normal saline 20 mL/kg in 1 hour = 200 mL (sodium given = 31 mEq)
- Remaining fluid deficit is 800 mL (1,000 − 200 mL) sodium required = deficit (135 mEq) + ongoing losses (80 mEq) + maintenance (3 mEq/kg/day) = 135 + 80 + 27 = 242 mEq

  sodium already given = 31 mEq

  Balance 242 − 31 = 211 mEq
- Total fluid required for next 1 day = 900 + 800 + 360 = 2060 mL.

  Therefore, 2,060 mL of fluid and 211 mEq sodium need to be given in next 24 hours, which can be provided as 800 mL N/2 glucose saline in 7 hours and 1,260 mL N/2 glucose saline in next 16 hours.

Outcome: At the end of 8 hours, the patient was well hydrated, skin normal, but not accepting orally therefore intravenous fluids continued for next 16 hours.

CASE 2

A 1-year-old weighing 9 kg, presented with vomiting and loose stools for 3 days. The child had been passing 3–4 watery stools every day.

Examination: The child was moderately dehydrated, skin turgor was lost, eyes sunken, dry mouth, and irritable. He had passed urine about 1 hour back. Pulse rate 106/min, low volume, BP 90/60 mmHg, bladder not palpable. As per record his previous weight was 10 kg.

Investigations: Hemoglobin 10.5 g/dL, TLC 8,200/cm³, BUN 40 mg/dL, serum, creatinine 0.5 mg/dL, serum sodium 125 mEq/L, and serum potassium 3.9 mEq/L.

Diagnosis: Acute gastroenteritis with moderate dehydration with hyponatremia.

Treatment:
- Bolus fluid 20 mL/kg/h, i.e., 200 mL of normal saline in 1 hour
- Calculation of sodium deficit:
  - Sodium deficit from isotonic fluid deficit = 1 L × 135 mEq = 135 mEq (1 kg body weight has 1 L of fluid)
  - Hyponatremic sodium deficit (desired serum sodium − current serum sodium × 0.5 × weight) (135 − 125) × 9 × 0.5 = 45 mEq
  - Maintenance sodium required at 3 mEq/kg/day = 30 mEq
  - Maintenance sodium required for 2 days = 30 × 2= 60 mEq
  - Ongoing diarrheal losses of sodium = 80 mEq per day, and for 2 days 160 mEq
  - Sodium loss in vomiting = 0 (as no further vomiting)

  Total sodium required i + ii + iv + v = 135 + 45 + 60 + 160 = 400 mEq.
- Sodium already given in bolus 200 mL normal saline = 31 mEq
- Fluid already given in bolus = 200 mL
- Balance of sodium 400 − 31 = 369 mEq
- Total fluids needed for next 2 days = 800 mL (remaining fluid deficit) + 2,000 mL (maintenance fluid for 2 days) + ongoing loses 720 mL (10 mL/kg for each episode of diarrhea for 2 days = 10 × 9 × 4 × 2) = 3,520 mL
- Half isotonic saline (N/2 glucose saline) at 80 mL/h × 40-hour would fulfil the requirements.

Outcome: Serum sodium checked after 6 hours of treatment was 128 mEq/L which meant that the rise of was not very rapid. Serum sodium checked at 24 hours and 48 hours after treatment was 130 mEq/L and 138 mEq/L, respectively. At the end of treatment, the child looked well hydrated, had passed urine several times and his BUN was 10 mg/dL.

CASE 3

A 3-year-old boy, known case of nephrotic syndrome presented with fever, laziness, and not accepting orally.

Examination: Child had edema ++, throat congested, temp 38°C, pulse rate 90/minutes, BP 90/70 mmHg, weight pre-edema 12 Hg, weight at the time presentation 13 kg.

Investigations: Hemoglobin 10.0 g/dL, BUN 20 mg/dL, serum creatinine 0.6 mg/dL, serum sodium 125 mEq/L, serum potassium 4 mEq/L.

Diagnosis: Nephrotic syndrome with upper respiratory tract infection, with edema and hyponatremia.

Treatment: Restricted intravenous fluid (half of normal requirement), i.e., 600 mL of N/3 glucose saline was given in 24 hours (it had provided 30 mEq of sodium).

Outcome: Repeat serum sodium at 12 and 24 hour was 128 mEq/L and 135 mEq/L, respectively.

CASE 4

A 2-year-old child weighing 9 kg presented with loose stools and vomiting for 3 days. Parents were giving plain water as the child was not taking oral rehydration solutions (ORS). He develops seizures and altered mental status prior to admission to the hospital. The child had continued to void urine several times prior to admission.

Examination: Child is moderately dehydrated, BP 90/55 mmHg, eyes are sunken, pulse 108/min, regular. As per records, previous weight 10 kg, temperature 38°C, RR 30/min, color pale, skin turgor poor.

Investigations: Hemoglobin 10.0 g/dL, TLC 9,200 cm³, BUN 40 m/dL, serum creatinine 0.5 mg/dL, serum sodium 115 mEq/L.

Diagnosis: Dehydration with severe hyponatremia with seizures.

Treatment:
- 20 mL/kg 3% saline in 1 hour
- Calculation of sodium deficit
  - Sodium deficit from isotonic fluid deficit 1 L × 135 = 135 mEq/L
  - Hyponatremic sodium deficit = desired serum sodium − current serum sodium × 0.5 × weight = 135 − 115 × 9 × 0.5 = 90 mEq
  - Maintenance sodium required at 3 mEq/kg/day = 30 mEq (for 2 days 60 mEq)
  - No ongoing losses: Total sodium deficit a + b + c (135 + 90 + 60) = 285 mEq
- Sodium already given in bolus = 200 mL of 3% saline = 93 mEq
- Fluid already given in bolus = 200 mL
- Balance sodium 285 − 93 = 192 mEq
- Total fluid need for next 2 days = 800 mL (remaining fluid deficit) + 2,000 mL (maintenance fluid for 2 days) = 2,800 mL
- 800 mL of N/2 glucose saline is given in next 7 h, with sodium being 62 mEq
- Total sodium given by now is 93 + 62 = 155, balance of sodium to be given = 285 − 155 = 130 mEq
- Half isotonic saline (N/2 glucose saline) at 45 mL/h × 40 hours could fulfil the requirements.

Outcome: Serum sodium checked after 6 hours of treatment was 120 mEq/L and after 24 hours and 48 hours was 135 mEq/L and 140 mEq/L, respectively. The child was well hydrated, had passed urine several times and his BUN was 10 mg/dL.

CASE 5

A 1-year-old child developed diarrhea, vomiting, and fever for 3 days. He had been refusing feed for 2 days. He has received ORS by parents without supervision. He has passed urine 1 hour prior to admission to hospital.

Examination: Weight 10 kg, temperature 38°C, pulse rate 110/min, RR 40/min, BP 95/65 mmHg.

Investigations: Hemoglobin 10.0 g/dL, TLC 9,200/cm³, serum sodium 160 mEq/L, K 4.0 mEq/L, BUN 40 mg/dL, serum creatinine 0.5 mg/dL.

Diagnosis: Acute gastroenteritis with hypernatremia.

Treatment: For a 10 kg child having plasma sodium of 160 mEq/L, water replacement is as follows:

Total body water (TBW) = 10 × 0.6 = 6 liters

$$\text{Current required body water} = \frac{\text{Actual plasma Na}}{\text{Desired plasma}} \times \text{TBW}$$

$$\frac{160}{140} \times 6\,L = 6.8\,L$$

Therefore, 6.8 L − 6.0 L, i.e., 800 mL positive water balance will correct plasma sodium concentration.

One half of 800 mL (i.e., 400 mL) + maintenance fluid for 24 hours (1,000 mL) = 1,400 mL was given as N/3 glucose saline in 24 hours. No more sodium was needed as there were no ongoing losses. The remainder 400 mL + maintenance fluid for 24 hours (1,000 mL) was given in next 24 hours.

Once urine output was established, potassium 40 mEq/L was added to the fluids.

Outcome: Serum sodium checked after 6 hours of treatment was 156 mEq/L, after 24 hours and 48 hours. The levels were 148 mEq/L and 138 mEq/L.

CASE 6

A 10-year-old child presents with edema and oliguria with history of sore throat 3 weeks back.

Examination: Weight 30 kg, pulse rate 100/minutes, RR 20/minutes, BP 100/70 mmHg, height 125 cm, edema over eyes and feet present.

Investigations: Hemoglobin 10.0 g/dL, TLC 10,500/cm^3, serum sodium 140 mEq, potassium 6.8 mEq/L, serum creatinine 1.5 mg/dL, anti-streptolysin O 400 units, electrocardiogram (ECG) normal.

Diagnosis: Poststreptococcal glomerulonephritis with acute kidney injury with hyperkalemia.

Treatment:
- Restricted fluids 400 mL/m^2/day + urine output of 24 hours
- Salbutamol 5 mg in nebulized form
- Intravenous Na bicarbonate 1 mEq/kg over 15 minutes
- Calcium gluconate (10%) 1 mL/kg over 15 minutes with infusion pump and cardiac monitoring
- Kayexalate (sodium polystyrene sulfonate) orally 1 g/kg with sorbitol.

Outcome: Serum potassium checked after 2 hours was 5.5 mEq/L and after 24 hours 4.5 mEq/L.

CASE 7

A 1-year-old child, weighing 10 kg, presented with history of loose stools and vomiting for 3 days. The child has passed urine 1 hour back.

Examination: Child has moderate dehydration, pulse 100/minutes, BP 90/60 mmHg.

Investigations: Hemoglobin 10.5 g/dL, TLC 8,700/cm^3, BUN 40 mg/dL, serum creatinine 0.5 mg/d, serum sodium 135 mEq/L, serum potassium 2.5 mEq/L, ECG flat T waves.

Diagnosis: Acute gastroenteritis with moderate dehydration with hypokalemia.

Treatment: Calculation of potassium infusion (rapid correction with concentrated potassium chloride is attempted) 25 mEq/L at a rate of 0.5 mEq/kg/dose in 1 hour, i.e., 10 kg × 0.5 = 5 mEq.

Fluid to be given in first hour 20 mL/kg normal saline = 200 mL

Potassium to be given in first hour = 5 mEq (2.5 mL of 15% KCl)

Outcome: Serum sodium repeated after 1 hour was 3.5 mEq/L. Electrocardiogram also reverted to normal. Further potassium was supplemented according to the maintenance required, i.e., 2 mEq/kg/day.

CASE REVIEW IN A NUTSHELL

Case 1

A 1-year-old child presents with diarrhea and has features of moderate dehydration. His serum sodium and potassium are normal. The child receives a bolus of normal saline 20 mL/kg in 1 hour and looks better hydrated and passes urine freely. His deficit fluid (including bolus) is given in first 8 hours and then the maintenance fluid along the losses in diarrhea (fluid and electrolyte) is given in next 16 hours. For each diarrheal stool, additional 10 mL/kg of fluid is given.

Case 2

A 1-year-old child develops hyponatremia (serum sodium 125 mEq/L) after loose stools and vomiting. The child is dehydrated and has a low volume pulse. The child does not have symptoms of central nervous system (CNS) involvement. As the child had features of moderate dehydration with a low volume pulse, he received a bolus of normal saline in first hour followed by administration of fluids and sodium as per recommendations. The child showed improvement in 48 hours.

Case 3

A 3-year-old child, known case of nephrotic syndrome with edema presents with hyponatremia. The child has hypervolemic hyponatremia and by correction of water balance, the sodium level improved in 48 hours.

Case 4

A 2-year-old presents with acute gastroenteritis and hyponatremia which is severe (serum sodium 115 mEq/L) and has CNS symptoms. Such children require administration of 3% saline initially for rapid correction of hyponatremia.

Case 5

A 1-year-old child develops hypernatremia following acute gastroenteritis and faulty administration of ORS by the mother. As serum sodium is high due to water deficiency, current required body water is calculated which when given corrects the sodium imbalance.

Case 6

A 10-year-old develops hyperkalemia following AKI and poststreptococcal glomerulonephritis. As ECG is normal, the child is not shifted to pediatric intensive care unit. With administration of salbutamol inhalation, intravenous sodium bicarbonate, intravenous calcium gluconate, and potassium exchange resins, the serum potassium could be controlled without resorting to use of insulin, glucose or dialysis. Serum potassium needs to be repeated 2–3 times after it has reached normal levels.

Case 7

A 1-year-old child develops acute gastroenteritis, moderate dehydration, and has hypokalemia with ECG changes. Potassium is corrected in a dose of 0.5 mEq/kg in the first hour when ECG changes are present. In a peripheral vein, the concentration should not exceed 40 mEq/L.

INTERACTIVE TOPIC REVIEW

Q. How exactly is rehydration therapy given?

Oral rehydration therapy (ORT) is the preferred treatment of fluid and electrolyte imbalance caused by diarrhea in children with mild to moderate dehydration. Oral rehydration therapy is as effective as intravenous fluids in rehydrating a child with mild to moderate dehydration. In addition, ORT has many advantages as it can be administered at home and requires no involvement of emergency facilities. Oral rehydration therapy is considered to be unsuccessful if vomiting is severe and persistent. Such cases and those with severe dehydration and shock require intravenous therapy. Treatment of such cases should include 20 mL/kg of isotonic saline over 30–60 minutes. No other fluid type is recommended for children for volume resuscitation. Treatment should be repeated as necessary with monitoring of the vital signs. Electrolyte measurement should be done in all children who have moderate to severe dehydration. These patients should be offered ORT as soon as they are able to take orally without vomiting.

Q. How is the fluid requirement calculated?

Fluid requirements can be calculated as per Holliday-Segar method (Table 1) or if possible according to the actual weight loss of the child. Holliday-Segar method estimates calorie expenditure in fixed weight categories, it assumes that for each 100 calories metabolized, 100 mL of water will be required specifically for each 100 Kcal expended. About 50 mL of fluid is required to provide for skin, respiratory tract and basal stool loses, and 50 mL is required for the kidneys to excrete an ultrafiltrate of plasma at 300 mosm/L without having to concentrate urine.

Deficit therapy: A precise method for assessing the fluid deficit is based on preillness weight, if this is not possible, clinical observations may be used as described in table 2.

Fluid deficit is calculated as (L) = preillness weight (kg) – illness weight (kg)

$$\text{Dehydration} = \frac{\text{Preillness weight} - \text{illness weight} \times 100\%}{\text{Preillness weight}}$$

Q. What are the clinical disorders associated with hyponatremia?

Hyponatremia is defined as serum sodium less than 130 mEq/L. Approach to hyponatremia in patients with either normal or impaired renal function begins with consideration of serum osmolality to determine whether the low serum

TABLE 1: Holliday-Segar method

Body weight	Water (mL/kg/day)	Electrolytes (mEq/100 mL of H_2O)
First 10 kg	100	Na: 3
Second 10 kg	50	Cl: 2
Each additional kg	20	K: 2

TABLE 2: Clinical observations in dehydration

Weight loss	Older child 3% (30 mL/kg)	6% (60 mL/kg)	9% (90 mL/kg)
	Infant 5% (50 mL/kg)	10% (100 mL/kg)	15% (150 mL/kg)
Dehydration	Mild	Moderate	Severe
Skin turgor	Normal	Tenting	Lost
Buccal mucosa	Normal	Dry	Parched
Pulse rate	Normal	Slightly increased	Increased
Capillary refill	Normal	2 s	3 s
Urine output	Normal	Decreased	Oliguria

sodium level is associated with hypotonic state; hypotonic hyponatremia is further subdivided into hypovolemic, isovolemic and hypervolemic forms according to the volume status.

In the beginning, it is important to determine whether hyponatremia is real. Circulating plasma is composed of 93% water and 7% protein and lipids (solid portion). The solid portion of plasma is expanded in hyperproteinemia and hyperlipidemia, and the aqueous phase to which sodium is confined shrinks. Since sodium is distributed in the aqueous phase, the amount of sodium in that aliquot of serum will be less and a reduced serum sodium concentration will be measured. This is called pseudohyponatremia. However, osmolality of the serum will remain normal.

Patients with isotonic hyponatremia incur none of the ill effects of hypotonic hyponatremia per se. No treatment is necessary.

Hypertonicity of the body fluids is recognized by the finding of hyponatremia. All hypotonic patients are hyponatremic, not all hyponatremic patients are hypotonic. Measurement of serum osmolality distinguishes hypotonic hyponatremia from isotonic and hypertonic varieties.

Hyponatremia can also occur because of fluid shifts from the intracellular to extracellular compartment because of nonsodium effective osmoles in the ECF space. These effective osmoles cause an osmotic gradient for water movement from the intracellular space to extracellular space with resultant dilution of serum sodium. Diabetic hyperglycemia and therapeutic administration of mannitol or glycerol are the usual clinical situations in which hypertonic hyponatremia appears.

The presence of hypertonicity despite hyponatremia is established by measurement of serum osmolality which is high. For every 100 mg/dL rise in glucose or mannitol, the serum sodium concentration declines by 1.6 mEq/L. A high measured osmolality resulting from ineffective osmoles such as urea does not cause redistribution of water. Unless symptomatic, no specific treatment is needed except to correct the causative factor.

Hypotonic hyponatremia is the most common cause of hyponatremia. It occurs when water intake is in excess of kidney's ability to excrete water. All such patients except with primary polydipsia have inappropriately concentrated urine. Total body sodium content is not reflected by the serum sodium concentration. It can be low, normal, or high in hyponatremic states and is best assessed by clinical evaluation of ECF volume. It is useful to further subdivide hypotonic hyponatremia according to patients hydration and assumed total body sodium stores.

Hyponatremia with edema: The edematous states of congestive heart failure, cirrhosis, and in some cases nephrotic syndrome, have in common a shrunken effective arterial blood volume that starts the pathophysiologic effects observed with contracted ECF volume. Antidiuretic hormone (ADH) levels are elevated despite the hypo-osmolar state and thirst is increased. Unless diuretics have been administered, the urine demonstrates a low sodium concentration and relatively high osmolality indicating ability of the kidney to conserve salt and water, but poor diluting ability.

Hyponatremia without edema (isovolemic hyponatremia): The syndrome of inappropriate secretion of ADH (SIADH) is the most common condition characterized by hyponatremia, hypo-osmolality, inappropriately concentrated urine, high urine sodium, normal renal and adrenal function, and euvolemia. The persistent excretion of a relatively high sodium in the urine, along with water retention, contributes to the hyponatremia of SIADH.

Hyponatremia with dehydration (hypovolemia): Loss of salt from gastrointestinal tract (GIT) skin, or kidneys results in a sequence of hormonal and hemodynamic factors that lead to renal water retention. The decreased effective blood volume leads to decreased delivery of salt and water to the diluting segments of the kidneys, increased ADH levels and thirst. Patients present with the findings of a shrunken ECF volume. In the absence of renal or adrenal disease, the urinary sodium concentration is low. Other causes of hyponatremia with hypovolemia could be mineralocorticoid deficiency and salt losing nephropathy.

Approach to a child with hyponatremia in depicted in flowchart 1.

Q. How is hyponatremia managed?

- The principal danger of hyponatremia relates to effects on CNS function due to changes in brain size. Hyponatremia initially leads to cell swelling driven by the higher intracellular osmolality. When treating a patient of hyponatremia, the sodium concentration should be raised at the rate at which it decreased. Sudden return of ECF osmolality to normal values leads to cell shrinkage, neurological symptoms, and brain damage central pontine myelinolysis has been associated with rapid correction. In a patient who loses sodium rapidly, neurological symptoms are usually present due to cerebral edema
- Patients with hypovolemia and asymptomatic hyponatremia should receive normal saline as initial bolus, while further maintenance and deficit therapy can be managed with half normal saline
- If a child has symptomatic hyponatremia, e.g., convulsions and altered sensorium, then 3% saline at rate of 3–5 mL/kg over 1 hour is used. In case there is no clinical improvement, another such bolus is given. 3% saline infusion is discontinued if child becomes asymptomatic or when serum sodium reaches 125 mEq/L. Correction of hyponatremia should not be more than 0.5 mEq/h or 10–12 mEq/day. Serum sodium should be monitored every 4–6 hours to avoid sudden and rapid changes in serum sodium.

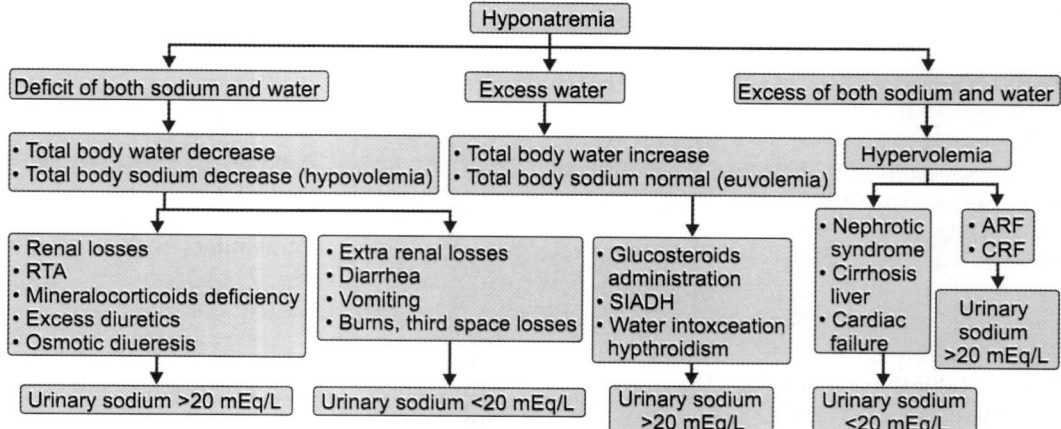

RTA, renal tubular acidosis; SIADH, syndrome of inappropriate secretion of antidiuretic hormone; ARF, acute renal failure; CRF, chronic renal failure.

Flowchart 1: Algorithmic approach to hyponatremia

The total body sodium deficit (mEq/L) is calculated as:
(Desired serum sodium − present serum sodium) × 0.6 × body weight
- In edematous patients (hypervolemia with decreased extracellular volume) efforts are made to improve the underlying condition. In addition, water restriction allows slow restoration in the balance between the preexisting total body sodium and water overload and prevents further exacerbation of clinical symptoms.

Q. How do you manage hypernatremia?

When serum sodium exceeds 150 mEq/L, it is called hypernatremia. Clinical signs manifest when serum sodium exceeds 160 mEq/L. Hypernatremia occurs less frequently than hyponatremia. Hypernatremia is a state of water loss and the overall sodium of the body can be high, normal or low. Causes of hypernatremia can be divided into 3 categories:
1. Normal total body sodium, with pure water loss
2. Low total body sodium with hypotonic loss
3. High total body sodium with pure salt gain.

All instances of hypernatremia are associated with hypertonicity. The primary defence against hypernatremia is thirst. Those patients who have intact thirst mechanism and who have access to water, usually do not become hypertonic and hypernatremic.

Hypovolemic hypernatremia

Hypernatremia is due to shrunken ECF volume, indicating loss of both salt and water, but water to a greater extent. Mostly, this loss of hypotonic fluid occurs through GIT.
Renal loses occur in osmotic diuresis or hyperglycemia

Hypervolemic hypernatremia

There is gain of both salt and water, but the gain in sodium is greater. This situation can occur with excessive administration of sodium bicarbonate in cases of acidosis or with administration of hypertonic saline.

There is expansion of ECF space in primary aldosteronism and serum sodium concentration can often reach 148–150 mEq/L.

Isovolemic hypernatremia

Pure water loss, from kidneys or insensible losses lead to isovolemic hypernatremia. Due to the free permeability of membranes to water, water loss is only one-third from ECF impartment and two-thirds from within the cells.
Renal water losses occur in central or nephrogenic diabetes insipidus.

Treatment of hypernatremia

The treatment of hypernatremia depends on (i) ECF volume status and (ii) rapidity of development of hypernatremia. If extracellular osmolality is returned rapidly to normal during treatment, the intracellular osmoles pull water into the brain cells, causing cerebral edema. Therefore, it is recommended that hypernatremia be corrected slowly at a rate that leads to half correction in 24-hour or the level should be reduced not exceeding a rate of 0.5 mEq/L/h (10–12 mEq/day). First, amount of water is calculated, which is the positive water balance to correct plasma sodium concentration. This is achieved by providing hypotonic fluid such as N/3 or N/4 saline. Blood levels are estimated every 4–6 hours so as to avoid sudden reduction however, acute hypernatremia associated with neurologic features should be corrected rapidly.

Q. How is potassium metabolism regulated?

The total body K is approximately 50 mEq/kg, so that 500 mEq of potassium could be found in a 10 kg child; of this, 98% is contained in intracellular and 2% in ECF compartment. The serum levels of potassium are controlled by renal excretion, gastrointestinal losses and uptake of potassium into the cells.
Excretion of potassium is increased by aldosterone, alkalosis also increases the excretion of potassium. About 90–95% of the potassium intake is excreted by the kidneys.

Q. What are the causes of hypokalemia?

The causes of hypokalemia are depicted in box 1.

Q. How is a patient of hypokalemia evaluated?

Spurious hypokalemia is always without any ECG changes and it can be avoided if plasma is rapidly separated from the cells and the blood is stored at 4°C. Along with checking of blood pressure, blood pH, electrolytes, BUN, serum creatinine and urinary potassium concentration are useful tests (Flowchart 2).

BOX 1: Causes of hypokalemia
- Redistribution:
  - Activation of β2 adrenergic receptors
  - Insulin, aldosterone
  - Hypokalemic periodic paralysis
  - Metabolic alkalosis
  - Increased mineralocorticoid activity
- Renal losses:
  - Renal tubular acidosis
  - Bartter syndrome
  - Gitelman syndrome
  - Mineralocorticoid excess
  - Diabetic ketoacidosis
  - Diuretics
  - Recovery from acute kidney injury
- Potassium depletion:
  - Malnutrition
  - Gastrointestinal losses
  - Skin losses

Q. Discuss the management of hypokalemia.

The treatment of hypokalemia depends on the severity and etiology. Unlike hyponatremia where, total body sodium deficit can be estimated easily, serum potassium value may not reflect the total body stores accurately.
- Mild hypokalemia: Serum potassium 3.0–3.5 mEq/L, usually asymptomatic
- Moderate hypokalemia: Serum potassium 2.5–3.0 mEq/L, may be symptomatic
- Severe hypokalemia: Serum potassium <2.5 mEq/L usually symptomatic

Patients who have mild to moderate hypokalemia (2.5–3.5 mg/L) and are asymptomatic can be managed with oral potassium chloride.

Dose 0.5–2 mEq/kg oral every 12 hours [20 mL of KCl (15%) contains 15 mEq of potassium]

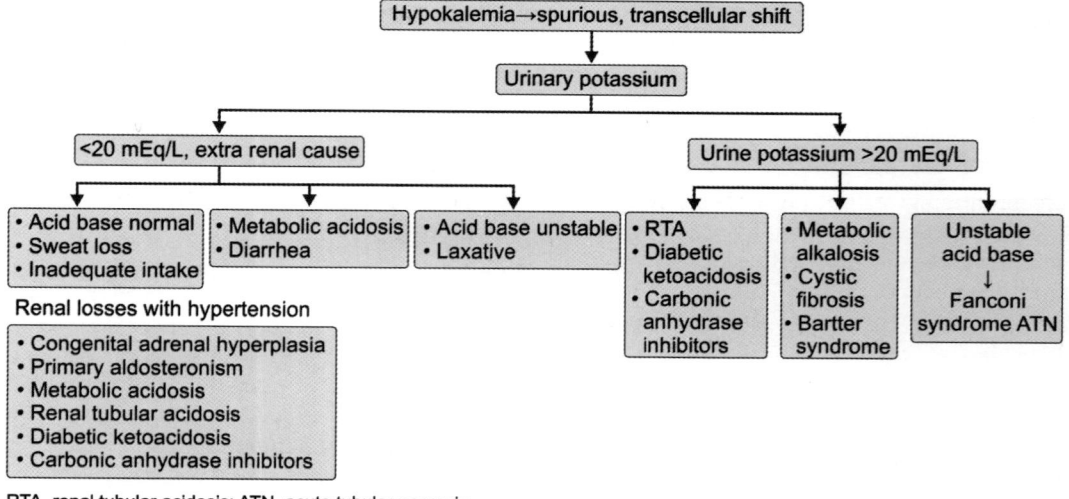

RTA, renal tubular acidosis; ATN, acute tubular necrosis.

Flowchart 2: Algorithmic approach to evaluation of hypokalemia

In severe hypokalemia (<2.5) or symptomatic patient, intravenous correction is required. The concentration of potassium in intravenous fluid should not exceed 40 mEq/L if given through a peripheral vein and 60 mEq/L if given in a central line. Higher concentrations in peripheral vein result in phlebitis.

Approximately 0.5–1.0 mEq/kg/dose of potassium can be given in the first hour with further treatment guided by laboratory results.

Q. What are the causes of hyperkalemia and how do you manage such patients?

Hyperkalemia is defined as serum potassium level above 5.5 mEq/L. For infants, the cut off level is 6.0 mEq/L.

Causes of hyperkalemia are given in flowchart 3.

Pseudohyperkalemia or spurious hyperkalemia occurs as a result of release of intracellular potassium and occurs following difficult blood collection with hemolysis. A light tourniquet with movement of hand clinching while collecting a blood sample can elevate the plasma potassium by 2.5 mEq/L. Also improper storage of blood (in a cold environment for prolonged periods) causes hyperkalemia.

Leucocytes and platelets which are rich in potassium may release their intracellular stores of potassium during the clotting process.

Evaluation

The cause of hyperkalemia is judged from the clinical presentation and tests of renal function. If renal function is normal, estimation of transtubular gradient of potassium (TTKG) helps in assessing the renal response to hyperkalemia. Transtubular gradient of potassium is accurate till the urine osmolality exceeds the serum osmolality and urine sodium >25 mEq/L.

$$TTKG = \frac{Urine\ K \times Serum\ osmolality}{Serum\ K \times urine\ osmolality}$$

A TTKG value below five indicates an inadequate aldosterone effect. Serum aldosterone level helps in differentiating hyperaldosteronism and renal resistance to aldosterone.

Management

Pseudohyperkalemia should be diagnosed and excluded promptly so that treatment of other conditions does not get delayed.

The basic aim of treatment is to counteract the cardiac toxicity and to shift potassium into intracellular spaces and lastly to effect a net loss of potassium from the body.

- Treatment with no changes in potassium balance:
  ○ The immediate treatment of life-threatening hyperkalemia is administration of calcium in the form of calcium gluconate

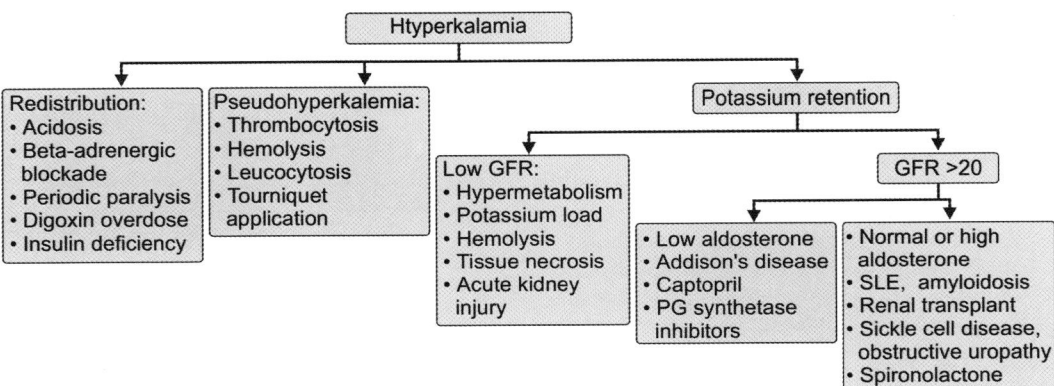

GFR, glomerular filtration rate; prostaglandin; SLE, systemic lupus erythematosus.

Flowchart 3: Causes of hyperkalemia

10% intravenous in a dose of 1 mL/kg with cardiac monitoring over a period of 5-10 minutes. Calcium reduces the threshold potential and reduces the propensity for cardiac arrhythmia. The presence of ECG changes, e.g., increase in pulse rate interval or widening of QRS complex always warrants treatment with calcium
- Treatment with potassium movement into the cells:
  - Insulin is usually given in a dose of 0.1 units/kg with 0.5 g/kg (2 mL/kg) of 25% glucose solution over 30 minutes. It may be repeated after 1 hour
  - Sodium bicarbonate administration causes expansion of ECF compartment and results in dilution of serum potassium level. Also potassium is shifted into the cells. These effects last for about 1 hour. Sodium bicarbonate can be given in a dose of 1 mEq/kg over 15 minutes
  - Beta-agonists: Salbutamol 5 mg in saline sodium can be given in nebulized form
- Treatment to decrease total body potassium:
  - The effect of calcium, bicarbonate glucose, insulin, and β-agonists are temporary. To reduce the total body potassium, sodium polystyrene sulfonate (kayexalate) can be given orally 1 g/kg with sorbitol or as retention enema. Potassium removal begins in 30-60 minutes when given as enema, 0.5 mEq of potassium is bound for every gram of resin, however, when resin is given orally, 1 mEq of potassium is bound for every 1 g of resin and action starts in 3-4 hours
  - When serum potassium is rising rapidly or there is associated renal failure, hemodialysis is usually required in addition to the abovementioned therapy. Hemodialysis can remove 25-30 mEq of potassium per hour. Peritoneal dialysis is less efficient but is still effective.

CONCLUSION

A thorough knowledge about management of fluid and electrolytes is necessary to save many a life. Management of hyponatremia does not always mean correction by deficit therapy. Dilutional hyponatremia is managed by fluid restriction. Disturbance of sodium levels are in many cases deficit of water metabolism.

KEY LEARNING POINTS

- Correction of fluids and electrolytes is a lifesaving procedure and therefore a thorough knowledge about management is mandatory
- The evaluation of the patients with complex fluid and electrolyte problem requires serial biochemical monitoring and also clinical evaluation
- Fluid requirements of a child can be determined by Holliday-Segar method
- The clinician should be well versed with the formulas available to correct fluids and electrolytes
- Disturbance of sodium levels are in majority of cases defects of water metabolism
- All hypotonic patients are hyponatremic but not all hyponatremic patients are hypotonic
- Rate of sodium correction should depend on the rate of its fall or rise
- Anticipate hypokalemia in patients with diarrhea or those receiving diuretics and during treatment of diabetic ketoacidosis
- Uncommon causes of hypokalemia should also be considered, e.g., Bartter syndrome and renal tubular acidosis, also look for clues in the history and examination
- Intravenous route of potassium is required if serum potassium is <2.5 mEq/L or when symptoms are present.

SUGGESTED READINGS

1. Bagga A, Sinha A, Gulati A. *Protocols in Pediatric Nephrology.* New Delhi: CBS; 2012.
2. Canavan A, Arant BS. Diagnosis and management of dehydration in children. *Am Fam Physician.* 2009;80:692-696.
3. Custer JW, Rau RE. The Harriet Lane Handbook. New York: Mosby/Elsevier; 2012.
4. Lien YH, Shapiro JI. Hyponatremia clinical diagnosis and management. *Am J Med.* 2007;120:653-658.
5. Raserger A, Soleimani M. Hypokalemia and hyperkalemia. *Postgrad Med J.* 2001;77:759-764.
6. Roberts KE. Pediatric fluid and electrolyte balance critical care case studies. *Crit Care Nurs Clin North Am.* 2005;17:361-373.
7. Stems RH, Hix JK, Silver S. The treatment of hyponatremia. *Semin Nephrol.* 2009;29:282-299.

SECTION 13
Rheumatology

CHAPTER 44

Vasculitis Syndrome

Abhilasha Singh, Anjul Dayal

INTRODUCTION

Childhood vasculitis is a challenging and complex group of conditions that are multisystem in nature and often require integrated care from multiple subspecialties. Vasculitis is defined as the presence of inflammation in the blood vessel wall. The site of vessel involvement, size of the affected vessels, extent of vascular injury, and underlying pathology determine the disease phenotype and severity.

The annual incidence of primary vasculitis in children and adolescents younger than 17-year-old is approximately 23 per 100,000. Primary vasculitis accounts for approximately 2–10% of all pediatric conditions evaluated in pediatric rheumatology clinics. Of the primary vasculitides, Henoch-Schönlein purpura (HSP) and Kawasaki disease (KD) are the most common accounting for 49% and 23% of all childhood vasculitis, respectively. Vasculitis can be secondary to infection, malignancy, drug exposure, and other rheumatic conditions such as systemic lupus erythematosus and juvenile dermatomyositis. Other theories of pathogenesis include humoral factors, as manifest by antineutrophil cytoplasmic antibodies (ANCA)-associated vasculitides. Abnormal regulation of immune complex formation may be contributory, as in HSP. Impaired lymphocyte regulation, specifically T-regulatory cell dysfunction, may also be involved. Antecedent infections, particularly streptococcal infections, have been implicated in many of the vasculitides including HSP, granulomatosis with polyangiitis (GPA) and polyarteritis nodosa (PAN).

CASE 1

A 12-year-old male presented with fever and sore throat for 5 days. He was given oral penicillin by his primary care doctor. After a day, he developed an erythematous, nonpruritic rash which progressed proximally from both feet to thighs and upper extremities including palms and soles. Later the feet became swollen with moderately intense burning pain, aggravated by ambulation.

On physical examination, there was pharyngeal erythema, petechiae on the soft palate, cervical lymphadenopathy, and a nodular, nontender, nonblanching purpuric rash involving both upper and lower extremities with nonpitting pedal edema. Penicillin was stopped and antiallergics were started for him as primary care doctor thought it to be penicillin allergy. Two days later, the patient developed abdominal pain involving the right and left upper quadrant which was constant, colicky in nature, aggravated with meals, and associated with hematemesis and watery stools.

Laboratory tests showed leukocytosis (WBC: 16,900/µL); Hb: 14 g/dL; Hct: 41.2%; serum creatinine: 0.9 mg/dL; urinalysis: no hematuria or proteinuria; erythrocyte sedimentation rate (ESR): 58 mm/hr; antistreptolysin O (ASO) titer: 823 IU/L; C3:125 mg/dL; C4: 11 mg/dL; antinuclear antibodies (ANA): Negative; stool for occult blood: positive. Esophagogastroduodenoscopy showed multiple erosions in the duodenum and antrum. Histopathology of the small bowel showed preserved villous architecture, and neutrophilic and eosinophilic infiltrates with leukocytoclastic vasculitis. Warthin-Starry stain was negative for *Helicobacter pylori*. There was no evidence of epithelioid granuloma. Colonoscopy showed erythema and inflammation in the terminal ileum and cecum. Cecal biopsy also showed leukocytoclastic vasculitis. Skin biopsy showed pustular leukocytoclastic fibrinoid vasculitis with microabscess.

The patient was diagnosed as HSP. He was treated with intravenous fluids, oral prednisone twice a day with resolution of his symptoms and a decrease in ESR and C-reactive protein (CRP). His diet was advanced to regular diet on the fourth hospital day.

This child was suffering from vasculitis, precisely HSP. Children usually present with rash, predominantly affecting the lower limbs but occasionally much more widespread, stomach pain, arthritis and joint pains. The most severe complication is kidney involvement (glomerulonephritis), affecting about a quarter of patients, albeit usually only mildly. Less than 10% develop more severe kidney involvement, sometimes requiring kidney biopsy and more intensive therapy and monitoring. Here initial symptoms of rashes were wrongly diagnosed as allergy to medications. But, onset of stomach pain, hematemesis and features of leukocytoclastic vasculitis on biopsy clinched the diagnosis. Initiation of steroids helps to prevent the onset of renal involvement.

INTERACTIVE TOPIC REVIEW

Q. What is vasculitis?

The vascular system refers to the collection of all blood vessels in the body. Vasculitis is the term used for a group of diseases characterized by the inflammation of and damage to the blood vessels or the blood vessel walls. Vasculitis (plural vasculitides) can be a primary disease or a secondary condition related to another underlying disease.

Different types of vasculitis have certain patterns of distribution that may affect particular organs, certain types of vessels or specific vessel sizes.

Q. What are the etiology and types of vasculitis?

The causes of vasculitis diseases are largely unknown. Immunologic abnormalities (auto-immune disorders) seem to be the underlying cause for many vasculitic disorders, leading to inflammatory changes in the blood vessels walls.

Vasculitis diseases can involve certain blood vessel types or sizes. They may also involve certain organs. The most common classification system is based on blood vessel size. European League against Rheumatism (EULAR) and the Pediatric Rheumatology European Society (PReS) has given the classification based upon size of affected vessels and the presence or absence of granuloma (Box 1).

Vasculitis affecting large blood vessels: Vasculitis affecting large blood vessels is called large vessel vasculitis and may include Takayasu arteritis and giant cell arteritis. Takayasu arteritis typically involves the aorta and its main branches. Giant cell arteritis or temporal arteritis generally affects the branches of the aorta that supply blood to the head.

Medium-vessel vasculitic disorders: Medium-vessel vasculitic disorders include PAN, KD, and vasculitis of the central nervous system. PAN classically affects the medium- to small-sized arteries, and it mainly involves the vessels of the kidneys (renal vasculitis) and the gut. A variation of this condition may affect smaller vessels and is called microscopic polyangiitis or microscopic polyarteritis.

Kawasaki disease is a type of medium- and small-vessel vasculitis affecting the arteries of the heart (coronary arteries) in children. It is associated with a generalized febrile infection of the children, which can cause vasculitis of the heart in the convalescence period of the illness.

Small-vessel vasculitic diseases: There are several types of small-vessel vasculitic diseases. Churg-Strauss arteritis is an uncommon small-vessel disease, which mainly affects the skin

BOX 1: European League against Rheumatism/The Pediatric Rheumatology European Society classification of vasculitis

Vasculitis category
- Predominately large vessel
  - Takayasu arteritis
- Predominately medium vessel
  - Childhood polyarteritis nodosa
  - Cutancous polyarteritis
  - Kawasaki disease
- Predominately small vessel
  - Granulomatous
    - Wegener's granulomatosis*
    - Churg-Strauss syndrome
  - Non-granulomatous
    - Microscopic polyangiitis
    - Henoch-Schönlein purpura
    - Isolated cutaneous leucocytoclastic vasculitis
    - Hypocomplementemic urticarial vasculitis
- Other
  - Behcet disease
  - Vasculitis secondary to infection, malignancy, drugs
  - Vasculitis associated with connective tissue disease
  - Isolated vasculitis of the central vervous system
  - Cogan syndrome
  - Unclassified

Hypersensitivity vasculitis is the term used for types of small-vessel vasculitis that may be related to an allergic insult to blood vessels. The main areas of involvement of these conditions are cutaneous (affecting the skin) as they damage the small vessels of the skin, and, therefore, they may also be called predominantly cutaneous vasculitis or cutaneous leukocytoclastic vasculitis.

Small- and medium-vessel vasculitis can also be caused by certain viruses. The most common viruses associated with vasculitis are hepatitis B, hepatitis C, human immunodeficiency virus (HIV), cytomegalovirus (CMV), Epstein-Barr virus and parvovirus B19.

Q. What are the symptoms of vasculitis?

Manifestations of vasculitis can be very vague, generalized, and nonspecific because of the complexity and variability of the different types of vasculitic diseases.

Vasculitis, as a whole, is a rare condition compared to other common conditions that may also cause similar signs and symptoms.

Most of the manifestations of vasculitis are related to the inflammation of the blood vessels that results in impaired or complete lack of blood flow to the specific organ(s).

Box 2 presents the common signs and symptoms of vasculitis.

BOX 2: Manifestations of vasculitis
- Central nervous system (CNS) vasculitis: Headache, confusion, or focal neurologic problems
- Churg-Strauss vasculitis: Symptoms similar to asthma
- Henoch-Schonlein purpura or anaphylactoid purpura: Purpura (small raised purple areas under the skin due to hemorrhage), abdominal pain or nausea and vomiting, joint pain, or blood in the urine (hematuria) because of its systemic involvement
- Temporal arteritis: Headache; tender, thick blood vessels on the side of the forehead
- Cutaneous vasculitis: Purpura, urticaria (hives), or ulcers of the skin

(cutaneous vasculitis) and the lung, although it rarely can involve other organs.

Wegener's granulomatosis is vasculitis of small arterioles and venules. It can affect many organs of the body (systemic vasculitis), but it usually involves the kidneys, the lungs (pulmonary vasculitis) and upper respiratory tract (nasal cavity and sinuses). Certain antibodies (ANCA) are associated with Wegener's disease and may be detected in the blood of these patients.

Henoch-Schonlein purpura is another small-vessel vasculitis which also affects many different organs (systemic vasculitis). This vasculitis is seen in infants, children and adults, but it is more common in children between 4–7 years of age.

Q. How do we diagnose vasculitis?

Diagnosis of vasculitis may be challenging because of significant overlap of signs and symptoms with other more common conditions. A careful medical history and complete physical examination are the initial steps if the diagnosis of some type of vasculitis is suspected.

The laboratory evaluation for vasculitis should include a complete blood count and acute phase reactants such as the ESR and CRP, which can be markedly elevated. Liver enzymes, blood urea nitrogen and creatinine, and urinalysis will evaluate for hepatic and renal involvement. Specific antibody testing such as ANA and ANCA and complements should be sent depending on the vasculitis being considered.

When clinical suspicion is high, imaging such as CT angiography, MR angiography, or conventional angiography may help detect blood vessel abnormalities. Imaging may demonstrate prototypical patterns of vessel involvement, such as beading and aneurysms in PAN and TA, respectively. Typically, imaging is most useful when there is suspicion for medium or large vessel disease.

The diagnostic gold standard for diagnosis, however, is tissue biopsy. The biopsy is typically done from the skin, kidneys, or the lungs. Brain biopsy can be performed if brain vasculitis is suspected.

Diagnosis of the retinal vasculitis may trigger an investigation to find a systemic cause including lupus vasculitis, temporal arteritis, PAN, Wegener's disease, or Behcet's disease.

Medications

The medical treatment of vasculitis largely depends on the severity of disease and the organs involved. In general, treatment is directed toward stopping or slowing the inflammatory process going on in the blood vessels. The most common medications used are the steroid-based anti-inflammatory medications, such as prednisone.

Other immunologic medications may also be used in the treatment of vasculitis, such as cyclophosphamide, azathioprine, or methotrexate.

Q. What are the various types of vasculitis?

Henoch-Schönlein purpura

Henoch-Schönlein purpura is a leukocytoclastic vasculitis that predominantly affects the small blood vessels. It is also known as anaphylactoid purpura or purpura rheumatic. This is the more common form of vasculitis in children, affecting between 10 and 20 per 100,000 children every year. Around 50% of cases present before the age of 5 years.

The classic presentation of HSP includes lower extremity purpura, arthritis, abdominal pain, and renal disease. The purpuric rash is usually on dependent areas but may be seen on the arms, face and ears. The purpura may be preceded by a maculopapular or urticarial rash that usually disappears within 24 hours. The rash may appear as bullae, necrotic lesions or deep bruising.

Arthritis affects three-quarters of children and the most commonly affected joints are the knees and ankles. The arthritis is usually oligoarticular, self-limited and nondestructive. It is the presenting symptom in 15% of patients.

The gastrointestinal manifestations of HSP affect 50–75% of children and may include bleeding, intussusception and abdominal pain. Gastrointestinal (GI) manifestations may precede the purpura by up to 2 weeks.

The most severe complication is renal involvement. Less than 10% will develop more severe kidney involvement; most common manifestation is microscopic hematuria with or without proteinuria. Children may present with nephritic or nephrotic syndrome, or rarely renal failure.

Henoch-Schönlein purpura must be distinguished from other causes of purpura in childhood including acute hemorrhagic edema of infancy, immune thrombocytopenic purpura, acute poststreptococcal glomerulonephritis, hemolytic-uremic syndrome, disseminated intravascular coagulation, infections and hypersensitivity vasculitis.

Therapy for mild HSP cases is primarily supportive with analgesics and nonsteroidal anti-inflammatory drugs. However, current literature supports that the early use of corticosteroids for HSP is associated with improved outcomes particularly GI comorbidities.

In life-threatening cases or acute renal failure, plasmapheresis followed by a more potent immunosuppressive agent such as cyclophosphamide, azathioprine, or cyclosporine, should be considered.

Kawasaki disease

This is the second most common vasculitic condition of childhood, affecting approximately 8 per 100,000 children under the age of 5 years. It affects primarily medium-sized blood vessels and is also known as mucocutaneous lymph node syndrome. The disease presents with prolonged fever, typically longer than 5 days, sometimes much longer, unusual rashes taking many forms. Conjunctivitis affects 85% of children and is bilateral and nonexudative ring. Oral mucosal changes may include dry and cracked lips and strawberry tongue. Cervical adenopathy is the least common of the diagnostic criteria. The rash associated with KD is typically nonpruritic, macular red lips and tongue, swellings of the palms and soles. Sheet-like desquamation on the fingers and toes occurs toward the end of the acute phase.

Cardiovascular disease during the acute phase may include valvulitis, myocarditis, and pericarditis. Around 25% of untreated children develop coronary artery aneurysms; prompt treatment with intravenous immunoglobulin (IVIG) combined with high-dose aspirin reduces this severe complication to approximately 4%; low-dose aspirin in the convalescent phase may prevent thrombotic complications. The criteria to diagnose KD are given in box 3.

The goal of treatment in KD is to reduce inflammation and prevent the formation of coronary aneurysms. The American Heart Association (AHA) recommends treatment with high-dose aspirin (80-100 mg/kg/day) and IVIG (2 g/kg) within the first 10 days of disease. Approximately 10-15% of patients

> **BOX 3: Classification criteria for Kawasaki disease**
>
> **Fever that persists for at least 5 days plus at least four of the following:**
> - Bilateral conjunctival injection
> - Changes of the lips and oral cavity
> - Cervical lymphadenopathy
> - Polymorphous exanthem
> - Changes in the peripheral extremities or perineal area

fail to respond to initial IVIG therapy; failure is defined as persistent fever or recurrence of fever within 36 hours of IVIG therapy. Current AHA guidelines recommend redosing IVIG at least once in the event of IVIG failure. If two or more doses of IVIG are ineffective then corticosteroid pulse therapy (30 mg/kg for 1-3 doses) or treatment with infliximab (5 mg/kg) should be considered.

Polyarteritis nodosa

This is a rare but serious form of vasculitis, involving predominantly medium and small-sized arteries. PAN can affect the vascular supply to any organ, although the lungs are typically spared. Vascular insufficiency is most common to the skin, muscles, kidneys and GI tract. Involvement of the heart, peripheral and central nervous systems are less common. Children may have fever, malaise, weight loss, myalgias and arthralgias at presentation. Depending upon the distribution of involved vessels, children may have hypertension, ischemic heart disease, testicular pain, abdominal pain, hematuria or proteinuria. Neurologic involvement may include mononeuritis multiplex with both sensory and motor deficits. Inflammation of the small arteries leads to vasculitic skin rashes including livedo reticularis, purpura, necrosis and possibly digital gangrene.

Such special tests as skin/other tissue biopsy, nerve conduction studies, and imaging (including various forms of angiography) may be indicated to secure the diagnosis.

In a proportion of children may develop a predominant cutaneous form of the disease that requires less aggressive approaches to treatment.

Aggressive therapy with high doses of corticosteroids and immunosuppressants such as cyclophosphamide to induce remission is indicated in severe forms of the illness. Subsequently, after 3-6 months, therapy with lower doses of corticosteroids and maintenance agents such as azathioprine, methotrexate, IVIG, mycophenolate mofetil (MMF), etc. suffices.

Recent additions to the therapy of vasculitis include biologics, especially rituximab, a chimeric monoclonal antibody of human and mouse origin.

ANCA-associated vasculitis

The ANCA-associated vasculitides (AAV) are a group of pediatric conditions classified by small- and medium-vessel inflammation, multiorgan system involvement, and potentially life-threatening disease. Granulomatosis with polyangiitis (GPA, formerly Wegener's granulomatosis) occurs in children much more commonly than microscopic polyangiitis (MPA). The third variation is Churg-Strauss syndrome (CSS).

The clinical features of GPA in children are virtually identical to those affecting adults with ear, nose and throat inflammation, airway involvement, lung involvement and renal vasculitis amongst other symptoms.

Microscopic polyangiitis is a necrotizing, nongranulomatous, pauci-immune disease that affects the small vessels. The most common features of MPA include pulmonary capillaritis and necrotizing glomerulonephritis. CSS is a granulomatous vasculitis of small- and medium-sized vessels that primarily affects individuals with severe asthma or allergies. The most common features in children at diagnosis are asthma (91%), pulmonary infiltrates (85%), sinusitis (77%), skin involvement (66%), cardiac disease (55%), gastrointestinal symptoms (40%), peripheral neuropathy (39%) and kidney disease (16%).

The current approaches to treatment in children include induction of remission with high-dose corticosteroids combined with cyclophosphamide, rituximab or MMF. Maintenance therapy is typically with MMF or azathioprine for 18-24 months. Infliximab (5 mg/kg twice a month), rituximab (375 mg/m^2/week for 4 weeks) and IVIG (2 g/kg/month) are options for refractory disease.

Takayasu arteritis

This is the only recognized large vessel vasculitis affecting children. The disease is very rare, probably affecting less than one in 1 million children per year. The disease presents very nonspecifically with symptoms such as fevers, headache, fatigue, aches and pains. Hypertension may be the first indication of a problem in children. The most common complaints at diagnosis are headache (84%), dizziness (37%), abdominal pain (37%), claudication of the extremities (32%), fever (26%) and weight loss (10%). Other early indicators of disease are night sweats, back pain, myalgias and arthralgias. Hypertension is present in approximately 90% of children at diagnosis. If left untreated more specific disease manifestations develop such as involvement of the aortic arch or its major branches is associated with CNS symptoms, claudication and absent peripheral pulses. CNS involvement may include headache, ischemic strokes, cerebral aneurysms and seizures. Cardiac manifestations may include cardiomyopathy congestive heart disease and valvular disease. Involvement of the mid-aorta is associated with hypertension, abdominal pain and lower extremity claudication.

Imaging, especially angiography, is the key to securing the diagnosis.

Therapy with corticosteroids along with another immunosuppressant (say, cyclophosphamide, methotrexate, MMF) is needed for inducing remission. For maintaining remission, tapering of corticosteroids, usually combined with methotrexate, or azathioprine is appropriate.

Antitumor necrosis factor (TNF) and anti-interleukin (IL)-6 treatments may be tried in resistant cases.

Unclassified forms of vasculitis

At times, vasculitis affecting children may not fit into any single entity. Even in such cases with severe vasculitis, therapy must not be delayed.

CONCLUSION

Pediatric vasculitis is a challenging and complex group of conditions. The site of vessel involvement, size of the affected vessels, extent of vascular injury, and underlying pathology determine the disease phenotype and severity. The most common vasculitides are HSP and KD. Early diagnosis, which requires a high level of clinical suspicion, may help to improve outcomes. Pediatricians should consider vasculitis as part of the differential diagnosis in children with evidence of systemic inflammation and multisystem disease that cannot be otherwise explained. Therefore, there needs to be increased awareness particularly of the rarer and more serious forms of vasculitis that can affect children as particular diagnostic delay is still contributing to poor outcomes.

KEY LEARNING POINTS

- Vasculitis should be considered in differential diagnosis in children with multiorgan dysfunction and systemic inflammation
- Treatment with biologic agents and disease modifying drugs is increasingly being explored in vasculitis
- Early diagnosis and initiation of treatment help to improve outcomes.

SUGGESTED READINGS

1. Cellucci T, Benseler SM. Central nervous system vasculitis in children. *Curr Opin Rheumatol.* 2010;22:590-597.
2. Chen KR, Carlson JA. Clinical approach to cutaneous vasculitis. *Am J Clinc Dermatol.* 2008;9:71-92.
3. Natter M, Winsor J, Fox K. Rheumatology ACo. The Childhood Arthritis & Rheumatology Research Alliance Network Registry: Demographics and characteristics of the Initial 6-month cohort. *Proceedings of the Pediatric Rheumatology Symposium (PRSYM);* Miami, Florida. 2011;43-44.
4. Ozen S, Pistorio A, Iusan SM, Bakkaloglu A, Herlin T, Brik R, et al. EULAR/PRINTO/PRES criteria for Henoch-Schonlein purpura, childhood polyarteritis nodosa, childhood Wegener granulomatosis and childhood Takayasu arteritis: Ankara 2008. Part II: Final classification criteria. *Ann Rheum Dis.* 2010;69:798-806.
5. Ozen S, Ruperto N, Dillon MJ, Bagga A, Barron K, Davin JC, et al. EULAR/PReS endorsed consensus criteria for the classification of childhood vasculitides. *Ann Rheum Dis.* 2006;65:936-941.
6. Ozen S. Problems in classifying vasculitis in children. *Pediatr Nephrol.* 2005;20:1214-1218.
7. Peco-Antic A, Bonaci-Nikolic B, Basta-Jovanovic G, Kostic M, Markovic-Lipkovski J, Nikolic M, et al. Childhood microscopic polyangiitis associated with MPO-ANCA. *Pediatr Nephrol.* 2006;21:46-53.
8. Peru H, Soylemezoglu O, Bakkaloglu SA, Elmas S, Bozkaya D, Elmaci AM, et al. Henoch Schonlein purpura in childhood: clinical analysis of 254 cases over a 3-year period. *Clin Rheumatol.* 2008;27:1087-1092.
9. Roane DW, Griger DR. An approach to diagnosis and initial management of systemic vasculitis. *Am Fam Physician.* 1999;60:1421-1430.
10. Sundel RP. Update on the treatment of Kawasaki disease in childhood. *Curr Rheumatol Rep.* 2002;4:474-482.

SECTION 14
Sleep Disorders

CHAPTER 45

Obstructive Sleep Apnea

Anjul Dayal, Nalini Nagalla

INTRODUCTION

Obstructive sleep apnea (OSA) in children has emerged not only as a relatively prevalent condition but also as a disease that imposes a large array of morbidities, some of which may have long-term implications, well into adulthood. The major consequences of pediatric OSA involve neurobehavioral, cardiovascular, endocrine and metabolic systems. The underlying pathophysiological mechanisms of OSA-induced end-organ injury are now being unraveled, and clearly involve oxidative and inflammatory pathways. However, the roles of environmental and lifestyle conditions (such as diet, physical and intellectual activity), may account for a substantial component of the variance in phenotype. Moreover, the clinical prototypic pediatric patient of the early 1990s has been insidiously replaced by a different phenotypic presentation that strikingly resembles that of adults afflicted by the disease.

CASE 1

A 6-year-old girl was brought with a longstanding history of snoring with off and on cold and cough. She was brought to the hospital with sudden cessation of breathing in the night and followed by a seizure lasting for few seconds. The child was rushed to the hospital and on arrival, she was drowsy but responding to verbal commands. Of late, her snoring has worsened over 4 days due to associated cold and congestion. She was investigated for sepsis and meningitis and the tests were all negative.

Her electroencephalography (EEG) on arrival in the hospital was found to be normal. On examination, she had enlarged adenoids and tonsils and she was mouth breathing.

She was on antiallergic treatment for past 6 months. Yet, she had several episodes of waking up in the night.

She underwent polysomnographic evaluation in the sleep laboratory and was diagnosed to have severe sleep apnea and had high apnea-hypopnea index score (>30) with oxygen saturation level of less than or equal to 79%.

She underwent adenotonsillectomy and her symptoms of snoring and frequent waking in nights dramatically reduced and she is doing well of follow-up.

CASE REVIEW IN A NUTSHELL

This child, who was brought in for seizures, appeared to be having obstruction in sleep leading to hypoxia and seizures. She had family history of asthma and was suffering from repeated episodes of cold and cough. She was having the history of daytime sleepiness and irritability with frequent waking episodes. In view of this degree of obstruction, she underwent the sleep study. In view of severe degree of obstruction and symptomatic hypoxia during sleep, she underwent adenotonsillectomy. In case of suspected obstructive sleep apnea, doing a sleep study (polysomnography) was done which is diagnostic of the disorder and also helps in gauging the severity of obstruction. Surgery is generally curative.

INTERACTIVE CASE REVIEW

Q. What are the causes of obstructive sleep apnea?

Most common cause of childhood OSA is enlargement of the tonsils and adenoids. Tonsils and adenoids grow most quickly in the preschool years, sometimes outstripping growth of the bony pharynx and leading to airway obstruction. Other risk factors include obesity in older children, nasal allergy or hay fever, underlying medical conditions that cause low muscle tone, or abnormal craniofacial structure with small airway size, such as Down syndrome or achondroplasia.

Box 1 lists the disorders associated with childhood OSA.

Q. What are the signs of obstructive sleep apnea?

The clinical presentation of a child with OSA is nonspecific and requires increased awareness by the primary care physician. OSA symptoms in children can include the following:
- Abnormal breathing during sleep
- Frequent awakenings or restlessness
- Frequent nightmares
- Enuresis
- Difficulty awakening
- Excessive daytime sleepiness
- Hyperactivity/ behavior problems
- Daytime mouth breathing
- Poor or irregular sleep patterns.

Q. What is the age group distribution for obstructive sleep apnea?

Obstructive sleep apnea is observed in children of all ages and may develop even in infancy.

BOX 1: Disorders associated with childhood obstructive sleep apnea
- Adenotonsillar hypertrophy: Most common cause of OSA in children (however, the size of the tonsils and adenoids alone does not predict the presence or severity of OSA)
- Chronic nasal obstruction including choanal stenosis, severe septal deviation, allergic rhinitis, nasal polyps and rare nasal and/or pharyngeal tumors
- Down syndrome
- Pierre Robin anomaly
- Crouzon syndrome
- Treacher Collins syndrome
- Klippel-Feil syndrome
- Beckwith-Wiedemann syndrome
- Apert syndrome
- Prader Willi syndrome
- Morbid obesity
- Marfan syndrome
- Achondroplasia
- Laryngomalacia
- Mucopolysaccharidoses
- Conditions involving neuromuscular weakness, including Duchenne muscular dystrophy, Werdnig-Hoffman disease, late-onset spinal muscular atrophy, Guillain-Barré syndrome, myotonic dystrophy and myotubular myopathy
- Chiari malformation
- Cerebral palsy
- Sickle cell diseases
- Hypothyroidism
- Hallermann-Streiff syndrome
- Osteopetrosis
- Oropharyngeal papillomatosis.

Retrospective studies note that a large number of parents with children in whom OSA is diagnosed recall that their child's snoring began within the first months of life. Preterm babies are at risk for more obstructive events while supine, but some have suggested that they are still at a lower risk of death from sudden infant death syndrome. However, Moon et al., citing three studies, report that premature infants may be at 4 times increased risk for sudden infant death syndrome compared with term infants, with the risk increasing at lower gestational age and birth weight.

Most children with OSA are aged 2–10 years (coinciding with adenotonsillar lymphatic tissue growth). Children with severe obstructive apnea are likely to present when aged 3–5 years. The mean age at diagnosis has been reported to be 14 months, plus or minus 12 months.

Q. How is obstructive sleep apnea diagnosed?

Currently, the only available tool for definitive diagnosis of OSA is an overnight polysomnographic evaluation (Fig. 1) in the sleep laboratory. Ideally, polysomnography should be performed overnight and during the patient's usual bedtime.

Q. What does polysomnography measure?

Polysomnography provides the measures listed in box 2.

Polysomnography is necessary to document OSA and gauge its severity. A history of snoring alone is not adequate for making a diagnosis of OSA or for determining its seriousness.

Some children with OSA have primarily obstructive hypoventilation in which repetitive partial obstructions occur with some degree of relative oxygen desaturation and hypercapnia. Because of this, pediatric polysomnographic testing should include some means of determining CO_2 levels, such as end-tidal (ET) CO_2 monitoring or transcutaneous CO_2 monitoring.

Polysomnographic normal standards differ between children and adults. In the pediatric age range, abnormalities include oxygen desaturation under 92%, more than one obstructive apnea per hour, and elevations of ET CO_2 measurements of more than 50 mm Hg for more than 9% of sleep time or a peak level of greater than 53 mm Hg. (Table 1).

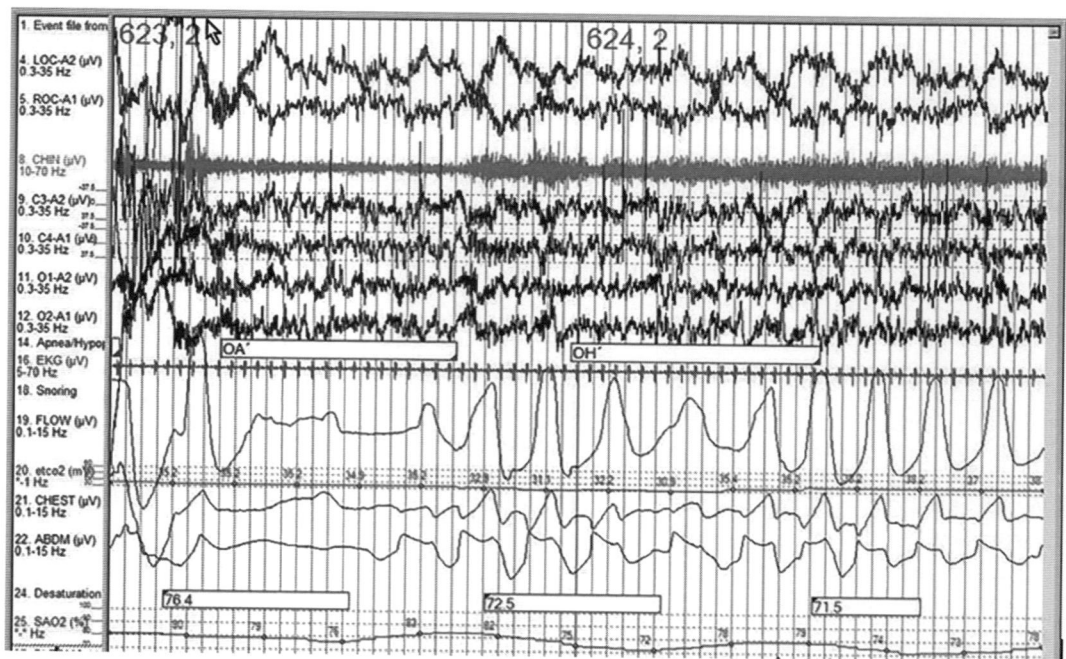

Figure 1: Polysomnographic evaluation for obstructive sleep apnea *(For color version, see Plate 4)*

BOX 2: Measures provided by polysomnography
- Sleep state (≥2 EEG leads)
- Electro-oculogram (right and left)
- Submental electromyogram (EMG)
- Airflow at nose and mouth (thermistor, capnography, or mask and pneumotachograph)
- Chest and abdominal wall motion (impedance or inductance plethysmography)
- Electrocardiogram (preferably with R-R interval derivation technology)
- Pulse oximetry (including a pulse waveform channel)
- End-tidal carbon dioxide (side stream or mainstream infrared sensor)
- Video camera monitor with sound montage (analog or digital)
- Transcutaneous oxygen and carbon dioxide tensions (in infants and children <8 years)

TABLE 1: Normal parameters for sleep gas exchange in children

Criteria	Normal values
Sleep latency	>10 m
TST	>5.5 h
% REM sleep	>15% TST
% stage 3–4 non-REM sleep	>25% TST
Respiratory arousal index (#/h TST)	<5
Periodic leg movements (#/h TST)	<1
Apnea leg movements (#/h TST)	<1
Hypopnea index (nasal/esophageal pressure catheter, #/h TST)	<3
Nadir oxygen saturation	>92%
Mean oxygen saturation	>95%
Desaturation index (>4% for 5 s; #/h TST)	<5
Highest CO_2	52 mmHg
CO_2 >45 mmHg	<20% TST

TST, total sleep time; REM, rapid eye movement.

Q. What are the complications of obstructive sleep apnea?

Morbidities can generally be divided into the four following immediate consequences of upper airway obstruction during sleep:
- Sleep fragmentation
- Increased work of breathing
- Alveolar hypoventilation
- Intermittent hypoxemia.

Q. What are the treatment modalities for obstructive sleep apnea?

Continuous positive airway pressure

Continuous positive airway pressure (CPAP) is the mainstay of therapy for most adults with OSA, as well as a large number of children and adolescents. However, it is often difficult for children to adhere to the therapy regimen.

Continuous positive airway pressure devices can be uncomfortable and inappropriately fitting masks can leak, leading to the development of pressure sores on the bridge of the nose. Air leaks can also irritate the conjunctiva, causing increased lacrimation and eye discomfort. Also, midfacial hypoplasia may develop with long-term use, particularly in children with neuromuscular weakness.

Surgical intervention

Although OSA has multiple etiologies in children, once the diagnosis has been established and its severity assessed, adenotonsillectomy is usually the first line of treatment. Tonsillotomy, rather than tonsillectomy, has been recently advocated as equally effective with less postoperative morbidity.

Adenotonsillectomy should be implemented along with weight normalization in obese children. Caloric intake limitation and dietary counseling are necessary if obesity complicates OSA. Children and adolescents with significant sleep apnea should avoid eating large amounts just before bedtime.

Q. What is the role of medications in treatment of obstructive sleep apnea?

In general, medical therapy is of limited value in the typical pediatric patient with OSA. Oxygen therapy should not be prescribed as the primary therapy for OSA.

Antihistamine or antimuscarinic therapy may lead to relief in cases of nasal congestion, although sustained benefit is uncertain. For allergic rhinitis or conditions associated with decreased nasal airflow, efforts to improve nasal patency may be beneficial.

An oral leukotriene modifier may eliminate residual OSA following surgery, and these agents may have a role in improving clinical outcomes without surgery.

Nasal fluticasone administered daily for 6 weeks is shown to ameliorate the frequency of obstructive events in children with mild-to-moderate OSA due to tonsil or adenoid hypertrophy.

Q. What is the prognosis after the surgery in children?

Surgical treatment of severe OSA warrants an overnight observation, especially if the child is younger than 3 years or has concomitant cardiopulmonary disease, morbid obesity, hypotonia or craniofacial anomalies.

The major determinants of surgical outcome include the apnea hypopnea index (AHI) and obesity at the time of diagnosis. The AHI is the total number of apneas and hypopneas that occur divided by the total duration of sleep in hours. An AHI of 1 or less is considered to be normal by pediatric standards. An AHI of 1–5 is very mildly increased, 5–10 is mildly increased, 10–20 is moderately increased, and greater than 20 is severely abnormal.

In children with enlarged tonsils and adenoids that lead to OSA, an adenotonsillectomy usually results in complete cure, although no definitive studies have clearly demonstrated this issue.

The outcome of patients who require extensive surgical management obviously depends on the severity of the condition that leads to upper airway compromise. With the emergence of noninvasive ventilation as an alternative option for these children, upper airway obstruction during sleep can be conservatively and successfully managed in most children.

CONCLUSION

The spectrum of disease that encompasses habitual snoring and OSA in children is associated with increased prevalence of a variety of morbidities spanning the central nervous system (CNS) and the cardiovascular and endocrine systems. The coexistence of obesity and OSA appears to yield not only increased morbidity rates and poorer responses to therapy, but is altogether associated with a distinct and overall recognizable clinical phenotype. Therapeutic options have somewhat expanded since the initial treatment approaches were conducted, to include not only surgical extraction of hypertrophic adenoids and tonsils, but also nonsurgical alternatives such as CPAP. Early recognition, diagnosis and treatment may prevent the majority of complications in pediatric age group.

KEY LEARNING POINTS

- Polysomnography is the diagnostic tool of choice for OSA
- Apnea-hypopnea index is important tool to assess the requirement of surgery
- CPAP has emerged as the alternative for surgery in children with obstructive sleep apnea.

SUGGESTED READINGS

1. Aurora RN, Zak RS, Karippot A, Lamm Cl, Morgenthaler TI, Auerbach SH et al. Practice parameters for the respiratory indications for polysomnography in children. *Sleep.* 2011; 34:379-388.
2. Perfect MM, Archbold K, Goodwin JL, Levine-Donnerstein D, Quan SF. Risk of behavioral and adaptive functioning difficulties in youth with previous and current sleep disordered breathing. *Sleep.* 2013;36:517-525.
3. Section on Pediatric Pulmonology, Subcommittee on Obstructive Sleep Apnea Syndrome, American Academy of Pediatrics. Clinical practice guideline: Diagnosis and management of childhood obstructive sleep apnea syndrome. *Pediatrics.* 2002;109:704-712.
4. Tsubomatsu C, Shintani T, Abe A, Yajima R, Takahashi N, Ito F, et al. Diagnosis and treatment of obstructive sleep apnea syndrome in children. *Adv Otorhinolaryngol.* 2016;77:105-111.
5. Verhulst SL, Van Gaal L, De Backer W, Desager K. The prevalence, anatomical correlates and treatment of sleep-disordered breathing in obese children and adolescents. *Sleep Med Rev.* 2008;12:339-346.
6. Whitla L, Lennon P. Non-surgical management of obstructive sleep apnoea: a review. *Paediatr Int Child Health.* 2016;14:1-5.

Index

Page numbers followed by *b* refer to box, *f* refer to figure, *fc* refer to flowchart, and *t* refer to table.

A

Acidosis 48, 169, 216
Acquired
  bleeding disorders 281
  coagulation factor
    deficiencies 281
  hypopituitarism 40
Acquired immune deficiency
  syndrome 262
Activated partial thromboplastin
  time 280, 282
Acyclovir 86
Addison's disease 56
Adenotonsillar hypertrophy 309
Adenoviruses 154, 161
Adipsic diabetes insipidus 42
Adrenal
  crisis 46, 48-50
    acute 46
    suspect 48
  hyperplasia, congenital 43, 56
  insufficiency 47, 50
    causes of
      primary 48
      secondary 48
    diagnosis of 49
    secondary 48
    types of 47
Aedes aegypti 199
Aerosolized therapies 172*t*
Airborne transmission 219
Airway 71, 86*fc*
  management of 54
  pressure, continuous
    positive 311
  pressure-release ventilation 149, 150
  secretions 162
Akinetic seizure 78
Alanine transaminase 201, 203
Albuterol 157
Aldosteronism, primary 187
Allopurinol 288
Alveolar diseases 142

Ambulatory blood pressure
  monitoring 186
Amikacin 137
Aminoacidogram 133
Amnesia 55
Amoxicillin 161, 217
Amoxicillin-clavulanic acid 144
Amphetamines 178
Ampicillin 24
Amrinone 195
Analgesics, role of 72
Anaphylactic
  reactions 238
  shock 2
Anaphylaxis 1-3, 5, 6, 288
  causes for 3
  diagnosis of 4
  episodes of 6
  mimics of 4
  refractory 6
  signs of 3*f*
  symptoms of 3*f*
Anatomic defects, congenital 39
Androctonus australis 230
Anemia, severe 271
Anesthetics, role of 72
Anesthetizing drugs 96, 97*t*, 98
Angiotensin
  converting enzyme 196
    inhibitors 3, 11, 12
  receptor blockers 11
Annular pancreas, embryology
  of 65
Anorexia 155, 271
Antibiotic therapy 137, 157
  duration of 275
Anticipated intraoperative
  complications 62
Antidiarrheal agents 243
Antidiuretic
  effect 38
  hormone 37, 39, 295
Antiemetics 224
Antiepileptic drug 81, 83, 86, 98
  therapy 85

Antihypertensive drug 189*t*
  treatment 184
Antimalarial
  chemotherapy 211
  drugs 211
Antineutrophilic cytoplasmic
  antibodies 22
Anti-seizure prophylaxis, role of 72
Anti-snake venom 238
  treatment, stop 238
Antistreptolysin O 21
  antibodies 30
Antitumor necrosis factor 306
Antiviral
  agents 222, 222*t*
  drug 223
  therapy 223
  therapy 157
Anxiety 55
Aortic arch sidedness 195
Apert syndrome 309
Aphasic seizure 78
Apnea hypopnea index 312
Appetite test 271, 272*t*
Aquaporin 39
Arboviral encephalitis 112
Arboviruses 112
Arginine vasopressin 37
Arginosuccinic acid 133
Artemisinin 211
Artemisinin-based combination
  therapy 116
Arterial blood
  gas 131, 195
    analysis 130
    oxygen saturation 143
  pressure 104
Arterial pressure, mean 69
Artesunate 212
Arthralgia 264
Arthritis 29, 264
Ascorbic acid 27
Aspartate aminotransferase 201
Aspartate transaminase 262
Aspiration pneumonia 165

Astatic seizure 78
Asthma 3, 155, 168, 174
  acute severe 168
  pathophysiology of 169
  severe 173t, 174
  severity, classification of 170t
Astrovirus 241
Ataxia 55
Atonic seizure 78
Atrial septal defect 142, 193
Atrioventricular valve
  regurgitation 194
Atropine sulphate 237
Autoimmune
  adrenal insufficiency 48
  anemia 264
  disorders 302
  encephalitis 117
    syndrome 118t
  hepatitis 255, 264
Autonomic nervous system 55
Avian influenza viruses 219
Azithromycin 144
Azotemia, prerenal 10

B

Bacterial meningitis 135, 138, 139fc
  antibiotics in acute 137b
Bacterial pneumonias 162
Barbiturate coma, role of 73
Barbiturate, high-dose 73
Barium meal 65f
Battle's sign 71
B-cell lymphoma 286
Beckwith-Wiedemann
  syndrome 56, 309
Benzodiazepines 72, 84, 87, 93, 94, 215
Bernard-Soulier syndrome 283
Beta-blockers 55
Bezold-Jarisch reflex 2
Bickerstaff encephalitis 127
Bilious emesis 65
Bilirubin load, increased 263
Biphasic anaphylaxis 4
Bleeding
  local 235f
  severe 208b
Bleomycin 15
Blindness, cortical 216
Blood 12
  counts, routine 142
  glucose 32, 131
  pressure 62, 135, 182, 186, 207, 236
    controlling 138
    management of 183
  measurement 185
  monitoring 186
  products, transfusion of 208
  sugar 83, 86
  test 227, 232
  transfusion 208
  urea 30
    nitrogen 290
  vessels, large 302
Blood-brain barrier 108
Body mass index 52
Body temperature
  management 107
Botulism 122, 125
Bradypnea 141
Brain
  abscess 76
  herniation
    infections 93
  injury
    primary 68
    secondary 68
  tissue oxygen 72
Brainstem reflexes 119
Breakbone fever 199, 262
Breastfeeding 240
Breath-holding spells 78
Breathing 54, 71, 86fc, 242
  increased work of 155
Broken neck sign 235, 236f
Bronchial mucosa 169
Bronchiolitis 145, 154, 155
  acute 153
  diagnosis of 155
  obliterans 158
  severe 153, 157, 158
Bronchitis
  epidemiology of 154
  etiology of 154
  severe 158
Bronchodilators 157, 158
Bronchopneumonia 155, 161
Buccal mucosa 295
Budd-Chiari syndrome 255
Bungarus caeruleus 234f
Burkitt's lymphoma 285

C

Cairo-Bishop scoring 287, 287t
Calcineurin inhibitors 178
Calcium channel blockers 62
Calicivirus 241
Campylobacter jejuni 127, 241
Capillary blood glucose 52, 54
Capillary refill 242, 295
  time 207
Captopril 196
Carbon dioxide, end-tidal 99
Cardiac arrhythmias 84
Cardiogenic syncope 78
Cardiomegaly 194
Cardiomyopathy 62
Cardiopulmonary disease 153
Cardiotoxin 225
Cardiovascular
  disease 3, 305
  system 178, 185
Carnitine palmitoyl synthase 133
Carvedilol 196
Causative organisms 249
Cefotaxime 116, 146
Ceftazidime 137
Ceftriaxone 110
  injection 86
Cefuroxime 144
Central airway obstruction 142
Central diabetes insipidus 37, 41
  causes of 39b
Central nervous system 84, 100, 130, 142, 178, 185, 201, 303, 312
  infection, cause of 136
  signs 226
  symptoms of 293
Cerebral
  autoregulation curve 104f
  blood
    flow 72, 100
    volume 70, 106
  edema 35
    signs of 35
  glucopenia 55
  malaria 112, 210, 211, 214, 213-216
  monitoring
    multimodal 104
  palsy 79, 309
  perfusion pressure 67, 69, 99, 105
Cerebrospinal fluid 70, 88, 91, 110, 117, 123, 135, 136, 139
Cervical lymph nodes 220
Charcot's triad 263
Chediak-Higashi syndrome 281
Chest
  discomfort 221
  retraction 140, 141
  wall retractions 145
Chiari malformation 309
Child's immune status 145
Childhood
  obstructive sleep apnea 309b
  vasculitis 301
Chlamydia 161
Chloramphenicol, combination of 137

Index

Chlorpheniramine maleate,
  injection of 224
Cholestatic liver disease 255
Churg-Strauss
  arteritis 302
  vasculitis 303
Churg-Strauss syndrome 306
Ciprofloxacin 24
Cisplatin 15
Clevidipine butyrate 180
Clonic seizure 78
Clonidine 189
Clopidogrel 15
Clostridium difficile 241
Clot formation time 270
Cloxacillin 144
Coagulation cascade 282*fc*
Coarctation of aorta 178, 187
Cocaine 178
Common cobra 233*f*
Common cold 221*t*
  differ 221
Community acquired
  pneumonia 161
  antibiotics in 163
Complete blood
  count 131
  picture 285
Congenital heart defects, repair
  of 197
Congestive heart failure 192-195, 197*t*
  causes of 193
  pathophysiology of 194
  treatment of 197
Conn's classification 258
Convulsive status epilepticus 83, 88
Coral snakes 233
Corpus callosotomy 97
Corticosteroids 137, 187
Cough 72, 192, 221
Counterregulatory hormone 55, 55*t*
  deficiency of 56
Cranial nerve 135
  signs 226
C-reactive protein 302
Crescentic glomerulonephritis 22
  disorders with 22*b*
Crouzon syndrome 309
Cryptosporidium 241, 244, 263
Cushing's disease 178
Cushing's reflex 261
Cushing's syndrome 187
Cushing's triad 72
Cutaneous vasculitis 303
Cyanosis 155
Cyclic adenosine
  monophosphate 39

Cyclosporine 15
Cystic fibrosis 217
Cytoadherence 213
Cytokine releasers 225
Cytomegalovirus 126, 261

D

Daboia russelii 234*f*
Deafness 39
Decompensation, management of
  acute 197
Deep vein thrombosis 37
Deficit therapy 294
Dehydration 48, 242, 273, 276, 295,
  295*t*
  degree of 242*t*
  grade 241
  in gastroenteritis, management
    of 246*fc*
  mild 241
  mild-to-moderate 242
  moderate 243, 291
  severe 40, 242, 243, 271
  treatment of 241
Dengue 200, 204, 208
  diagnosis of 204
  disease 199
  fever 200, 203
    control in 203
    derangements in 202
    stages of 202
  hemorrhagic fever 200
  infection 203, 204*f*
  severe 199, 200, 208
    risk factors 202*f*
  shock syndrome 200, 201
  virus 199
Dengue-related hepatic
  involvement 203
Dexamethasone 137, 173
Diabetes 217
  insipidus 37, 39, 42
    diagnosis of 40
    types of 39
  mellitus 39, 53
Diabetic ketoacidosis 31, 33, 34, 36
  classified 33
  complications of 35
  resolution of 35
Dialeptic seizures 78
Diarrhea 49, 241
  acute 245, 246*b*
  causes of acute 241
  complications of acute 241
  episode of 248
  negative 16

positive 16
  role of
    antibiotics in 244
    prebiotics in 245
  therapy of acute 245
Diarrheal
  dehydration, grading of 242*t*
  diseases 240
Diastolic blood pressure 177, 182
Diazepam 88, 94, 228
Digoxin 196
Diphenhydramine 1
Diphtheria 122
Disopyramide 55
Disseminated encephalomyelitis,
  acute 112, 116
Disseminated intravascular
  coagulation 225, 267, 282
Diuretic therapy, adverse effects
  of 196
Dizziness 55, 59
Dobutamine 195
  injection 224
Dopamine 195
  infusion 2
Dorsal root ganglia 122
Down's syndrome 309
Dravet syndrome 79
Drugs
  first line 85*f*
  second line 85, 94
  third line 85
Duodenoduodenostomy 66
Duodenojejunostomy 66
Duodenum, surgical bypass of 66
Dysarthria 55
Dysentery 249, 249*f*
  acute 248, 250
  complications of 249
Dysphagia 227
Dysplastic kidneys 178
Dyspnea 154
Dystonia 133
Dysuria 29

E

Ebstein's anomaly 193
Echis carinatus 234*f*
Elapidae 233
Electrographic seizures 96
Electrolyte imbalance 84, 290
  correct 274
Emergency room, stabilization
  in 71*t*
Enalapril 196
Encephalitis 112
  syndrome, acute 110, 112, 113

Encephalopathy 221
Endocrine 178
 disorders 187
 disturbances 60
Endogenous toxins 11
End-organ damage 184
Endoscopic
 sclerotherapy 256, 257, 258*t*
 variceal ligation 256, 258*t*
Endotracheal intubation, role of 174
Entamoeba histolytica 249
Enteric adenovirus 241
Enteroviral illness including
 polio 124
Enterovirus 112, 116, 154
Envenomation 224
 degree of 236, 236*t*
 local 237
 mild 227
 moderate 227
 signs of 234
 site of 225
Enzymes 54
Epilepsy, history of 83
Epileptic
 encephalopathy 79
 seizure 78
Epithelial cells 154
Epstein-Barr virus 126, 261
Erythromycin 144
Escherichia coli 14, 135, 136, 161, 249
 infection 135
 vaccines 245
Esmolol 189
Esophageal
 atresia 64
 balloons 257*f*
Extensive superficial infection 271
Extracorporeal carbon dioxide
 removal 152
Extracorporeal membrane
 oxygenation 150, 151
 role of 151
Extrahepatic portal venous
 obstruction 254
Extremities 207
Eye 178, 220, 242
 movement, nonrapid 79
 opening 119
Eyelid
 myoclonia 78
 swelling of 4

F

Facial dysmorphism 52, 79
Falciparum malaria, severe 211

Familial dysautonomia 187
Fang marks 234*f*
Fat necrosis 267
Fatty acid oxidation disorder 133
Febrile
 encephalopathy, acute 110, 112,
  113, 115, 117
 phase 202
 seizures 93
 status epilepticus 93
Feeding in gastroenteritis,
 management of 246*fc*
Fenoldopam 180
Fever 220, 221, 271, 288
 mild 223
Fibrinolysis inhibitors 283
Flaccid paralysis, acute 121, 122,
 122*t*, 123, 126, 127
Fluid 290
 redistribution of 11
 status, management of 16
Food
 allergy 43
 and drug administration 288
Foreign body in airway 155
Fosphenytoin 89, 94
Four-lumen minnesota tube 257*f*
Free fatty acids 57, 225
Fresh frozen plasma 278
Functional residual capacity 141
Furosemide 24, 180, 196
 injection of 224

G

Gallop rhythm 194
Gas
 chromatography mass
  spectrometry 114
 exchange goals 28, 149
Gastric
 hyperdistention 227
 leiomyosarcoma 60
 varices 258
Gastroenteritis 245
 acute 240, 244, 291, 293
Gastroesophageal
 reflux 43, 155
 varices 258
Gastrointestinal
 bleeding 267, 278
  causes of 251, 254t
  mid 254
 signs 227
 tract 296
Gaucher's disease 254
Gelastic seizure 78

Genetic
 defects 39
 epilepsy 79
 testing 283
Genitourinary signs 227
Gentamicin 137
G-glutamyl transpeptidase 260
Giardia lamblia 241
Gingival sulci, bleeding from 235*f*
Glanzmann thrombasthenia 283
Glasgow Coma Scale 99, 114, 119,
 210, 260
 modified 101*t*
Glomerular
 abnormalities 20
 filtration rate 10, 299
Glomerulonephritis
 acute 11, 18, 19, 178
  poststreptococcal 19
 chronic 187
 primary 19
Gluconeogenic enzymes 55
Glucose 57
 homeostasis 52
 insulin infusion 44
Glucose-6-phosphate
 dehydrogenase 262
 deficiency 288
Glutamic acid decarboxylase 114
Glycogenolytic enzymes,
 activating 55
Glycoprotein 219
Glycosaminoglycans 225
Gram-negative
 bacilli 165
 orgainisms 136, 164
Gray hepatization 166
Growth
 failure 195
 hormone 57
  deficiency 56
Grunting 155
Guillain-Barré syndrome 122, 124,
 126, 127, 127*t*, 187
 management of 127
 pathogenesis of 127
 subtypes of 126

H

H1N1-influenza 151
Haemophilus influenzae 126, 135-
 138, 146, 154, 160, 161, 164
 meningitis 137
 vaccine 135
Haemophilus pertussis 154, 158
Hallermann-Streiff syndrome 309

Index

Head injury 72
  management of severe 105
  severity of 68, 69t
Headache 55, 220, 221, 288
  children experience 59
Heart
  failure 187
    acute decompensation of 193
    category of 194
    treatment of acute 195
  rate 62, 192, 207, 242
Helium-oxygen mixture 174
Hemagglutinin 218
Hematological signs 227
Hematuria 26-28
  diagnosis of 30fc
  glomerular 29t
  management of 30fc
  nonglomerular 29t
  pathophysiology of 27
Hemiparesis 216
Hemiscorpius lepturus 224
Hemodynamic monitoring 207t
Hemoglobin 135, 199, 270, 285, 290
Hemogram 188
Hemolysis 288
Hemolytic toxin 225
Hemolytic uremic syndrome 11, 14-16, 178, 304
  atypical 15, 16t
  typical 16t
Hemophagocytic lymphohistiocytosis, primary 262
Hemophilia 279
Hemorrhage 187
Hemostasis
  defects in primary 283
  primary 279, 280f
  secondary 279
Hemostatic disorders 280
Henoch-Schönlein purpura 11, 301, 303, 304
Hepatic
  dysfunction 263
  failure 290
  venous pressure gradient 251
Hepatitis
  A viruses 203
  acute 260, 261b, 264, 265
  B 126
    viruses 203
  C viruses 203
  causes of acute 263
  setting of acute 263
Hepatorenal syndrome 252
Hermansky-Pudlak syndrome 281

Herniation 103
  syndromes 102t
Herpes simplex
  encephalitis, treatment of 116, 116t
  virus
    encephalitis 116
    polymerase chain reaction 110
Herpesvirus 154
Hirschsprung disease 64
Histamine 225
Holliday-Segar method 294, 294t
Hormonal tests, essential 44
Horn cell, anterior 122
Hospital acquired pneumonia 161, 164
  antibiotics in 165
  antimicrobials in 164b
Human immunodeficiency
  virus 19, 126
Hyaluronidases 225
Hydralazine 180, 189
Hydrochlorothiazide 195
Hydronephrosis 187
Hydrophiidae 233
Hyperaldosteronism 178
Hyperammonemia 132, 133fc
  cutoff value for 132
  management of 132
Hyperekplexia 79
Hyperglycemia 73, 225, 267
  correlation of 73
Hyperinflated lungs 153
Hyperinflation 153
Hyperinsulinemia 53, 57
Hyperinsulinism 56
Hyperkalemia 12, 48, 50, 225, 294
  causes of 299, 299fc
  management of 289
Hyperlucent lung syndrome 158
Hypernatremia 77, 187, 297
  managed 41
  treatment of 297
Hypernatremic dehydration 243
Hyperosmolar therapy 70
Hyperphosphatemia, management of 288
Hypersensitivity vasculitis 303
Hypertension 29, 59, 62, 177, 178, 184, 185, 187, 188b
  acute severe 184
  causes of 186
  chronic 187b
  malignant 177, 178b
  portal 252, 253f, 254t
  transient 187b
  diagnosis of severe 185

essential 187
malignant 176, 177, 179b
pharmacotherapy for
  malignant 180t
severe 184, 185, 187, 189, 189t
stages of 177t
treat 62
treatment in severe 189
Hypertensive
  crisis 179b
  emergency 176, 177, 185, 185b
  manifestations of 178t
  encephalopathy 21
  retinopathy 187
  urgency 177
Hyperthermia 84
Hyperthyroidism 178
Hypertonic saline 70
  nebulization, role of 158
Hyperventilation
  role of 72
  severe 72
Hypervolemic hypernatremia 297
Hypocalcemia 75, 77, 267
Hypocarbia 73
Hypoglycemia
  acute episode of 57b
  drugs causing 55
  pathological 56, 57
  prevent 272
Hypoglycemia 48, 50, 52, 54, 55, 55b, 55t, 56, 57, 62, 75, 84, 215, 235, 271, 276
  in emergency room,
    pathological 56fc
  to maintain sugars 54b
Hypokalemia 123
  causes of 298, 298b
  evaluation of 298fc
  management of 298
  mild 298
  moderate 298
  severe 298
  treatment of 298
Hypokalemic periodic paralysis 125
Hyponatremia 48, 75, 77, 291, 294-296, 296fc
  with edema 295
Hypotension 1, 48, 62, 73
  manage 73
Hypotensive shock 209
Hypothermia 98, 271, 276
  prevent 272
Hypothyroidism 309
Hypotonic hyponatremia 295
Hypovolemia 62, 215
Hypovolemic hypernatremia 297

Hypoxemia 73
 in children 73
Hypoxia 73, 169
 sign of severe 141
Hypoxic ischemic insult 75

I

Immunodeficiency 162
Immunoglobulin 23
Immunomodulatory therapies 97, 98
Impending herniation 101
Infection
 related causes 93
 serious secondary 223
 treatment of 274
Infectious
 diseases 153, 199
 gastrointestinal disorder 248
Infective pathologies 115t
Inflammatory bowel disease 264
Inflammatory demyelinating
  polyneuropathy, acute 121
Influenza 112, 126, 136, 161, 217, 219-221, 221t
 diagnostic test 221
 prognosis in 222
 uncomplicated 220b
 vaccine 217, 222b
 virus 154, 218, 219
  replication 218f
  survival of 219
  types of 218
Inherited bleeding disorder 281t
Inspiratory pressure, maximum 150
Insulin 52, 57, 300
 dependent diabetes 264
 infusion therapy 33
 secretion 225
Insulin-like growth factor binding
  protein-1 57
Intensive care unit 127
Interstitial nephritis, acute 11, 24
Intestinal
 obstruction 43, 267
 perforation 267
Intracranial
 hypertension 69, 71
 mass 187
 pressure 69, 99, 110, 215
  acute surges in 107t
  controlling raised 138
  increased 187
  monitoring 71, 104, 105f
  volume curve 103f
 temperature 139
Intravascular volume depletion 11

Intravenous
 acyclovir 110, 116
 calcium gluconate 294
 fluids 144
 immunoglobulin 88
 infusion 238
 rehydration 273
Ipratropium 173
 bromide 172
Irritability 155
Ischemic infarct 75
Isolated gastric varices 258
Isovolemic hypernatremia 297
Isradipine 180

J

Japanese B encephalitis 116
Jugular venous distention 195

K

Kawasaki disease 301, 302, 305
 classification for 305b
Kayser-Fleischer ring 255
Ketamine 96, 97
 role of 174
Ketogenic diet 97, 98
Ketones 57
Ketotic hypoglycemia 56
Kidney 178
 disease
  acute 9
  chronic 15, 178
 injury
  acute 9, 10, 11b, 12b, 12t, 13, 14, 252
  causes of acute 10
  intrinsic acute 11, 11t
  network, acute 10
  prerenal acute 11, 11t
  treatment of acute 12
 malformations of 187
King cobra 233f
Klebsiella 161, 164, 165
Klippel-Feil syndrome 309
Krait 233, 234f, 236f
Kussmaul's breathing 215

L

Labetalol 179, 180, 189
Lacosamide 94, 95
Lactic acidosis 133
Leiurus quinquestriatus 230
Lennox-Gastaut syndrome 78
Leptospirosis 112
Leukemia 285

Leukocyte, differential 135
Levetiracetam 89, 94
Life-threatening emergency 1
Listeria meningitis 137
Listeria monocytogenes 136
Live attenuated influenza
  vaccine 223
Liver
 cell failure 56
 disease, chronic 256, 264
 dysfunction 203
 failure
  acute 261b, 263, 265
  chronic 203
 function test 227
 in sepsis, causes of 263b
 involvement, etiology of 263
 transplantation 203
Lobar pneumonia, stages of 166
Loeffler pneumonia 165
Loeffler syndrome 165
Lorazepam 88, 90, 93, 94, 215
Losartan 196
Lower gastrointestinal bleeding 254
Lower osmolarity oral rehydration
  salts 244
Lower
 pontine 102
 respiratory tract 153
Lumbar puncture 113
 second 137
Lung injury 147
 acute 151
Lupus anticoagulant 282
Lupus nephritis 178
Lyme's disease 112, 126
Lyme's serology 126
Lymphangitis 235f
Lymphoblastic leukemia,
  acute 285, 286, 287
Lymphocytes 91

M

Macrolides 144
Magnesium sulfate 174
Malaria 210
 complicated 211
 detection of 214
 development of severe 213
 manifestations of severe 210
 negative rapid 111
 severe 211, 211b, 212t
 tests for 214
Malnutrition, severe acute 112, 270, 271, 272, 275, 276
Mannitol 70

Index

Maple syrup urine disease 130, 133
Marfan's syndrome 309
Massive cell damage 148
Measles 112
  infection 112
Medullary carcinoma thyroid 60
Meningism 214
Meningitis 136, 138
Meningococcal meningitis 136, 137
Meningoencephalitis 76
Mental
  confusion 55
  status 242
Metabolic
  acidosis 31, 84, 133, 210
  cause 131
  crisis 129, 132
  disorders 133t
    classification of 132
  disturbances, acute 93
  signs 227
Metastatic spread 163
Methemoglobinemia 288
Methicillin 24
Methicillin-resistant
  staphylococcus 144
Methylprednisolone 173
Metoclopramide 217
Metoprolol 196
Microcytic hypochromic cells 270
Micronutrient
  supplementation 245, 274
Microvascular blood flow 213
Midazolam 82, 88, 94, 93, 96, 97, 215
  infusion 91, 92, 110
Midbrain 102
Miller fisher variant 127
Milrinone 195
Minoxidil 189
Mitochondrial disorders 60
Mitomycin 15
Monro-Kellie doctrine 103
Morbid obesity 309
Motor response 101
Mouth 242
Mucocutaneous bleeding 279
Mucosal neuromas 60
Mucous membranes 220
Multicystic kidney 187
Multiple organ dysfunction
  syndrome 204
Mumps 112
Myalgia 220
Myasthenia gravis 117
Mycobacterium tuberculosis 161
Mycoplasma 158

Mycoplasma pneumoniae 116, 126, 154, 161, 165
Myelogenous leukemia, chronic 286
Myeloid leukemia, acute 286, 287, 287
Myocardial
  depression 267
  function 2
Myocarditis 221
Myoclonic 78
  absence 78
  atonic 78
  jerks 78
  seizures 78
Myoclonus, negative 78
Myositis 122, 221

N

N-acetyl cysteine, infusion of 203
Nasal
  congestion 223
  obstruction, chronic 309
National Anti-malaria Program 211, 212t
National polio surveillance
  project 123
Nausea 55, 136, 227, 288
Nebulizer solution 172
Neck rigidity 135
Neisseria meningitides 136
Neonatal pneumonia 164, 166
Nephritic, disorders with acute 24
Nephritis
  acute 19
    etiology 19b
Nephritogenic streptococci 19
Nephrotic syndrome 264, 290, 293
Nephrotoxin 225
Nerve conduction study 121
Netilmicin 137
Neuraminidase 218
  inhibitors 223
Neuroblastoma 178, 187
Neurocutaneous syndromes 79
Neurocysticercosis 75, 76, 115
Neurological
  emergency 100, 110
  sequelae 216
  signs 226
Neurologically injured child 104
Neurometabolic disorders 79, 129
Neuromuscular junction 122
Neuroprotective measures 103
Neurotoxic snakebite 237
Neurotoxin, concentrations of 225
Neutropenia 288

Nicardipine 179, 180, 189
Nifedipine 189
Nitazoxanide 244
Nitric oxide, inhaled 146
Nitroblue tetrazolium test 137
Nitroglycerine 189
N-methyl-D-aspartate 114
Nonallergic anaphylaxis 2
Nonbilious emesis 65
Nonconvulsive status
  epilepticus 84, 88, 95
Nonglomerular hematuria 28
Non-Hodgkin lymphoma 286, 287
Noninvasive
  positive pressure ventilation 174
  ventilation 174
  role of 168
Nonketotic hyperglycinemia 133
Non-neurological systemic signs 226
Nonpoisonous snake 233
Nonradiopaque foreign bodies 163
Nonrespiratory causes 142
Nonsteroidal anti-inflammatory
  drugs 4, 11, 12, 24, 203, 269
Nonstructural protein 218
Normoglycemia, restoration of 215
Normovolemia 104
Norwalk virus 241
Nucleoprotein 218
Nutrition 73, 126
  role of 151
Nutritional edema 271
  classification of 271t

O

Obstructive sleep apnea 308, 310
  causes of 309
  complications of 311
  signs of 309
  treatment of 311
Obstructive uropathy 178
Ophiophagus hannah 233, 233f
Optic atrophy 39
Oral
  fludrocortisones 50
  hydrocortisone replacement 50
  hypoglycemic agent 54
  medications, dosage of 196t
  nifedipine 180
  rehydration 273
    salt 243, 244
    solution 240, 242, 244t, 273t
    therapy 241, 243, 294
Organic
  acidemia 133

diagnosis of 133
treatment of suspected 133
personality changes 55
Ornithine transcarbamylase
  deficiency 133
Oropharyngeal papillomatosis 309
Oscillatory ventilation, high
  frequency 146, 149, 150
Oseltamivir 217, 222
Osmolarity 70
Osmotic agent 107
Osteopetrosis 309
Oxygen 157, 197
  prongs 144
  role of 171
  saturation 150, 171
    maintain 149
  supplementation 145
  levels of 144

P

Pain
  management 126
  severe abdominal 249
Palmar pallor, severe 271
Palpitation 55, 59
Pancreas
  annular 64, 66
  embryology of 65
Pancreatic infection 269
Pancreatitis
  acute 266
    causes of 267
  complications of acute 267*b*
  management of severe 268
  severe acute 266, 267
Pandemic influenza 217
Papilledema, bilateral 176
Paracetamol 203
Paragangliomas 59
Parainfectious myelitis 122
Parainfluenza 158
  viruses 154, 161
Parasitemia, levels of 216
Parasympathetic signs 226
Parathyroid hyperplasia 60
Parental hydrocortisone 50
Parenteral antibiotics 144
Paresthesias 55
Paroxysms 59
Parvovirus 241
Patch test 5*f*
Patent ductus arteriosus 142
Pathogen antimicrobial 164

Pediatric
  acute hypertension 183
  acute liver 263*b*
    failure 260, 263
  hypertension, pharmacotherapy
    in 191*f*
  hypoglycemia 57
  intensive care unit 100, 146, 168,
    170, 228
    team 67
  status epilepticus, drugs in 94*t*
Penicillin hypersensitivity 164
Penicillinase-resistant penicillin 164
Pericardial effusion 267
Pericarditis 221
Perinorm 217
Peripheral
  airway obstruction 142
  edema 195
  nerves 122
  pulse 207
Persistent
  hypoglycemia, causes for 56*b*
  pneumonia 161
  vomiting 271
Perspiration 55
Pertussis 161
Phenobarbital 89
Phenobarbitone 84, 94, 97
Phentolamine 62, 180, 189
Phenytoin 24, 88, 94
  sodium 84, 85
Pheochromocytoma 58-61, 178, 187
  diagnosis of 60
  management of 61
  surgery in 62*t*
  symptom triad of 59*f*
  treatment of 61*fc*
Phosphodiesterase inhibitors 195
Phospholipases 225
Phosphor diesterases 225
Pierre Robin anomaly 309
Piperacillin 137
Pit viper 233
Plasma
  ammonia 131
  renin activity 188
Plasminogen activator inhibitor 282
Plasmodium falciparum 210, 213
  asexual parasitemia 211
Platelet function
  analyzer 283
  defects 281
  disorders 278
    treatment for 283
Pleural effusion 267
  complication of 166

Pneumococcal
  meningitis 136, 137
  pneumonia 164
  vaccine 160
Pneumococcus 136, 138, 154, 161
Pneumocystis carinii 161, 165
Pneumocystis jiroveci 161
Pneumonia 144, 160-162
  chronic 162*b*, 164
  classification of 161
  complications of 163
  congenital 161
  diagnosis of 163, 166
  primary atypical 165
  recurrent 161
  severe 271
  signs of 165
  symptoms of 165
  thrush 165
  type of 163
Poisonous snakes 233
Poliomyelitis 187
Polyarteritis nodosa 301, 305
Polycystic kidney disease 255
Polymerase chain reaction 214, 250
Polymorphonuclear neutrophils 135
Poor feeding 155
Porphyria 126
Portal
  circulation, anatomy of 253*f*
  hypertension 251, 255*b*
  vein thrombosis 254
Positive end-respiratory
  pressure 150
Postcoarctation repair 187
Postdiphtheritic
  polyneuropathy 124
Postencephalitic sequelae 79
Potassium metabolism 297
Prader Willi syndrome 309
Prazosin 228
Prednisolone 116
Prodrug 89
Prophylactic hyperthermia 70
Prophylaxis 217
  role of secondary 258
Propofol 72, 97
Prostaglandin 299
Protein 204
Prothrombin time 280, 282
Pseudohyperkalemia 299
Pseudohypoaldosteronism 44
Pseudomonas aeruginosa 164, 165
Pseudomonas meningitis 137
Pseudomonas pneumonia 165
Ptosis 235*f*

Index

Pulmonary
  candidiasis 165
  chondroma 60
  congestion
    signs of 195
    symptoms of 195
  diseases, chronic 162
  edema 62, 197, 215, 225
    management of 193
    venous connection 193
Pulse 135
  oximeter 143
    estimate 143
  quality of 242
  rate 295
Pyelonephritis, chronic 187
Pyloric stenosis 43
Pyogenic meningitis, age-wise etiology of 136*b*
Pyruvate dehydrogenase deficiency 133

Q

Quinine 55, 211, 212*t*
  salt 212

R

Rabies 112, 124
Raccoon eyes 71
Raised intracranial pressure 99, 178
Ranitidine 224
Rapid sequence intubation 114
Rasburicase 288
Rash 29, 288
Red blood cell 11, 26, 29, 30, 213, 256
Red cell deformability influence severity 214
Red hepatization 166
Reflex anoxic seizure 79
Refractory status epilepticus 91, 92, 93, 97*t*
  causes of 93
Rehabilitation phase 274
Rehydration therapy 294
Renal
  arteritis
    with aortitis 187
    without aortitis 187
  artery 178
    stenosis 187
  biopsy 12
    indications of 12
  cell carcinoma 60
  disorders 187

failure 216
  acute 8, 9, 21, 296
  chronic 296
  function test 188
    abnormal 227
  histology 24
  injury, acute 8, 12
  tubular acidosis 296, 298
  tumors 187
  ultrasonography 188
  vasculitis 302
  vein thrombosis 187
Renovascular disorders 187
Respiration 135
Respiratory
  acidosis 84
  causes 142
  distress 140-145, 288
    assessment instrument 156*t*
    causes of 142, 142*b*
    development of severe 153
    diagnose 142
    management of 193
    signs of 141*t*, 171
    symptoms of 141*t*, 171
    syndrome, acute 28, 142, 146, 147*f*, 148, 152, 267
    treatment of 145
  emergency 145
  failure 141, 174
  malformations, congenital 162
  rate 1, 140, 153, 207, 236, 270
    age-related 140*t*
    signs 227
  status 143
  syncytial virus 141, 154, 161
  system 224
Retinal angiomas 60
Reye's syndrome 56, 221, 264
Rhabdomyolysis 84
Rheumatology 301
Rhinorrhea 192, 223
Rickettsial 161
Rifampicin 24
Ringer's lactate 240
Roseola 112
Rotavirus 241, 245
Russell's viper 233, 234*f*
  injects 238

S

Saccharomyces boulardii 245
Safe food 244
Salbutamol 1, 2, 157, 173
  nebulization 145

Salicylates 55
Salmonella 241, 249
Salmonella typhi 245
Salt craving 49
Sanitation 244
Sarin's classification 258
Saw-scaled viper 233, 234*f*
Scorpion
  antivenom 230
    role of 229
  envenomation, pathophysiology of 225
  manifestations, system of 226
  sting 224, 227, 230
    cause of death in 230
    envenomation, signs of 226*b*
Sea snake 233, 233*f*
Seasonal influenza 222*t*, 223
  vaccines 222
Segmental hypoplasia 187
Seizure
  acute 75, 79
  causes of acute 76
  classification of acute 77
  controlling 138
Sengstaken-Blakemore tube 256, 257*f*
Sensorium 207
Sepsis 43, 263
Septic shock 275, 276
  treatment of 273
Serotonin 225
Serum
  antiganglioside antibodies 127*t*
  creatinine 30, 123, 290
  electrolytes 30, 188
  glutamic
    oxaloacetic transaminase 199
    pyruvic transaminase 199
  N-methyl D-aspartate 111
  osmolality 40, 42
  potassium 290
  sickness reactions 239
  sodium 290, 291, 293
Shiga toxin 249
Shigella 241, 248
  dysenteriae species 249, 250
  organisms 245
Shock 205*fc*, 215, 235, 267
  decompensated 205, 206*fc*
Sialyl-galactosyl moieties 219
Sickle cell diseases 309
Skeletal muscle breakdown 235
Skin 220
  allergy testing 5*f*

fold 242
rashes 264
reactions 4
turgor 295
Small-vessel vasculitic diseases 302
Snakebite 232, 233
  complications of 239
  effects of 239
  first aid for 236*f*
  symptoms with 233
Sodium
  bicarbonate 294
  morrhuate 257
  nitroprusside 179, 180, 189
  succinate 173
  tetradecyl sulfate 257
  valproate 94, 95
Sodium-water balance
  maintained 38
Somatic signs 226
Somatosensory 77
Sore throat 221, 223
Spinal cord 122
  hemangioblastomas 60
Spironolactone 195, 196
Splanchnic arteriovenous
  fistula 254
Splenic
  infarct 267
  vein thrombosis 254
Spurious hypokalemia 298
Staphylococcal
  meningitis 137
  pneumonia 163, 163*b*, 164
Staphylococcus aureus 164
  pneumonia 164
Status epilepticus 83, 84, 86-88, 92, 93, 93*t*, 98, 215
  management of 86, 86*fc*, 96*f*
  pathophysiology of 85
  stages of 85
Steroids 157, 158, 173, 178
  course of 137
Storage disorders 254
Streptococcus hemolyticus 136
Streptococcus pneumoniae 15, 138, 160, 161, 164
Stuffy nose 221
Sturge-Weber syndrome 79
Subcutaneous
  emphysema 163
  insulin therapy 35
Subfalcine 102*f*
Sublingual nifedipine 180
Sulfonylureas 55

Super-refractory
  epilepsy, management of 90
  status epilepticus 88*fc*, 90, 92, 95, 97*t*
  management of 86
Surfactant replacement therapy 146
Swyer-James syndrome 158
Sympathetic signs 226
Synacthen doses 49*t*
Syncope 49
Systemic
  envenomation 237
  glucocorticoids 6
  hypotension 73
  illness 56
  vasculitis 19
  venous congestion
    signs of 195
    symptoms of 195
Systemic lupus erythematosus 11, 299
Systolic blood pressure 177, 182

T

Tachycardia 1, 55, 194
Tachypnea 1, 141, 153, 195
Tacrolimus 15
Takayasu arteritis 306
Tandem mass spectrometry 114, 130
Tap sign 226
Temporal arteritis 303
Tendon reflexes 135
Therapeutic hypothermia 98
Thiazide diuretics 41
Thiopentone 96, 97
Thoracic chest wall defects 142
Thrombin time 282
Thrombocytopenia 281
Thrombotic thrombocyt 11
Thyroid stimulating hormone 57
Thyroiditis 264
Thyroxine 57
Ticarcillin 137
Tick bite 112
  paralysis 125
Tick-borne encephalitis 112
Ticlopidine 15
Tonic-clonic seizures 78
Topiramate 94, 95
Toxic
  encephalopathy 142
  fumes, inhalation of 158
  metabolites, formation of 129
Transient
  hypoglycemia, causes for 55*b*
  pseudohypoaldosteronism 43

Transjugular intrahepatic
  portosystemic shunt 256, 259
Transverse myelitis 221
  acute 124
Traumatic brain injury 67, 70-73
  management of severe 67
  severe 73, 100
Treacher Collins syndrome 309
Tremulousness 55
Tricuspid regurgitation 193
Trivalent influenza vaccine 222
Tryptophan 225
Tuberculoma 75, 76, 115
Tuberculous pneumonia 165
Tubular necrosis, acute 11, 267, 298
Tumor 115
  lysis syndrome 285, 286, 286*t*, 287, 288*fc*, 289
  necrosis factor-α 203
Typhoid hepatitis 262
Typical hemolytic uremic
  syndrome 15

U

Umbilical artery catheterization 187
Upper gastrointestinal
  bleeding 254
  endoscopy 256
Upper pontine 102
  herniation syndromes 101
Urea cycle
  defect 133, 133*fc*
  disorder 130
    diagnosis of 129
Urethral valves, posterior 178
Uric acid 57
Urinary
  catecholamines 188
  electrolyte 188
  tract infection 29, 44
    severe 45
Urine 12
  analysis 188
  culture 188
  output 242, 295
  test 227

V

Valproate 89
Vancomycin 144
Variceal bleed 251
  acute 254, 256*fc*, 258, 259
  control 257
Variceal hemorrhage 251

Varicella zoster 112
  encephalitis 116
Varices
  endoscopic grading of 258*b*
  endoscopic management of 258*t*
Vascular
  aneurysms 267
  endothelium 213
Vasculitic
  diseases, types of 303
  disorders 302
    medium-vessel 302
Vasculitis 302
  category 303
  diagnosis of 304
  diseases, causes of 302
  manifestations of 303*b*
  symptoms of 303
  syndrome 301
  types of 302, 304
  unclassified forms of 307
Vasopressin synthesis 39
Vein thrombosis 178
Ventilation 169, 174

Ventricular septal defect 142, 192
Verbal response 101
Versive seizure 78
Vesicoureteral reflux
  nephropathy 187
Vibrio cholerae 245
Viperidae 233
Viral 161
  infections 136
  myositis 125
  pneumonia 165
  respiratory infection 264
  shedding 219
Virologic tests 157
Visual disturbances 55
Vitamin
  B_{12} 123
    deficiency 126
  K antagonists 282
Vitiligo 49, 264
Voltage gated potassium
  channel 114
Vomiting 48, 59, 136, 155, 227, 288
von Hippel-Lindau syndrome 60

von Willebrand
  disease 278, 282
  factor antigen 278

W

Waterhouse-Friderichsen
  syndrome 136
Wegener's granulomatosis 303
Weight loss 49
Wheezing 155
White blood cell 11, 206, 285, 287
White-coat hypertension 185
Wilson's disease 255, 262, 263
Wiskott-Aldrich syndrome 281

X

Xanthine oxidase 288

Y

Yersinia enterocolitica 241

Z

Zanamivir 217, 222